ANAESTHESIA AND THE
AGED PATIENT

Anaesthesia and the Aged Patient

EDITED BY

HAROLD T. DAVENPORT
FRCPC, FFARCS (Eng)
Consultant Anaesthetist
Northwick Park Hospital
and Clinical Research Centre
Harrow
Middlesex

Blackwell Scientific Publications

OXFORD LONDON EDINBURGH

BOSTON PALO ALTO MELBOURNE

© 1988 by
Blackwell Scientific Publications
Editorial offices:
Osney Mead, Oxford OX2 OEL
  (*Orders*: Tel. 0865 240201)
8 John Street, London WC1N 2ES
23 Ainslie Place, Edinburgh EH3 6AJ
3 Cambridge Center, Suite 208
  Cambridge, Massachusetts 02142, USA
667 Lytton Avenue, Palo Alto
  California 94301, USA
107 Barry Street, Carlton
  Victoria 3053, Australia

First published 1988

Set by Times Graphics
Singapore
Printed and bound
by Oxford University Press

DISTRIBUTORS

USA
  Year Book Medical Publishers
  200 North LaSalle Street,
  Chicago, Illinois 60601
  (*Orders*: Tel. 312 726-9733)

Canada
  The C.V. Mosby Company
  5240 Finch Avenue East
  Scarborough, Ontario
  (*Orders*: Tel. 416-298-1588)

Australia
  Blackwell Scientific Publications
  (Australia) Pty Ltd
  107 Barry Street
  Carlton, Victoria 3053
  (*Orders*: Tel. (03) 347 0300)

British Library
Cataloguing in Publication Data

Anaesthesia and the aged patient.
  1. Old persons. Anaesthesia
  I. Davenport, Harold T.
  617′.96′0880565
  ISBN 0-632-01947-6

Contents

List of contributors, vii

Acknowledgments, ix

Introduction, xi

1　An approach to the basic science of ageing, 1
M.J. HALSEY

2　The demography of ageing, 9
A.M. WARNES

3　The aged cardiovascular system, 27
T.P. CRIPPS

4　The aged pulmonary system, 47
J.G. JONES

5　The aged nervous system, 70
M. HILDICK-SMITH

6　Psychological changes with ageing, 89
C. TWINING

7　The extent, character and patterns of disease in the aged, 104
M.R.P. HALL

8　Mechanisms of altered drug effects in the aged, 126
G.T. TUCKER

9　The milieu interieur in the aged, 145
M.D.W. LYE

10　Surgical decisions in the aged, 168
K.J.D. VOWLES

11　Preparations for anaesthesia for the aged, 183
H.T. DAVENPORT

12 Modifications of general anaesthesia for the aged, 204
    M.E. DODSON

13 The place of regional anaesthesia for the aged, 231
    J.A.W. WILDSMITH

14 Postoperative complications in the aged, 242
    D.G. SEYMOUR & F.G. VAZ

15 Intensive care for the aged, 258
    R.B. HOPKINSON

16 Chronic pain in the aged, 285
    P.J.D. EVANS

17 Ethics of treatment and research in the aged, 308
    M.J. DENHAM

    Index, 321

List of contributors

T.P. CRIPPS MB, ChB, FFARCS, *Consultant Anaesthetist, Peel Hospital, Galashields*

H.T. DAVENPORT, MB, ChB, FRCPC FFARCS(Eng), *Consultant Anaesthetist, Northwick Park Hospital and Clinical Research Centre, Harrow, Middlesex*

M.J. DENHAM, MD, FRCP, *Consultant in Geriatric Medicine, Northwick Park Hospital and Clinical Research Centre, Harrow, Middlesex*

M.E. DODSON, MD, ChB, FFARCS, *Consultant Anaesthetist, Royal Liverpool Hospital, Liverpool*

P.J.D. EVANS, MBBS, FFARCS, *Consultant Anaesthetist, Charing Cross Hospital, and Royal Masonic Hospital, London. Clinical Teacher, University of London*

M.R.P. HALL, MA, BM, BCh, FRCP, *Emeritus Professor of Geriatric Medicine, Southampton General Hospital and University of Southampton, Southampton*

M.J. HALSEY, MA, DPhil, *Head of Research Group, Division of Anaesthesia, Clinical Research Centre, Harrow*

M. HILDICK-SMITH, MD, FRCP, *Consultant in Geriatric Medicine, Kent and Canterbury Hospital, Canterbury,*

R.B. HOPKINSON, MBBS, FFARCS, *Consultant Anaesthetist, Director of Intensive Care, East Birmingham Hospital, Birmingham*

J.G. JONES, FRCP, FFARCS, *Professor of Anaesthesia, University of Leeds, Leeds*

M.D.W. LYE, MD, MB, ChB, FRCP, *Professor of Geriatric Medicine, Royal Liverpool Hospital and University of Liverpool, Liverpool*

D.G. SEYMOUR, MB, ChB, MRCP(UK), *Senior Lecturer in Geriatric Medicine, University of Wales College of Medicine, Cardiff*

G.T. TUCKER, BPharm, PhD, *Professor of Clinical Pharmacology, Royal Hallamshire Hospital and University of Sheffield, Sheffield*

C. TWINING, MSc, PhD, *Top Grade Clinical Psychologist, Whitchurch Hospital, Cardiff*

F.G. VAZ, MBBS, MRCP(UK), *Senior Registrar in Geriatric and General Medicine, North Tees General Hospital, Stockton on Tees*

K.D.J. VOWLES, MB, ChB, FRCS, *Lately Consultant Surgeon, Royal Devon and Exeter Hospital, Exeter*

A.M. WARNES, BA, PhD, *Reader in Geography, Age Concern Institute of Gerontology, Kings College, University of London, London*

J.A.W. WILDSMITH, MD, FFARCS, *Consultant Anaesthetist, Royal Infirmary and University of Edinburgh, Edinburgh*

Acknowledgments

I wish to thank the contributors who have all shown great cooperation in this project.

I have made some changes in the manuscripts to stress the relevant needs of anaesthetists and I must therefore be responsible for any consequent imbalance of contents.

The diagrams were expertly produced by the Department of Medical Illustration at the Clinical Research Centre and at Blackwell Scientific Publications.

Messrs P. Saugman, E. Wates and N. Parsons provided invaluable assistance with my editorial duties. Also the contributors and my own secretaries deserve appreciation for the arduous task of transposing our drafts.

H.T.D.

Introduction

There is some antipathy to medical sub-specialization on the basis of
the age of patients but I would contend that anaesthetists, like physicians, surgeons, radiologists, pathologists, etc., are better prepared to
care for children, pregnant women and the aged if they are aware of
developments in paediatrics, obstetrics and geriatrics. This collection
of essays on aspects of geriatrics is designed to be of use to anaesthetists, who are increasingly involved in the care of the old.

Anaesthetists' involvement in intensive care and chronic pain relief
has reinforced the idea that they are the physicians of surgical teams.
As there is a limited number of physicians with geriatric training it is
sensible that the anaesthetist should become the geriatrician *manqué*
on each surgical team. Research in this field is rapidly expanding but it
is sometimes difficult for specialists in one area of medicine to understand those in another. Specialist writing on geriatrics, as on most
other subjects, addresses fellow specialists, so that it is often too ab-
struse to be assimilated by those outside the field. This is a two-way
process, of course, so that geriatricians also have misconceptions about
anaesthesia. It is the purpose of this book to try to overcome such
problems, presenting those aspects in the study of the aged which are
relevant to anaesthetists in the hope that this exchange of ideas between geriatrics and anaesthesia will be both informative and a stimulus to new research.

For modern anaesthetists, giving an anaesthetic, particularly in its
technological aspects, represents only a small part of the care of
patients. For this reason this book has little 'how to do' anaesthetic
advice. It concentrates, instead, on developing an understanding of old
patients and problems specific to their care. The definition of the elderly or aged patient is somewhat contentious and inexact. In these
chapters, when the age of patients is not specified, the terms elderly
and aged will be used to refer to those between 60 and 75 and those over
75 respectively. Patients in both groups are referred to as old, but it
should be noted that the majority of patients in geriatric care in this
country are in the aged group which, in the last years of this century,
will rapidly grow as a proportion of the population. At present it is this
group of which we know the least.

I hope that this book will stimulate interest in the exciting chal-
lenges involved in the care of the old, of which Sir Peter Medawar who
died in 1987 has written with characteristic elegance and perception:

The prolongation of a good life, happy and healthy, is fully in keeping with the spirit of medicine and is in a sense the very consummation of all that medical research has worked towards, *for all advances in medicine increase life-expectancy.* Even a couple of aspirin tablets taken daily might circumvent a platelet crisis and so be seen on an epidemiology scale to increase life-expectancy. The same would go for putting a plaster on a cut finger, something that will infinitesimally reduce the chances of septicaemia, and so on. The prolongation of life will increase the population size at a time when there are enough people in the world already, and although the people added will be post-reproductive in age they will eat and occupy space and consume energy. A graver problem is the burden upon a caring State of pensions and medical care, a burden falling disproportionately on the young. Moreover, working years and provisions for pensions will have to change. These are grave problems but they are not insoluble, for social changes of an essentially similar kind have happened over the past two hundred years, during which the mean expectation of life rose from about 30 to between 60 and 70, and anyhow the changes are not going to take place overnight. Consider the changes since Jane Austen's day. In her first novel *Sense and Sensibility* the elderly Colonel Brandon seeks the hand of a romantic young girl, Marianne Dashwood. In Marianne's view he is an old man who should be thinking not of matrimony but of woolly underwear and how best to avoid draughts. How old was this amorous old dotard? He was just over thirty-five, we read; and when the question arises of purchasing an annuity for Marianne's mother, a 'healthy woman of forty,' it is thought most unlikely that she will live until the age of fifty-five. Suppose now that some prescient man were to have told Jane Austen's characters that over the next century the mean expectation of life at all ages would double — something much more far-reaching than the modest 20–25 per cent we now have here in mind — would not Jane Austen's characters have been very mistaken to have been shocked by the riskiness and impiety of such a possibility? The great social adaptation was, however, made and there is no reason to think it cannot be made again. Let us take care that people as far distant from us as we are from the world of Jane Austen do not have reason to pity us for being so faint spirited. But there is an element of risk: we cannot foresee all the distant consequences of increasing life-expectancy, especially in respect of the risk of cancer and perhaps of Alzheimer's disease, senile dementia, and many may think this element of uncertainty should turn us away from our project. What I believe will happen is that some enthusiasts, especially in California, will go ahead with the longevity project to purchase extra years of life at the risk of contracting senile dementia and for its own reward. Francis Bacon, though pious and deeply religious, was the first advocate of just this kind of adventurousness in science, and would have approved: 'The true aim of Science,' he wrote in his little-known *Valerius Terminus,* 'is the discovery of all operations and all possibilities of operations from immortality (if it were possible) to the meanest mechanical practice.'

Bacon, then, was on my side. We already have a moral commitment to biomedical research which increases life-expectancy and I see no reason to think that the highway of medical melioration that has brought us so far already will now lead us into evil. We have long since been travelling that road and it is too late now to cease to be ambitious.*

H.T.D.

*Peter Medawar (1986) *Memoir of a Thinking Radish: An Autobiography.* (Oxford University Press, Oxford, pp. 199–200, with kind permission.)

1 | An approach to the basic science of ageing

M.J. HALSEY

Introduction

The basic science approach to gerontology attempts to answer two fundamental questions: What is the ageing process? and Why does ageing occur? These questions should not be confused with the description of the age relationships of physiological, pharmacological and pathological changes in living organisms. Such investigations have accumulated vast amounts of data which may or may not be relevant to answering the basic questions. The real difficulty is to sort out which changes are causes rather than consequences of ageing. This chapter is a selective summary of current views with the emphasis on underlying mechanisms. With few exceptions, it is based on the expositions of the authors referenced under 'Further reading' at the end of the chapter.

Variability of ageing

Many discussions on the biology of ageing start with the well established decrease in different cell functions and other variables (Fig. 1.1). The point is often made that this results in an inevitable reduction in reserve capacity (illustrated, for example, by the rapidity of pH correction) which in turn is related to biological and pathological ageing. The data in Fig. 1.1 illustrate a number of other important points which are relevant to the different viewpoints of the basic scientist and the clinician. Much of the data for the decrement estimations have come from longitudinal studies which are scientifically invaluable but of limited interest to clinicians. The problem is that the presentation of the results disguises the fact that there is a considerable variability in any one measurement and it is extremely difficult to produce a definitive 'normal' absolute value. Thus the figure has been compiled in terms of a 'normal' decrement in an 'average' male. However, individuals and the organ systems within them age at different rates. Physical ageing does not necessarily proceed at the same rate as chronological ageing. The extreme example is provided by progeria such as Werner's syndrome and, to a lesser extent, Hutchinson–Gilford syndrome. In addition, physical ageing, although inevitable, affects individuals with varying degrees of severity and may affect some parts of the body more than others.

Fig. 1.1 illustrates the variability of different cellular functions with

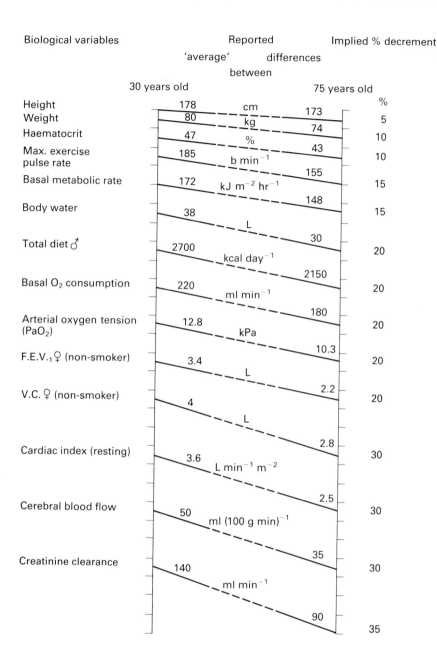

Fig. 1.1. Biological measurement related to age.

examples ranging from 5% to 35% decrements. Even a single variable such as weight loss can vary greatly for the different organs. Although this figure has selected two ages (30 and 75) for comparison, it should be noted that the biological ageing process is progressive over decades, as distinct from an acute step change over weeks. It is often noted that a particular illness apparently 'ages' an individual suddenly. However, this is the distinction between physiological changes, which are the normal biological ageing processes, and pathological changes which are the effects of disease or an unfavourable environment on the ageing process. It is clear that some diseases occur in the old either with a greater frequency or in a different form, or they may be exclusive to the old. In addition, the symptoms of the same disease can change. The latter aspects are covered by later chapters.

Physiological deterioration

A popular conception is that ageing is a form of inescapable deterioration which affects complex organisms in exactly the same way as mechanical breakdowns stop a machine. There are several arguments against this view in its simplest form. First, it seems extremely unlikely that an organism which is capable of the very much more difficult task of morphogenesis is nevertheless incapable of the apparently much simpler task of merely maintaining what is already formed. In fact, we are endowed with a multitude of mechanisms for self-repair which are not available to a machine. Second, ageing may not be intrinsic to all living organisms — bacteria, for example, can divide indefinitely — and thus there is no reason, in principle, why we should not exist in a physiological steady state. Third, it should be noted that some physiological functions can actually be improved by continued use. Athletic training and the associated cardiovascular improvements are good examples.

Early evidence for the importance of physiological deterioration, quoted in some of the textbooks, includes the observation that increasing the environmental temperature of poikilothermic animals significantly shortens their lifespan. The broad argument is that increasing ambient temperature increased the rate of metabolism which in turn accelerated physiological deterioration. However, it should be remembered that changing body temperature produces many perturbations in addition to simple metabolic effects.

A variation on the inevitable physiological deterioration hypothesis is the deleterious effect of accumulated stress. For example, it was postulated in the 1920s that people doing heavy manual labour were subjected to a greater degree of stress than others doing light work. However, it is now established that statistically there is no significant correlation between degrees of manual labour and life expectancy. In other studies it has also been found that repeated exposure to the stresses associated with infection does not significantly shorten lifespan. In summary, it is true that old people have a reduced ability to withstand stress and may succumb to a stress that would be tolerated by a younger person but there is no strong evidence that repeated stresses are the cause of ageing.

It is widely believed that the functioning of the nervous system (such as intermediate memory and learning of new tasks) deteriorates markedly with old age. One theory was that ageing is due primarily to lowered oxygen tension in critical areas of the brain. This hypoxia theory was based on the superficial resemblance between the symptoms of old age and those induced by breathing hypoxic gas mixtures. Changes in handwriting have been used as an example. However, there is no sound experimental or pathological evidence for this hypothesis. One of the complicating factors when considering physiological deterioration is the problem of age-related diseases. For example, Alzheimer's disease is increasingly common in older people above the age of 40. This does not mean, however, that it and other forms of dementia are part of the ageing process. There is strong evidence that intellectual functions remain essentially intact throughout life. Thus, Alzheimer's disease may start only at an advanced age because it requires the environment of an aged individual for its occurrence and progression.

Bioenergetics

It is well established in many animal species that the basal metabolic rates decrease with increasing age. A related, but not synonymous, observation is that an older person is less energetic. The simple hypothesis that this is due to general impairment of oxidative phosphorylation is both naive and untrue but a great deal of work has been carried out on the details of energy transducing pathways in the search for a biochemical basis underlying at least some of the physiological impairments of old age.

The current evidence is that mitochondria have substrate-specific decreases in activity with ageing that may be dependent on membrane permeability effects. This has led to studies in membrane composition changes which may inhibit active or passive transport processes. One speculation that is fashionable is that free radicals cause an increased lipid peroxidation in old age. However, defence mechanisms against radical induced damage are maintained in old age and there is no evidence that mitochondria of senescent animals cannot maintain cellular ATP when challenged. Mitochondrial turnover is of the order of days and this is known to be unchanged in a variety of mammalian tissues. It is conceivable that errors could accumulate if the mitochondrial protein synthesizing machinery was changed by peroxidative reactions but the evidence is against such damage because enzyme activities specifically dependent on protein synthesis are essentially unchanged in old age.

Nevertheless there are subtle and definite changes in catabolic metabolism which vary between different tissues. A classical view of these differences is to describe some as 'fixed postmitotic tissues', such as the central nervous system or the heart, and to contrast these with 'more rapidly dividing tissue', such as the liver or spleen. One of the interesting aspects of the mitochondrial work is that all tissues have a constant turnover with similar half-lives. However, the metabolic patterns of the tissues do vary and these do not all age at the same rate. For example, it is now established that some enzyme activities of the brain begin to decline earlier in the lifespan than do those of heart cells.

The biochemical and bioenergetic investigations may provide a link between the more molecular or genetic approaches and the gross physiological changes. However, to date the studies have revealed the enormous complexities of the ageing process and as yet there is no unifying concept which provides a satisfactory framework.

The evolution of ageing

The first attempt to explain the evolution of ageing was made by Weissmann in 1891. He, and subsequently others, argued that ageing was good for the species because it removed old and worn out individuals from the population, thus limiting overcrowding and promoting further evolution by accelerating the turnover of generations. The latter would increase the chance of a species adapting to a change in its environment. The flaws in these hypotheses are, first, that they presuppose what they set out to explain — namely that individuals wear out as they get older; second, that in the wild, animals normally die from predation, disease or starvation and thus old and worn out individuals are rarely encountered, with the result that the need and opportunity for an adaptive ageing process to have evolved would have been minimal; finally, the hypothesis depends on the advantages to a group rather than one individual. In a population of animals of that age, an individual with a mutation increasing longevity will have an advantage. Thus, any adaptive mechanism for ageing would be selectively unstable.

Age-specific genes

Medawar, when discussing 'an unsolved problem in biology' in 1952, proposed a fundamentally different hypothesis based on the time of expression of a harmful gene. He argued that selection would tend to defer the time at which the gene was expressed so that the potential for deleterious effects was minimized. However, the effect of mortality from other causes would reduce the force of natural selection in the later stages of life whether biological ageing occurred or not. Over a period of time a 'genetic dustbin' of late-acting deleterious genes would accumulate. In the wild, other causes of mortality would prevent these from being expressed but in a protected 'civilised' environment an individual would live long enough to encounter their detrimental effects. Another way of describing this hypothesis is to consider the failure to replace dead or damaged cells as being due to a preprogrammed, genetically coded failure. There are other versions of this hypothesis and the important concept is the effect of the passage of time on natural selection. However, it is not yet clear whether the accumulation of deleterious genes at the end of a lifespan is the actual cause of ageing or a reinforcing consequence of ageing.

Ageing versus reproduction

The previous hypotheses on age specific genes are based on the idea that natural selection is unable to prevent the deterioration of older organisms because it becomes attenuated with time. The alternative concept is that ageing is a by-product of selection for other beneficial traits. The latter idea led Kirkwood to develop the 'disposable soma theory' in the 1970s. Indefinite survival of an individual organism's body (the soma) is not necessary for the continuation of its genes, for which the body is merely a vehicle (see Fig. 1.2). All that is necessary is that the body should remain in good condition until an age after which most individuals would have died from accidental causes. The hypothesis argues that there is an optimum balance between the amount of energy that an organism allocates to maintenance and repair of its body and the amount used for survival, both in terms of defence against predators and most importantly in reproduction. There is no advantage in investing in a system which guarantees immortality of the body if the return from such an investment cannot be realized because of environmentally caused mortality.

These ideas were expressed by Kirkwood in mathematical models but can also be illustrated by a consideration of the specific lifespans of different species (Table 1.1). In general, we would expect a high risk of mortality and rapid ageing to be associated with large, frequent litters. This appears to be the case. Mice in the wild have many natural pred-

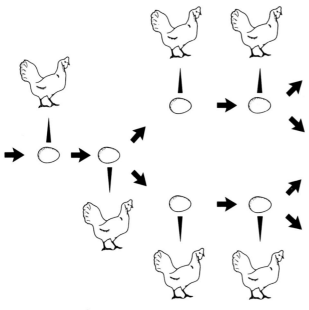

Fig. 1.2. Samuel Butler said that the chicken is the egg's way of making another egg. This neatly illustrates the distinction between germ-line (egg) and soma (chicken). (By courtesy of *New Scientist*.)

Table 1.1. Lifespan of a range of mammals

Species	Maximum lifespan (years)
Human	115
Indian elephant	70
Horse	46
Cat	28
Pig	27
Bat	24
Sheep	20
Dog	20
Rat	5
Mouse	3

ators and, as such, it is not worth investing much energy in offsetting the ageing process; it is more profitable instead to concentrate on producing as many offspring as cheaply and as quickly as possible — in their case approximately 45 offspring per female per year. On the other hand, another small mammal, the bat, has a dramatically longer natural lifespan and has adapted to maximize its survival; less energy is therefore needed, or is available, for reproduction — a female bat produces only one offspring per year. The elephant is the classic example of a species that reproduces slowly and therefore, Kirkwood would argue, has a longer lifespan. The female becomes sexually mature at 10–15 years of age, has a gestation period of about 620 days and produces not more than two offspring per decade.

There are special features of human ageing which distinguish it from that found in other animals. The first is that biological ageing carried through to the occurrence of natural death does occur in humans, whereas in most animals advanced ageing, in the absence of predation or disease, is extremely rare. A second feature is that human female reproduction is brought to a close by the menopause, whereas in the majority of animal species reproduction simply becomes irregular with increasing age. It has been argued that the menopause is a secondary adaptation in order to reduce the risk of the likelihood of parental death as a consequence of pregnancy being an excessive stress which cannot be tolerated in the older person. Thus, adaptation favours the situation in which the available resources are devoted to parental care and protection of children (which of course continues for a much longer period in humans).

The disposable soma theory is attractive because it has the advantage that it can be tested and if it is correct it would provide a coherent pattern for existing knowledge. For example, it makes the clear prediction that long-lived species should have higher levels of somatic maintenance and repair than short-lived species. Comparative studies should give a direct test of this prediction and, if it proves to be correct, a systematic comparison of different maintenance and repair mechanisms should help to identify those mechanisms which are primarily concerned in determining longevity. In addition, the theory defines a framework within which the huge variety of observations and hypotheses about ageing processes in animals can be brought together. Perhaps in this way future investigations into the biology of ageing will be able to provide more satisfactory answers to the question — what are the underlying principles of the ageing process and why does it occur at all?

Further reading

Physiological deterioration

Finch, C.E. & Schneider, E.L. (Eds)(1985) *Handbook of the Biology of Aging*, 2nd Edn. Van Nostrand Reinhold, New York.

Bioenergetics

Hansford, R.G. (1983) Bioenergetics in ageing. *Biochim. Biophys. Acta* **726**, 41–80.

Age-specific genes

Medawar, P.B. (1952) An Unsolved Problem in Biology. H.K. Lewis, London; reprinted in Medawar, P.B. (1981) *The Uniqueness of the Individual.* Dover, New York.

Ageing versus reproduction

Kirkwood, T.B.L. & Holliday, R. (1986). In *The Biology of Human Ageing* (Eds A.H. Bittles & K.J. Collins), pp. 1–16. Cambridge University Press, Cambridge.

Developmental biology

Kohn, R.R. (1978) *Principles of Mammalian Ageing.* Prentice-Hall, London.

2 | The demography of ageing

A.M. WARNES

Introduction

Awareness of the ageing of Britain's population has recently spread among politicians, service planners and the scientific community. In fact, demographic transition, whereby persons aged 60 years or more have increased from 1 in 20 to nearly 1 in 5 of the population, has been taking place in Britain since the beginning of the century. Unless fertility and mortality again fall substantially, the pensionable fraction of our population will not increase a great deal further. It is true, however, that until the end of the century the numbers in extreme old age (85+ years) will continue to increase but even for this age group the growth rates are likely to slacken. The basis for the concern of health and other service providers about the consequences of an ageing population is only partly demographic: it has much to do with the health expectations of a more affluent and better educated population.

If we are to arrive at worthwhile forecasts of health service demands from the older population, it will be valuable to address three interesting problems. Firstly, will mortality improve more rapidly than has been the case over the last 40 years, particularly among older people? Secondly, do improvements in life expectancy lead to a disproportionate growth of the population with disorders, or are they accompanied by improvements in morbidity or the delay of pathologies? In other words, what is the relationship between declines in mortality and the prevalence among people in their sixties and seventies of the most common physical and mental illnesses? Finally, what is the relationship between the rising income, housing and educational standards of the population and their health expectations?

This chapter will examine the latest demographic projections for Britain and the debate about the future needs and demands of old people for social and health services. Some space is given, however, to the general process of demographic ageing as it has affected Britain and other Western countries to date, and as it is likely to affect all regions of the world. This will put into global perspective the problems of improving the health and 'quality of life' of our own older population. It will show that the tasks which face the medical profession in Britain are less those of providing minimal or essential support and treatment to a rising total of aged people, but more those of influencing and responding to the economic and political choices concerning health priorities which are made by individuals and the government.

Demographic ageing

The age structure of a nation is a complex record of the demographic conditions which it has experienced over the previous century. It is influenced by the past and present schedules of fertility and mortality and by the record of net international migration. The northwest European history of fertility and mortality since the late 18th century can be simplified into a sequence of changes known as the demographic transition. Substantial falls in death rates during the middle decades of the 19th century were followed in its last quarter by a substantial decline in fertility, and it was the latter which rapidly reduced the relative presence of children and initiated growth in the relative share of aged people. As theoretical life-table analyses demonstrate, the level of fertility has a stronger influence on the age structure than life expectancy at birth (Clark & Spengler, 1980).

Throughout the late 19th century the pensionable age population of Great Britain remained around 6.1% although it increased each decade by 11–14% (Fig. 2.1). After 1911, the growth of the absolute pensionable population accelerated to its highest annual rates of over 2.2% during 1921–51. The total number of pensioners increased in the period 1931–51 by 2.4 million and by mid-century more than one in eight (13.6%) of the population was of pensionable age. Since 1951, the growth

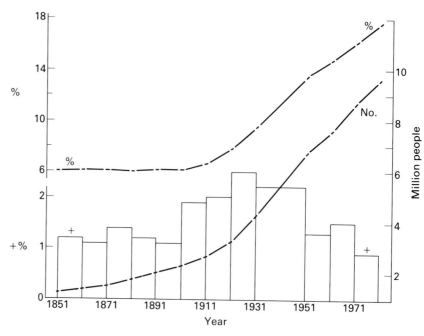

Fig. 2.1. The number, percentage share and mean annual growth rates of the pensionable population of Great Britain, 1851–1981. No. — millions of people aged 60+ (females) and 65+ (males); % — pensioners as a percentage of the total population; +% — average annual growth rate of the pensionable population. (From Census reports of Great Britain, 1851–1981.)

in the relative share has slowed although until the 1970s the absolute annual increase remained substantial. Not until the first decade of the next century, when the high post-1945 birth cohorts reach retirement, will there again be a substantial increase in the size of the aged population in Britain, and only if there are further substantial falls in fertility and late-age mortality will the aged share of the population increase substantially. Indeed it can be said that the demographic ageing of the Britain population extended from around 1900 until around 1970.

In common with its near neighbours in Europe, the UK has been in the vanguard of the ageing process. Several developed countries retain more rapid rates of relative and absolute growth of the elderly population. In the USA, for example, a continuous history of population growth by net immigration and high fertility currently supports annual old population increases of around 1.8%. This rate is moderating and the projections indicate an average annual growth of 0.4% during the 1990s. Concerned and even alarmist commentaries on ageing abound in the USA despite the nation's exceptional ability to adjust to an older population which derives from its general economic strength and from anticipated increases in its working population. In Australia too, high rates during the 1950s and 1960s and subsequent falls in both immigration and fertility have resulted in rapid rates of absolute and relative old population growth during the late 1980s (Hugo, 1986).

But the fastest growth of old populations and the most challenging problems of service provision in the next decade will occur in those less developed countries that since the 1960s have experienced marked fertility declines. Taking a global view, in 1980 the population aged 60 years or more ranged from 4.9% in Africa to 16.9% in Europe: among individual countries the range was from 3% in Kenya (and less than 4% in Malawi, Tanzania, Botswana and Nicaragua) to 21.9% in Sweden (and over 19% in Norway, East Germany, Denmark, the UK, Austria and Switzerland). Nearly a quarter (22%) of the world's elderly population lived in Europe. The global distribution shows a latitudinal arrangement with, in general, intertropical regions having the least old age structures (Fig. 2.2).

The United Nations Organization (UN) population projections suggest that from 1980 until 2000 the world's old population will increase by 66%, with a range from 95% in Central America to 2.7% in Northern Europe. For individual countries the probable range is from <1% in Sweden and Norway to >125% in Guatemala and Nicaragua. The global distribution is suggestive of an inverse correlation with the level of economic and social development (Fig. 2.3). The largest absolute increase was projected to occur in China, with an expectation that 62 million will be added to the old population between 1975 and 2000. Among the other countries faced with a combination of high absolute and proportionate increases are the Soviet Union, India, Brazil, Indonesia, Mexico and Bangladesh. Projections for 2025 suggest that 14% of

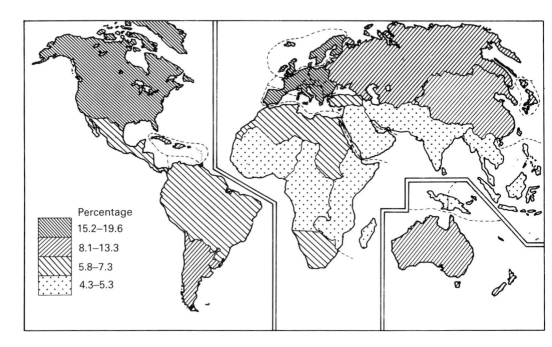

Fig. 2.2. The representation of old people (aged 60+ years) in the population of the world's major regions, 1980. (From United Nations Organization, Department of International Economic and Social Affairs (1985) *The World Aging Situation: Strategies and Policies.* UN, New York.)

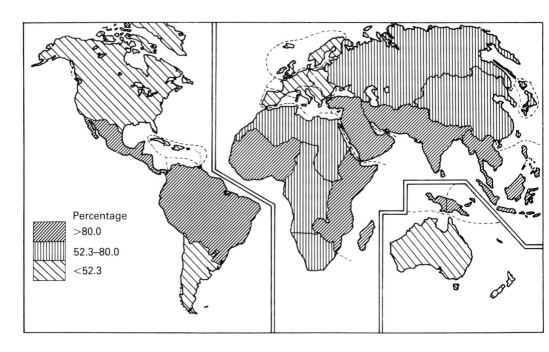

Fig. 2.3. Projected increases of the 60+ years population in major world regions, 1980-2000. (From United Nations Organization, Department of International Economic and Social Affairs (1985) *The World Aging Situation: Strategies and Policies.* UN, New York.)

the world's population will be aged 60+, that 71% of these 1135 million people will be living in the less developed regions and fewer than 12% in Europe.

While the remainder of this chapter will focus on our more immediate concerns and responsibilities in tackling the problems and demands of old people in Britain, it is salutary to note these wider implications of the process of demographic ageing (Myers, 1985; Warnes 1986). If the most common stereotype of an old person in the developed world is of a socially isolated and frail widow in an old, run-down house, by the end of the century sheer numbers will impress upon us another image of an indigent old person in a Third World country. Most of them will have no state income or social service support and little access to either acute or longstay medical facilities: many will be striving to survive in a bewilderingly changed society and living either in disorganized urban shanty towns or in neglected and economically retarded rural areas.

The sex and marital status of the older population

Marital status has important practical and social implications for the personal and household situations of older people. It is sometimes forgotten that among the principal providers of care and support to frail or sick old people are wives and husbands. Even when relatives, friends or neighbours are willing to offer support to people living alone, it is necessarily less intensive and responsive. There is therefore a relationship between the marital situation of a person and their reliance upon formal care and nursing support, as at times of convalescence. Aged people who are living alone or widowed concentrate, to a greater extent than do married old people, in industrial towns and in the inner city areas. These same areas sustain over-representations of poor housing, low income groups and educational disadvantages: the interactions among these generate taxing local concentrations of dependency upon the social and health services.

Improvements in mortality in Western countries during this century have disproportionately favoured females and produced strong sex differentials in life expectancy and an unbalanced sex ratio. An excess of females has also risen from losses during the First World War. Changing attitudes and customs with respect to marriage and divorce, as well as differential mortalities, have produced a marital status distribution of the older population which changes considerably from the younger to the oldest age groups. In Great Britain in 1981, among those aged 60–64 three-quarters were married and 13.6% widowed; however, these proportions reverse among people aged 90–94 years, of whom three-quarters were widowed and 9.8% married. Over half of the 75+ years old population were widowed and a third were married (Rees & Warnes, 1986).

In 1981, a surprising 10% of the 60+ years population were single, although this proportion had fallen since 1971. Only 2% were divorced, although this marital status had more than doubled during the 1970s. Males were much more likely to be married than females and as a result fewer were living alone. At the present time there is a simple, age-related decline in the prevalence of divorce up to the unusually advanced age of 95 years or more. It probably results from a combination of a strong cohort effect, reflecting the increase in the incidence of divorce in Britain since the late 1960s, and several ageing effects, e.g. those associated with differential mortality by marital status and the sex-specific propensities to divorce and remarriage at different ages.

Relatively little research or commentary has been devoted to trends in the marital status of the old population. One control will be the course of sex-specific differentials in mortality improvement. There is relatively little room for further declines among females in their fifties but male mortality at these ages continues to fall; however, there is no sign yet of the female advantage at advanced old ages ceasing to grow. Therefore, while the incidence of widowhood among women in their fifties might decline, a comparable change among women of pensionable age is unlikely in the near future. In any case, demographically based changes may be swamped by the trends in marriage dissolution. One result of spreading divorce in the early and middle adult years appears to be a widened age differential between husbands and wives in second and subsequent marriages. This may increase the late-age incidence of widowhood. The consequences of more common divorce in the late middle and old age groups remain unclear: the whole subject requires close study together with the course of mortality improvements.

The decline in late-age mortality

Mortality rates have been falling in Britain throughout this century although age-specific death rates in later life have fallen more erratically than all age mortality. Nothing comparable to the apparent irregular progress of mortality declines in the USA is evident in Britain (Brody, 1985). From 1961 until 1984 late-age mortality fell in the UK by about 20%. The improvement in survival chances between 1970 and 1980 has meant that life expectancy at birth has increased for males from 68.6 to 70.4 years and for females from 74.9 to 76.5 years, and that the life expectancy at 60 years has increased from 15.1 to 16.1 years for males and from 19.7 to 20.6 years for females (Rees & Warnes, 1986). There have been only minor differences in the recent mortality improvement at different ages among the older population (Fig. 2.4). On the other hand, recent mortality trends have shown interesting sex differentials, with the improvements among 'young' old males (aged 55–64 years) tending to reduce their differential disadvantage in comparison to females. Mortality among those 10 years older has improved faster for females and slower for males, resulting in an increasing sex differential until 1971. Since then there have been signs of a reversal. For the succeeding decennial age group (75–84 years), female mortality has been improving more rapidly than male mortality since at least 1931 (Anderson & Ashwood, 1985).

There are persistent regional and urban-rural differences in all-age and late-age mortality rates in the UK with, in general, the higher death rates being found in the climatically and economically harsher north. Scotland and Northern England have particularly high rates, more than 20% above the mean (Warnes, 1987). The most favourable regions are East Anglia, the South-West and the South-East of England. Death rates in the major urban areas are little above those for their containing regions, while among the 85+ population they are actually lower.

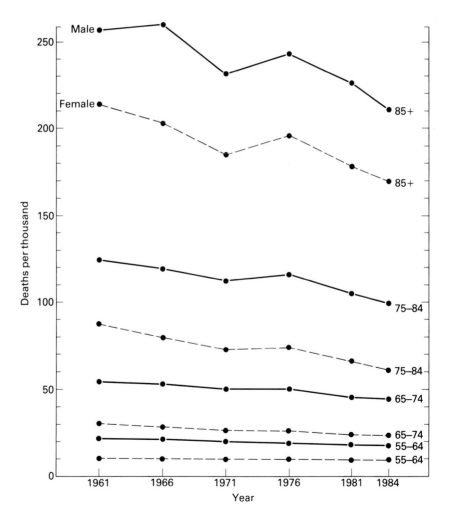

Fig. 2.4. Age-specific death rates per 1000, England and Wales, 1961–84. (From Office of Population Censuses and Surveys (1985) *Population Trends* **45**, Table 20.)

Aged population projections

Population growth during the late 19th century in Great Britain was sufficiently high to have produced a rising number of people reaching the old age groups until the 1970s. However, the annual increase in the size and share of the old population has been unsteady during the last 30 years and this will continue, largely as a consequence of the fluctuating annual totals of births during this century. Apart from the distortions associated with the two major European wars, economic growth during 1953–65 was associated with high birth rates, and the periods of recession during the interwar years and since the early 1970s have been associated with low fertility.

Official projections of the size, age and sex structure of the population of Great Britain are produced every two years by the Government Actuary in association with the Office of Population Censuses and Surveys (OPCS). These employ cohort-survival methods with conservative assumptions based on extrapolations of long-term mortality, fertility and net international migration trends (Daykin, 1986). Unlike UN or US Bureau of the Census projections, which offer alternatives based on higher or lower fertility assumptions, only one series is published in Britain. National projections of the old population are generally reliable for half a century ahead because they extrapolate age-specific mortality rates to an already born population, but in recent years revisions have been necessary because mortality assumptions have been too pessimistic (Benjamin & Overton, 1981; Warnes, 1983).

Recent OPCS projections indicate that the population of statutory pensionable age in England and Wales will increase from around 9 million in 1981 to around 10.8 million in 2021. The 1985 projections for Great Britain suggest modest growth of the 60+ years old population by 2006, comprising large increases of the smaller cohorts in extreme old age and a fall of approximately 11% in the population aged 65–74 years (Fig. 2.5; OPCS, 1985). The 85+ years old population has been growing during the 1980s at the exceptional annual rate of 3.8% but this will moderate to 2.2% during the 1990s and is likely to stabilize by the 2010s. It must be emphasized that the increases in the very old population are largely a function of the mortality assumptions built into the projections. Alternative projections by Rees in 1986, which are based on a constant mortality assumption, highlight this effect (Fig. 2.5). The post-1945 high birth cohorts will be reaching the old age groups after 2005 and the size of the pensionable population will once again increase more rapidly: the effect on the old share of the population will depend upon the course of fertility during the 1990s and beyond.

Regional and district projections

During the last decade the government's demographers have begun to publish age-structure projections for regions, counties, metropolitan districts and London boroughs (OPCS, 1986). At this scale migration flows are important influences and their instability and relationship to local employment, housing market and urban development factors must be appreciated. Even with the OPCS's conservative assumptions concerning the loss of population from urban areas with the growth of new suburbs, marked differences in area projections arise. During the 1980s the pensionable population of the Greater London County area is expected to decline annually by 0.5%, whereas in nearby Buckinghamshire it is expected to increase by 1.5% per annum. The prospects for any individual regional health authority may be quite different to that of the nation and should be given specific examination.

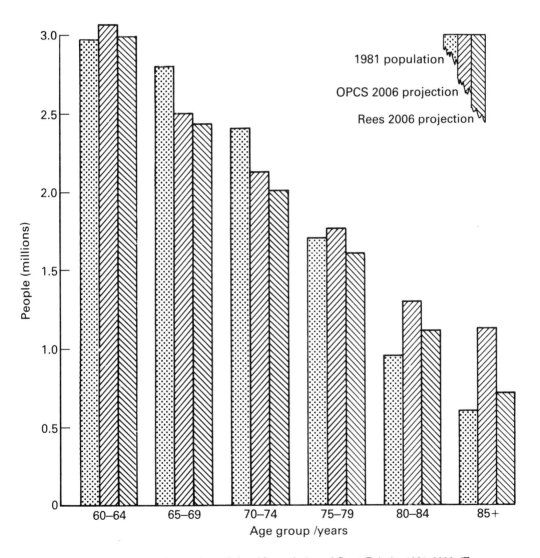

Fig. 2.5. Projections of the old population of Great Britain, 1981–2006. (From Office of Population Censuses and Surveys (1985) *Population Projections, 1983–2053,* Series PP2, No. 13. HMSO, London; Rees & Warnes (1986), Table 11.)

Rees has also produced projections for 20 regions of the UK, made up of Northern Ireland and the metropolitan areas and non-metropolitan 'remainders' of the regions of Great Britain (Table 2.1). He uses separate life-tables for each region and age-specific schedules for the migration flow from each origin region to each destination region. The method is therefore more sensitive than OPCS methods to regional patterns of migration, the effects of which are made clearer by the assumptions of constant fertility and mortality. The projections indicate that the 60+ years old population of the metropolitan regions will decrease by 10–20% between 1981 and 2006, with the largest falls likely to be in Greater London, Merseyside, Tyne and Wear (Newcastle and Sunderland) and Greater Manchester. On the other hand, most of the southern regions of England are likely to experience small increases of their old population, with the three most substantial gains being in the south-west (+6%), the Outer Metropolitan Area around London (+9%) and East Anglia (+12%). These three regions are precisely those which are receiving the greatest net migration gains of people aged 50+ years (Rees & Warnes, 1986).

Table 2.1. Projections of UK regional old populations, 1981–2006

Region	Population aged 60 and over (1000s)		
	1981	2006	Ratio
Non-metropolitan regions			
Outer south-east	1078	1083	101
East Anglia	403	453	112
South-west	1023	1083	106
East Midlands	755	777	103
West Midlands County remainder	466	484	104
Yorks and Humberside remainder	321	317	99
Wales	601	553	92
Northern Ireland	247	251	102
Scotland remainder	672	644	96
North-west remainder	480	451	94
North remainder	382	360	94
Metropolitan regions			
Outer London metro. area	902	1079	109
West Yorkshire	415	360	87
South Yorkshire	266	240	90
Greater Manchester	529	438	83
West Midlands metro. county	520	450	87
Tyne and Wear	240	196	82
Merseyside	308	246	80
Central Clydeside	312	276	88
Greater London	1448	1152	80
United Kingdom	11 457	10 875	95

From Rees & Warnes (1986, table 12).

Household projections

The household arrangements of old people are diverse, rapidly changing and inadequately studied. While the dominant forms of living alone, living with a spouse and living with children are clear, there is a daunting variety of combinations of relatives of different generation and of unrelated persons. Problems of classification and interpretation arise, e.g. in the case of a parent aged 85 years living with a child aged 62 years. Either the younger or the older person could be the head of a household or physically dependent upon the other. Recent studies using both the General Household Survey and the OPCS Longitudinal Study, which links records from the 1971 and 1981 censuses with registration information, are showing the dynamism of household changes among the old population and some of the characteristic transitions as people become widowed and aged (Dale *et al.*, 1987; Grundy, 1987).

In Western societies today an aged person is most likely to live either alone or only with spouse. There are variations among the developed countries but normally no more than 5% live in institutions (although a higher percentage pass the last months or weeks of their lives in these settings). In 1976, 30% of the non-institutional population aged 65 or more years in England lived alone, 44% lived with their spouse, 6% lived with a spouse and others and 3% lived with siblings only. Partly included in this third group were the 13% of the old who lived with their children and/or child's spouse (Hunt, 1978, Table 4.6.1). Reflecting the age and sex-related patterns of marital status, while a majority of women aged 85 or more years lived alone, only 14% of men aged 65–74 years were in this situation.

A strong social trend over recent years has been the decrease of household size. Ermisch has recently provided a substantial analysis for Britain since 1945 of the relationships between demographic trends and the demand for housing (Ermisch, 1983). Broadly, he finds that half of the increased demand for housing during this period has arisen from population growth and age-structure changes. The remainder must therefore be attributed to the population's increasing ability to express a preference for independent, small-household living. Many studies from several nations testify that there is a positive correlation between affluence and the propensity to live in small households. A similar point is that deterministic projections of the numbers living in institutions on the basis of demographic trends are of little value: the level of provision of such facilities is predominantly a reflection of health and social service policies and funding.

It is therefore difficult to forecast household arrangements of the old population and their use of domiciliary or institutional services. Demands will not be a question solely of the number of people living at different ages, their sex and marital status, but also a function of resources, preferences and supply. The Government Statistical Service

(1985), however, has published extrapolations of household headship rates based on the linear trend through the 1961, 1966, 1971 and 1981 census recorded rates (Table 2.2). These indicate a substantial increase in older males living alone during the 1980s but a moderation during the 1990s. While the number of females living alone will also continue to increase at a declining rate, other households containing females are likely to decrease substantially.

Table 2.2. Household projections for England and Wales, 1981–2001

Head of household	Number (1000s)			Average annual change (%)	
	1981	1991	2001	1981–91	1991–2001
Female, 60+ years					
One person	2057	2528	2734	+2.0	+0.8
All other	523	381	264	−3.2	−3.7
Male, 65+ years					
One person	483	667	766	+3.3	+1.4
Married couple	1939	2049	2025	+0.6	−0.1
All other	147	125	97	−1.6	−2.5

From Government Statistical Service (1985).

The distribution of the old population

The distribution of the old population of the nation and the directions of change provide a basis for predicting which districts will experience unusually rapid or slow rates of growth. Since the mid-century there has been a strong peripheral distribution in England and Wales of the areas with above average representations of older people (Warnes & Law, 1985). In Scotland a more intricate geography is found, with concentrations of the old in both the attractive upland areas to the north-west and south-east of the central, industrial lowlands, and in the much more remote highlands and islands (Fig. 2.6).

The mechanism which has brought about the peripheral distribution of the areas of over-representation of the old is age-selective migration. Large cities are, increasingly, areas of export of the late middle-aged and young elderly population, while non-metropolitan peripheral districts are areas of import. This pattern has arisen partly because of the size and topography of England and Wales: all coastal areas are now well serviced and accessible in no more than half a day's drive from the main metropolitan areas, and within the centre of southern Great Britain there are only a small number of non-industrial or urban areas attractive for retirement residence. As is the case in France, the phenomenon of retirement migration, of people moving from their districts of residence during working life, is most strongly associated with the capital. Both London and Paris have exceptionally high rates of out-migration among the retiring age group.

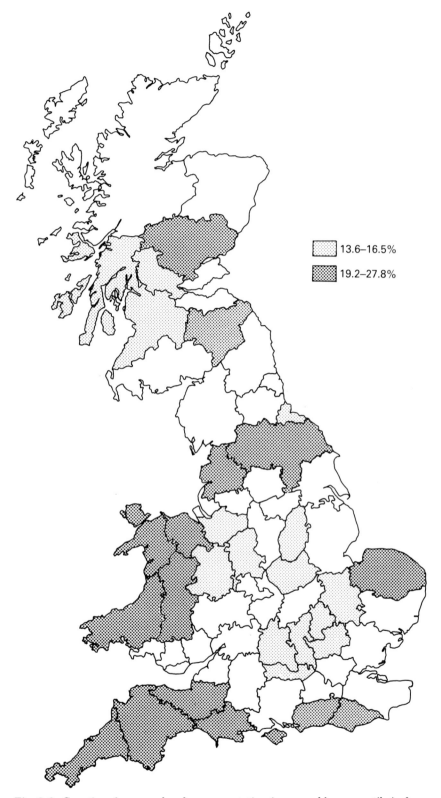

Fig. 2.6. Counties of over- and under-representation (upper and lower quartiles) of the pensionable population, Great Britain, 1981.

Whatever the interest in the evolution of the distribution of the areas of over- and under-representation of the old population, the great majority of Britain's old people live in the principal cities and industrial areas between Liverpool, Leeds, Bristol and the London region. Approximately a quarter of Britain's old in 1981 lived in Greater London and the six surrounding counties of Kent, Surrey, Berkshire, Buckinghamshire, Hertfordshire and Essex. Another quarter was found in the seven metropolitan counties of the West Midlands, Merseyside, Greater Manchester, West Yorkshire, South Yorkshire, Tyne and Wear and Strathclyde.

For the purposes of planning services, the critical demographic index may be the anticipated absolute increase of either the old population or a more finely specified sub-group such as those above a certain age or those living alone. Over the next decade the greatest increases of the old population will occur neither in the longest developed retirement resorts nor in the cities with the highest population density. Instead, they will occur in the suburbs and expanded towns which grew to a substantial size during the 1950s and 1960s (Fig. 2.7). The young adult population which moved into these areas a quarter of a century ago is now reaching or approaching the elderly age group. At the local level, variations in the age structure will therefore be most important in determining the rate of change of the old population for the remainder of this century, not least because the rate of migration has fallen by approximately one quarter since around 1971.

The debate on mortality improvement and morbidity

Since the late 1960s there has been a renewed period of declining mortality at later ages in Britain and the USA which has stimulated a lively debate among demographers, epidemiologists and clinicians about the future course of mortality and ageing. The opposing views are, on the one hand, that human life expectancy is unlikely to exceed substantially the 80 or so years presently attained in the healthiest and wealthiest regions of the developed world. Further progress in fighting cancers and heart disease will enable a larger percentage of future cohorts to reach their eighties but will not lead to a radical prolongation of life: essentially it is suggested that we are reaching the upper limit of survival potential. The result will be a reduction of both mortality and morbidity among people in their later sixties and seventies and an increase in the percentage of all deaths that occur to people in their eighties. The survival curve will become increasingly rectangular (Fries, 1980).

An alternative and more commonly held view is that further substantial increases in life expectancy are possible. The difference between average expectancy and the occasionally achieved span of 115–117 years can be cut much further. It is worth remembering that many data series aggregate all persons of 75+ years (or another

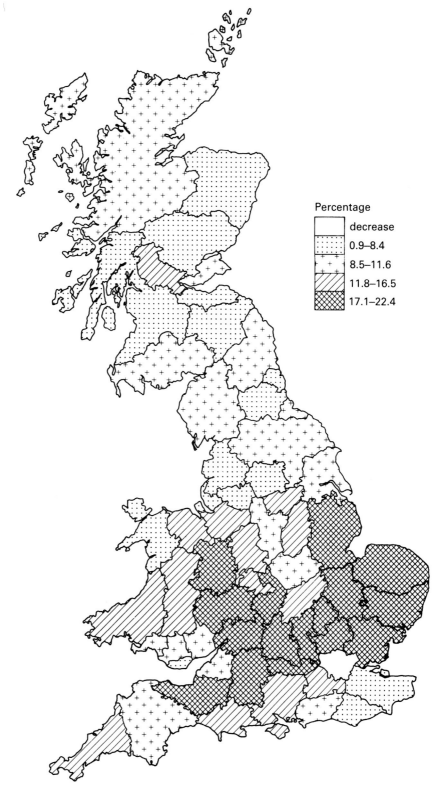

Fig. 2.7. The increase of the pensionable population of the counties of Great Britain, 1971–81.

Demography of ageing

number), and therefore have been insensitive to differential changes in mortality among the most advanced ages. Proponents of this view tend to be more cautious in foreseeing declining age-specific morbidity rates but draw attention to their expectation of higher survival rates into the eighties and nineties, ages with undisputedly high prevalence rates of physical and mental disorders.

The first view predicts a decreasing incidence of disabilities and widowhood among the retired population and therefore a growing proportion of healthy elderly people well able to support themselves. The alternative interpretation anticipates substantial increases of very old people and, in the most pessimistic appraisals, quite startling projections of the numbers who will be disabled, widowed, socially isolated, and suffering from specific disorders requiring either expensive surgery or long-term intensive care. Even the US Bureau of the Census published projections of the annual number of hip fractures in the USA rising from 0.2 million to nearly 0.7 million in 2050.

As is often the case with such debates, it has flourished partly because the evidence is unable to disprove conclusively one of the competing views, and partly because there is some basis for both. Many commentators recognize declines in mortality from the most common disorders, suggest that the lethality of certain diseases may be falling more quickly than their incidence or prevalence, and point to the complexities arising from the increasing reporting of multiple cause deaths (Anderson & Ashwood, 1985; Manton, 1982). For the USA, Brody (1985) has asserted that there are no data to establish age-specific declines in deafness, blindness, hip fracture, osteoarthritis or Alzheimer's disease and related disorders, and that 'there is at present no accepted scientific prospect that the net increase in healthy years will exceed the years of dysfunction'.

The importance of the issues for the planning and the financing of medical services and for the quality of older persons' lives has focused the attention of epidemiologists, demographers and actuarians on the inadequate data concerning the health of the older population. Excellent work is being done to assemble improved data sets and to adapt conventional life-table analysis to modelling relationships between age and incapacity, disease, referral and the need for intensive care (Manton & Soldo, 1985). This work is an essential prerequisite for the generation of indicative rather than primarily alarmist forecasts of the incidence of specific disorders 20 or more years ahead.

As shown in connection with several topics discussed in this chapter, while demographic events provide a numerical foundation to the ageing process, many of the attendant critical changes for old people and for the health and social services are strongly influenced by non-demographic trends. Growing and spreading affluence along with higher educational attainment is associated with rising health expectations and demands. Advances in medical practice and facilities not only respond to these demands but to an extent promote them. Just as no limit has yet been detected in people's capacity to consume material products, no reason exists to expect a finite demand for improved functioning and health in old age. The further elaboration of demographic ageing and its interactions with social and economic change will undoubtedly raise the demands upon the medical profession and its paymasters. But it is more appropriate to see this situation as a challenge than as a set of dismaying problems. Now that so many of the disorders of pregnancy and infancy have been conquered, the agenda for those concerned with promoting health increasingly focuses on the last decades of life. The multiplying demands to cope with the diseases and disorders of old age are a by-product of the extension of life expectancy. There is therefore a paradox in the concern and alarm which societal ageing attracts: one way to diffuse these reactions will be to gain more detailed knowledge of the relationships between an individual's age and the incidence, prevalence and functional impact of disease and physical and mental disorders.

References

Citations have been minimized, with a leaning towards articles in the more widely circulated journals. For further reading on the topics raised in this chapter, the reader is referred to the books by Clark & Spengler (1980) and Bogue (1969). Hunt's (1978) survey of the characteristics and situation of old people in Britain has not been superceded. Ermisch (1983) and Manton (1982) provide more up-to-date and technical studies.

Anderson, M. & Ashwood, F. (1985) Projections of mortality rates for the elderly. *Popul. Trends* **42**, 22–29.

Benjamin, B. & Overton, E.(1981) Prospects for mortality decline in England and Wales. *Popul. Trends* **23**, 22–28.

Bogue, D.J. (1969) *Principles of Demography.* Wiley, New York.

Brody, J.A. (1985) Prospects for an aging population. *Nature* **315**, 463–66.

Clark, R.L. & Spengler, J.J. (1980) *The Economics of Individual and Population Aging.* Cambridge University Press, Cambridge.

Craig, J.(1983) The growth of the elderly population. *Popul. Trends* **32**, 28–33.

Dale, A., Evandrou, M. & Arber, S. (1987) The household structure of the elderly population of Great Britain. *Ageing Soc.* **7**, 37–56

Daykin, C. (1986) Projecting the population of the United Kingdom. *Popul. Trends* **44**, 28–33.

Ermisch, J.F. (1983) *The Political Economy of Demographic Change.* Heinemann, London.

Fries, J.F. (1980) Aging, natural death and the compression of morbidity. *New Engl. J. Med.* **303**, 130–35.

Government Statistical Service (1985) *1981-Based Household Projections 1981–2001.* HMSO, London.

Grundy, E. (1987) Retirement migration and its consequences in England and Wales. *Ageing Soc.* **7**, 57–82.

Hugo, G.J. (1986) Population aging in Australia: implications for social and economic policy. *Papers of the East-West Population Institute* **98**, 47pp..

Hunt, A (1978) *The Elderly at Home: A Study of People Aged 65 and Over Living in the Community in England in 1976.* HMSO, London.

Manton, K.G. (1982) Changing concepts of morbidity and mortality in the elderly population. *Milbank Mem. Fund Quart.* **60**, 183–244.

Manton, K.G. & Soldo, B.J. (1985) Dynamics of health changes in the oldest old: new perspectives and evidence. *Milbank Mem. Fund Quart.* **63**, 206–85.

Myers, G.C. (1985) Aging and worldwide population change. In *Aging and the Social Sciences* (Eds R.H. Binstock & E. Shanas), 2nd Edn. Van Nostrand Reinhold, New York, pp. 173-198.

Office of Population Censuses and Surveys (OPCS) (1985) *Population Projections, 1983–2053,* Series PP2, No. 13 HMSO, London.

OPCS (1986) *Population Projections, Area, 1983–2001.* HMSO, London.

Rees, P.H. & Warnes, A.M. (1986) *Migration of the elderly in the United Kingdom.* Paper presented at the Katholicke Universiteit, Nijmegen, The Netherlands. School of Geography, University of Leeds, Working Paper No. 473.

Warnes, A.M. (1983) Migration in late working age and early retirement. *Socio-Econ. Plann. Sci.* **17**, 291-302.

Warnes, A.M. (1986) The elderly in less developed countries. *Ageing Soc.* **7**, 373-80.

Warnes, A.M. (1987) The ageing of Britain's population: geographical dimensions. *Espaces, Population, Sociétés* **1987/2**, 317-27.

Warnes, A.M. & Law, C.M. (1985) Elderly population distributions and housing prospects in Britain. *Town Plann. Rev.* **56**, 292-314.

3 | The aged cardiovascular system

T.P. CRIPPS

Introduction

There are three important factors to bear in mind when considering ageing of the cardiovascular system: firstly — the common caveat of all authorities on ageing — it is almost impossible to differentiate between the physiological changes associated with *age* and those caused by *pathological* changes which are common with increasing years. As far as possible these two factors will be separated, since this helps an understanding of the actual processes involved; however, it must be borne in mind that apparently fit, asymptomatic 'normal' subjects may in fact have hidden pathology. Secondly, many of the studies (particularly those concerning mechanical and biochemical *in vitro* properties) have been performed on the hearts of non-human animals; the assumption is that ageing in other species is the same as in humans. Thirdly, there are very few studies on humans over the age of 80 years; although the changes present in the 'young' aged are unlikely to regress, they may become more prominent — or different problems may arise in the older subject.

Structural changes in the heart associated with age

The heart of a healthy person increases in weight by 1–1.5 g per year; there is an increase in left ventricular (LV) wall thickness of up to 30%. This may be a response to an increase of blood pressure or output impedance which is usual with increasing years; certainly this change is small compared to increases in size brought about by pathological processes like hypertension. Probably much more important are changes in heart weight associated with a person's body mass; thus, fatter people will have heavier hearts, and the 'atrophic' heart which used to be associated with old age is purely a reflection of the number dying of chronic disease with weight loss.

Microscopically, there is an increase in the amount of fat in the myocardium, and of fibrous tissue, particularly in the interatrial septum and the wall of both atria; this is associated with a loss of pacemaker cells in the sinoatrial node (even in subjects with no evidence of ischaemic damage). The endocardium shows changes which can be explained by mechanical factors: it becomes thicker with age, and elastic collagen fibres proliferate and become disorganized; similarly the valves may become thickened, particularly on the left side of the heart. There may be foamy vacuolation in the valve cusps, and 'powdery' calcification is usually present by the sixth decade.

There are also two quite specific histological changes in the heart associated with age; the accumulation of lipofuscin and basophilic degeneration. Lipofuscin is a pigment, derived from lysosomes, which is absent in the young and invariably present at the poles of myofibre nuclei of an aged heart, although the quantity present in fit people does not seem to correlate well with any known demographic factors. Basophilic degeneration presents as masses of amorphous material (derived from an insoluble product of glycogen metabolism) within the muscle fibre and is also invariably present in the aged.

With age, there are important changes in the major arteries. Most vessels increase in both diameter and wall thickness; there is a loss of endothelial uniformity, fragmentation of elastin and an increase in the amount of collagen in the media. This is particularly important in the aorta and has major mechanical consequences. Epicardial vessels become tortuous even in subjects who do not develop atherosclerosis.

The significance of all these structural changes is debatable: while the increase in aortic size has inevitable mechanical implications, none of the other changes has been shown to be harmful. However, an exaggeration of these changes may be associated with *pathological* states. Examples of these are shown in Table 3.1. Table 3.2 lists some pathological conditions which, although not a feature of normal ageing, are mostly found in the old.

Electrical, biochemical and mechanical changes

Most of the data published on the effects of ageing on electrical and biochemical properties of the myocardium have been derived from work on rat tissue in the laboratory; however, where evidence is available from

Table 3.1. Structural changes in the heart associated with ageing, and associated pathological changes

Change (usually benign)	Associated pathology (if exaggerated)
Macroscopic	
Increased size; (weight increases by 1–1.5 g per year)	
Increased tortuosity of epicardial vessels (without atherosclerosis)	
Aorta dilates and unfolds	Aortic regurgitation
Microscopic	
Lipofuscin accumulation	
Basophilic degeneration	
Increased fibrous tissue (especially sinoatrial node and conducting system)	Heart block
Increased fat (especially in the interatrial septum)	Fatty 'tumour-like' mass in septum: dysrhythmias
Loss of pacemaker cells in sinoatrial node (? 80% lost by age 75 years)	?Sick sinus syndrome: atrial dysrhythmias
Amyloid (may be demonstrable in 40% of hearts)	Senile cardiac amyloidosis

Table 3.2. Pathological conditions seen only or predominantly in old hearts*

(i) Calcific degenerative disease
   Mitral ring calcification
   Aortic cusp calcification
   Calcific aortic stenosis (isolated, tricuspid aortic valve)

(ii) Mucoid degenerative valvular disease
   Mitral regurgitation and rupturerd chordae tendineae
   Aortic regurgitation

(iii) Senile cardiac amyloidosis

(iv) Conduction system disease
   Sclerodegeneration of the conducting system (Lenegre's disease)
   Fibrosis or calcification of the conducting system from adjacent structures
   (Lev's disease)

(v) External cardiac rupture (after myocardial infarction)

*After Williams (1985), adapted from Noble & Rothbaum (1981).

human tissue, it does not conflict with that presented below. The time taken to develop peak myocardial muscle tension and the duration of isometric contraction are prolonged by about 20% in senescent animals. This is evident in humans by prolongation of the pre-ejection period and the time from aortic valve closure to opening of the mitral valve in subjects aged 60–80 years compared to younger adults. The degree of peak tension developed is not affected, nor is the maximum rate of change of tension, so it appears that there is no defect at the myofilament level. There is evidence, however, that it may be related to changes in the ability of sarcoplasmic reticulum to release and take up Ca^{2+}, and possibly changes in the duration of the action potential. It is of interest that the increased duration of contraction may be reversed in senescent animals which have undergone exercise training.

Various biochemical changes have been documented in tissue homogenates from aged hearts, and *in vivo*. Myocardial oxygen consumption and substrate oxidation rates are usually found to decrease in the order of 20%, and there is a reduced specific activity of certain mitochondrial enzymes in addition to a change in their relative activities in aged animals. Unfortunately, the difficulties in standardizing these experiments in terms of the cardiac workload performed means that their significance is at present uncertain.

The important consequence of the changes described is that the mechanical properties of the heart and aorta change in old age:
(i) The ventricle becomes less compliant at all phases of the cardiac cycle; this actually improves the rate of development of tension during contraction, but will reduce the rate of filling during diastole.
(ii) The aorta becomes less extensible as well as dilated. This results in an increase in the ventricular output impedance and, consequently, the workload. Thus, the LV afterload increases even in the absence of an increase of blood pressure. Indeed, it has been suggested that the mod-

erate age-associated increase in myocardial mass discussed above is an adaptive change to this increased impedance.

Changes in control

At any instant, the performance of the heart is the result of (i) its intrinsic rhythmicity and contractility, (ii) preload and afterload, and (iii) the effects of neuronal and endocrine control. The system of control of the heart is shown in Fig. 3.1. In the aged normal human, there are important changes. The intrinsic heart rate (i.e. the rate when the sympathetic and parasympathetic nervous input is pharmacologically denervated) falls from 104 beats per minute in young adults to 92 in the aged. There is a marked increase in the threshold of stimulation of the cardiac autonomic nerves required to elicit a response, and the cardiac responses to hypoxia and hypercarbia (i.e. the chemoreceptor arcs) and to postural and blood pressure changes (baroreceptor) are all attenuated in the aged. In addition, the cardiac responses to prolonged handgrip and the valsalva manoeuvre are reduced in the normal aged compared to

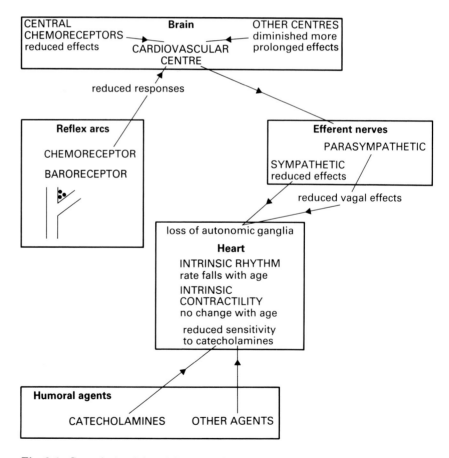

Fig. 3.1. Control of activity of the heart. Changes associated with ageing are shown in small letters.

younger adults, and there is a reduction in vagal influence, as demonstrated by a reduction in sinus arrhythmia associated with advancing age. Experiments demonstrate that in senescent animals stimulation of the hypothalamus (which has important input to the cardiovascular 'centre') causes diminished but more prolonged responses, in comparison to those in the young adult. The aged heart has a reduced sensitivity to both the inotropic and chronotropic effects of circulating catecholamines: it is well documented that the maximum exercise-induced increase in heart rate is attenuated (by about 30%), despite increased concentrations of circulating catecholamines, and the response to injected isoprenaline is reduced by 15%. Interestingly, although the vagolytic effects of atropine appear to be reduced, there is actually an increased sensitivity to injected acetylcholine; this phenomenon may be due to an increased sensitivity of the postsynaptic membrane in the presence of degeneration of vagal nerve endings (cf. postdenervation hypersensitivity).

The effect of all these age-related changes in the control of the heart is that the central influence becomes less reliable, with weakening of neural and humoral control. The heart of an aged person is less able to adapt to different conditions and it takes longer to reach equilibrium when the cardiovascular system is required to adapt to a change in demands.

The reader can also deduce from the above that the aged heart will respond differently to some drugs. While this results partly from differences in the control system, receptors, etc., many differences are due to different pharmacokinetics (see Chapter 8).

Function of the cardiovascular system in the aged

Although there have been many studies on the effects of age on the function of the cardiovascular system over the last 25 years, there is still controversy as to what actually happens. In a textbook published quite recently (Noble & Rothbaum, 1981), for example, it is stated that the cardiac output falls steadily with age so that at 61 years it is 25% less than at the age of 23. This is the conclusion of most published work up to this date, and it was commonly accepted that there is a linear decrease of approximately 1% per year. With exercise, cardiac output was found to increase by the same amount in all age groups so that it was lower at every workload in older individuals (by 1.5–2 l by the age of 70,) and the ejection fraction (EF) was found to decrease. In addition, it was observed that the maximum heart rate during exercise decreased with age from 180–200 beats per minute in a young adult to about 150 in 70–80 year olds. Part of this may be due to a lack of maximal effort: Shephard (1978) found a smaller decrease in maximum heart rate from 195 in young adults to 170 in 60–80 year olds.

Systolic (but not diastolic) blood pressure was found to increase with age, and the normal increase in blood pressure seen in exercise was exaggerated. An additional observation was that the Vo_2max decreases in a linear manner with age by approximately 0.5 ml kg^{-1} per year in men and slightly less in women. (Vo_2max is the maximum oxygen uptake, i.e. maximum cardiac output multiplied by difference in arteriovenous oxygen content. If a subject attempts to exercise above this, the maximum aerobic capacity, anaerobic metabolism and lactic acidosis will result.)

Many of these results are challenged by the recent study of Rodeheffer *et al.* (1984). Their subjects differed from those studied previously because they had been rigorously selected by history, clinical examination, resting and exercise electrocardiography, exercise thallium scintigraphy and exercise radionuclide ventriculography (RNV), to be free from ischaemic heart disease. In these people, who were also highly motivated volunteers and maintained a moderate level of physical activity, there was no age-related fall in cardiac output, nor in end-diastolic volume (EDV), end-systolic volume and ejection fraction (EF) *at rest* between the ages of 25 and 79 years. In addition, cardiac output during vigorous exercise was not related to age, but there was an age-related increase in EDV and stroke volume (SV), an age-related decrease in maximum heart rate, and the EF increased by a smaller amount in the older subjects. Systolic blood pressure at rest increased with age, but the increases during exercise did not vary significantly. Although it was not directly measured, a fall in Vo_2max with age was inferred from a decrease in maximum work load achieved in older subjects.

The conclusion of Rodeheffer *et al.* was that, in their carefully selected group there is no fall in cardiac output with age, but there is a change in the mechanism by which the heart achieves its maximum performance. As a person becomes older, their responsiveness to catecholamines is reduced and they rely more on the 'Frank–Starling' relationship — with an increased EDV and SV. This would explain a previous observation that those old people who achieved the highest cardiac outputs had the greatest increases in left ventricular filling pressures, even to values which would imply heart failure in a younger age group. The relative fall in EF with age during maximal exercise provides evidence that older subjects do have a decreased efficiency of ejection of blood; this might be due to the increased output impedance mentioned above which is present even in the absence of an increase in blood pressure.

With the caution that all the results presented above are based on *cross-sectional* studies of subjects aged less than 80 years, they can be interpreted as follows:

(i) In people who are free from all heart disease, there is no impairment of cardiac output with increasing age.

(ii) Maximum cardiac output is attained in these subjects by a mechanism which becomes increasingly dependent on increasing EDV and SV, as opposed to adrenergic stimulation (increased heart rate and contractility), as they grow older.

(iii) In the ageing population generally, i.e. one where subjects have been selected because history and clinical examination give no evidence of heart disease and are relatively sedentary, a fall in both resting and maximum cardiac output can be expected. This is because this population is likely to have a high incidence of asymptomatic (ischaemic) heart disease which will not be diagnosed without sophisticated investigations.

(iv) Maximum oxygen consumption falls with age in all populations studied (although there is considerable inter-subject variation so that some old people have a greater Vo_2max than others who are many years younger). This implies that there is either a fall in the oxygen saturation of arterial blood, or a decrease in the ability of an older individual to extract oxygen from blood — even when cardiac output is maintained.

Table 3.3 summarizes the haemodynamic changes which are to be expected in the aged, at rest and exercise, compared with those in the young.

The significance of changes in function, and effects of exercise and conditioning

The changes in anatomical, physiological and biochemical state presented above represent what might be considered an inevitable consequence of age on the cardiovascular system. It is worth attempting to

Table 3.3. Expected changes in haemodynamic variables associated with ageing

Measurement	Difference observed in subjects	
	Rest	Exercise
Heart rate		
Rest	No change	Decrease
Intrinsic	Decrease	—
Systemic arterial pressure		
Systolic	Increase	Greater increase than in young
Diastolic	No change	Slightly greater than in young
Cardiac output/index	Decrease (n/c*)	Decrease (n/c*)
Stroke volume	Decrease (n/c*)	No change (increase*)
Ejection fraction	No change	Reduction or less increase than in young*
Peripheral vascular resistance	Increase (n/c*)	Increase (n/c*) — but decreased from rest
Pulmonary arterial pressure		
Systolic	No change	Greater increase
Diastolic	No change	Greater increase
Capilliary	No change	Greater increase
Right ventricular EDP	No change	Increase

Data from various sources. *May relate to selection of subjects; results of Rodeheffer *et al.* (1984) (see text). (n/c — no change.)

assess their significance in terms of the ability of a person to live a normal existence, and also in comparison to pathological changes. Maximum oxygen consumption has been chosen as an indicator of cardiopulmonary 'ability' because it can be measured and compared far more easily than cardiac output. The reader should bear in mind that Vo_2max is also a reflection of pulmonary function, the tissues' ability to extract oxygen from blood, and the mass of active muscle, all of which can vary independently of the heart. In Fig. 3.2 the estimated oxygen cost of various everyday activities and medical events is shown beside curves respresenting the basal metabolic rate and Vo_2max as they change with age. The absolute values all represent the author's approximation, and are for illustrative purposes only.

Vo_2max has been found to decline by <0.4 ml kg^{-1} min^{-1} per year in some studies, and >1.0 in others. The reasons for this are partly explained by the growing number of studies of the effects of exercise on age-related changes. A physically fit but sedentary 20 year old adult male might have a Vo_2max 45 ml kg^{-1} min^{-1}, while it would be in the region of 70–80 in a highly trained athlete. At this age, complete bedrest for three weeks will result in a 30% fall in Vo_2max. The adoption of an inactive lifestyle results initially in a large rate of fall in Vo_2max in all individuals (initially at ≥1.0 ml kg^{-1} min^{-1} per year) but after a few years the fall is at a rate of about 0.4 ml kg^{-1} min^{-1} per year. The athlete who continues to train will decline only at this 'basal' rate. So the attainment of a high level of physical fitness (i) improves the absolute Vo_2max and (ii) maintains it at the 'basal' rate of decline. There are few studies of over 70 year olds, so extrapolation of the fall in Vo_2max for them is speculative. It seems clear that maintenance of physical fitness, or an exercise programme, can have beneficial effects upon the aged as increases in Vo_2max in the order of 10–30% are reported.

The thick line on Fig. 3.2 is derived from recent publications and gives a somewhat lower Vo_2max than the one of Dehn & Bruce (1972) shown as a thin line on the figure; it gives a linear decline of 1.0 ml kg^{-1} min^{-1} per year from the age of 25 to 40 years, with an intercept of 45 at the age of 25; this is followed by a linear decline of 0.4 ml kg^{-1} min^{-1} per year after the age of 40. In this hypothetical situation, the projected basal metabolic rate would be crossed at the age of 110 years — a situation presumably incompatible with life, and the Vo_2max would not support a major operation after the age of 102. (It should be noted that the 'reserve' of Vo_2max required over the oxygen demands of a major operation is not known. Possibly the suggestion (Shephard, 1978) that prolonged demands should be no more than 40% of Vo_2max is reasonable.) Whatever the actual situation may be in an individual patient, it is clear that the oxygen cost of a major operation is not great in comparison to even a relatively sedentary lifestyle: it is approximately equivalent to walking at 1.6 km h^{-1} (1 mph) or standing still; a patient who can walk about the ward probably has at least twice this capacity.

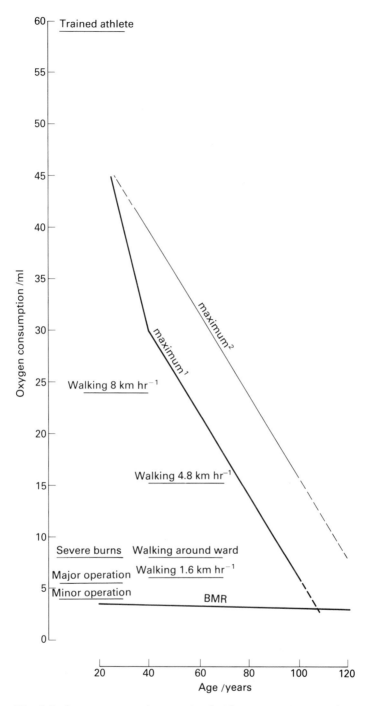

Fig. 3.2. Oxygen consumption associated with various activities and surgical conditions, also maximum oxygen consumption (VO₂max) and basal metabolic rate (BMR) as they change with age. Maximum[1] is derived from more recent publications (e.g. Buskirk and Hodgson, 1987), while maximum[2] is from Dehn & Bruce (1972). Values for the oxygen consumption associated with various activities are from Shephard (1985) and calculated from Vasilomanolakis *et al.* (1985). BMR is calculated from the Harris-Benedict equation (quoted by Long, 1984). The oxygen cost of surgical conditions is also calculated from Long (1984).

Aged cardiovascular system

Consequently it is unlikely that age-related changes in cardiovascular function will *in themselves* be responsible for an aged patient being unable to deliver an adequate quantity of oxygen to the tissues during anaesthesia or surgery except at the very extreme of senescence (for which data is not available). The effects of cardiac and respiratory pathology are likely to have far greater effect at any age. However, if the balance is critical or if considered desirable for other reasons, it is likely that a programme of exercise would improve the patient's aerobic capacity.

Assessment of the cardiac status of aged patients

Epidemiology

Those changes which are inevitable have been considered but most old patients will have pathological changes of the cardiovascular system which have been acquired over a lifetime or, more rarely, are congenital in origin. The actual prevalence of heart disease in a population depends on the nature of the population and, most importantly, the method of investigation. For example, a community survey in the Glasgow area gave a total prevalence of 43% for all types of heart disease in people aged 65 or over who were living at home (see Fig. 3.3a). The survey diagnosed an overall prevalence of ischaemic heart disease (IHD) of 20%, based on history and routine electrocardiography. However, a third of these people had no history of IHD, so the prevalence would have been 12.5% if the diagnosis was based on history alone, and electrocardiography without a history would have missed a quarter of the cases, giving the prevalence of IHD as 15% (Fig. 3.3b).

Undoubtedly, addition of the more specialized investigations which are discussed below will increase the apparent prevalence of disease in a given population. Prevalence of heart disease depends also on the characteristics of the population concerned, e.g. IHD is present in up to two-thirds of patients presenting for peripheral vascular surgery.

The prevalence of heart disease increases with age, mainly because of an increase in IHD; in the Glasgow study, for example, (Fig. 3.3c) it is present in about 20% more of the 75+ age group than those aged 65–74. In general, autopsy studies demonstrate a higher incidence of heart disease than those of live patients, but the distribution is similar, with the exception of those conditions which have little functional significance (e.g. most cases of senile cardiac amyloidosis). A representative autopsy series is shown in Fig. 3.4.

Investigations

In the old patient who presents for anaesthesia, pathological changes may be superimposed upon the inevitable results of ageing discussed

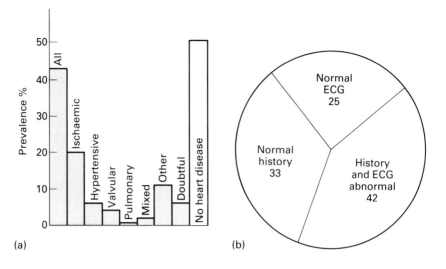

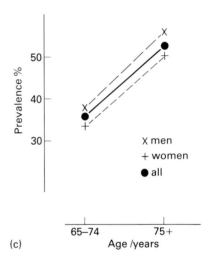

Fig. 3.3. The prevalence of heart disease in Scots over 65 years old (from a survey of 501 people living at home — Kennedy et al., 1977). (a) The prevalence of different sorts of heart disease. All — all patients with definite heart disease; Mixed — patients with hypertensive and ischaemic heart disease coexisting; Doubtful — possible heart disease. (b) The prevalence (%) of ischaemic heart disease according to the method of diagnosis. The circle represents all patients with ischaemic heart disease; of these, 25% have no electrocardiographic abnormality, and 33% have had no symptoms. (c) The prevalence of definite heart disease according to age.

above, so there is a frequent need to use various investigations which are available for assessing the circulatory system.

Investigating the patient's cardiovascular system in order to discover all the pathology present is a pointless exercise unless it can be demonstrated that this will have a beneficial effect on the outcome of surgery or anaesthesia. Such information may be useful in three ways:

(i) Assessment of operative risk.

(ii) Improving the patient's state preoperatively.

(iii) Planning peroperative management.

(i) Since the classic work of Goldman et al. (1977) there have been many attempts to use the results of preoperative investigations to assign to a patient a specific risk (probability) of cardiac complications when they

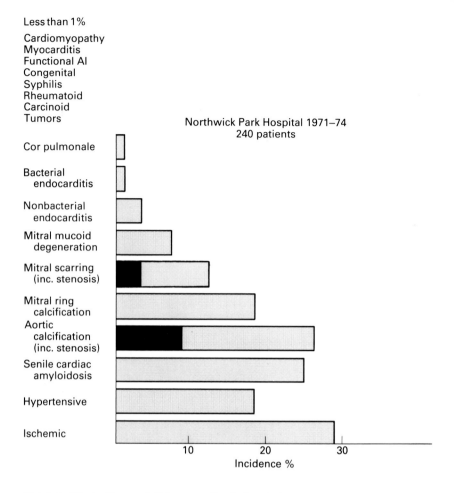

Fig. 3.4. The incidence of different cardiac lesions in hospital autopsies in patients aged over 65 years. The results of autopsy on 240 patients at Northwick Park Hospital, 1971–74 (from Pomerance, 1981).

undergo an anaesthetic and operation. This concept has not been investigated prospectively in old patients. Nevertheless, knowledge of the risk of peroperative complications is useful because it helps in deciding whether a procedure is justified. If the risk is considered unacceptable, the planned operation may be abandoned or replaced by a lesser one. Two different approaches have been tried. The first is the creation of a multifactorial risk index (MRI) where a number of preoperative factors (e.g. an abnormal electrocardiogram, history of myocardial infarction, heart failure and type of surgery) are processed to derive an index of peroperative risk. MRIs have been found to be rather unreliable when applied to institutions other than the one where they were created, and even to different subpopulations of patient within the same institution; indeed; frequently the ASA (American Society of Anesthesiologists' system) status has been found to have a predictive accuracy as high as MRIs. Another problem is that there are no published MRIs that deal specifically with an aged population: in Goldman's index, 'Aged over 70' is one of nine risk factors. A second approach to risk assessment is to use a single special investigation to estimate operative risk. This might be exercise electrocardiography or RNV, for example. The outcome of such a test is either the diagnosis of a specific pathology (e.g. IHD in the case of exercise electrocardiography) or an assessment of overall function. Two of the few published studies which specifically looked at aged patients are of this sort. Gerson *et al.* (1985) found that in patients aged over 65, an inability to achieve a specified exercise performance gave a useful indication of peroperative cardiac risk; this was of more value than the Goldman risk index, ASA status or rest and exercise radionuclide ventriculograms. Del Guercio & Cohn (1980) found that it was possible to predict operative mortality by assembling a 'physiological profile' with preoperative measurement of right-sided pressures, cardiac output and oxygen delivery; they also considered that they could improve outcome by treating haemodynamic abnormalities preoperatively. It should be noted that even in these two studies of 'geriatric' patients, the mean ages were only 73 and 68 years; there are no data available for the more aged patient. It is concluded that at present there is no evidence that the peroperative cardiac risk for an old patient can be estimated reliably. However, it is reasonable to assume that those factors which have been found to be associated with an increased risk in younger patients will still be so in the older population.

(ii) If the patient has any reversible conditions of the cardiovascular system, it is reasonable to assume that their correction will be beneficial. This may involve anything from the treatment of heart failure, arrhythmias or hypertension to coronary artery and valve surgery. Although it is difficult to demonstrate that this does improve outcome, even in young patients (since controlled trials have not been published and are probably unethical) most practitioners consider that it is desirable to use non-invasive ways of improving the patient's medical condition. The use of more aggressive treatment, such as coronary bypass surgery or haemodynamic 'fine tuning' with the aid of pulmonary artery catheters, is more controversial because any supposed benefit has to be weighed against the real risks of the treatment itself. There are again no data on the effectiveness of these interventions in an aged population. Finally in this category, is the use of exercise conditioning to improve cardiovascular reserve (see p. 34).

(iii) If the anaesthetist knows the state of a patient's cardiovascular system, it should be possible to plan the optimal anaesthetic management. In particular, specific techniques and drugs may be indicated or contraindicated and particular methods of monitoring can be chosen. For example, a patient with severe aortic stenosis is likely to react unfavourably to sudden decreases in afterload, while the hypertension associated with endotracheal intubation is harmful to a patient with coronary insufficiency. Foreknowledge of the pathology and use of appropriate monitoring for the recognition of such problems, followed by prompt treatment, are likely to improve outcome (Rao *et al.*, 1983).

Investigating the circulatory system

History and clinical examination

The tools available to investigate the heart of an old patient are the same as for younger people, although some of the results may require different interpretation. Investigation should always start with a detailed history and clinical examination, although obtaining a cardiac history may be difficult.

In contrast to the problems associated with history taking, there is little in the clinical examination which differs in the old from that of a young person. Inspiratory splitting of the second heart sound (S_2) is only audible in one-third of old people; a third heart sound (S_3) is always abnormal and frequently associated with heart failure, while a fourth sound (S_4) implies reduced ventricular compliance and may be present in many 'normal' old patients. Diastolic murmurs are always pathological, but up to 60% of old patients may have systolic murmurs; the majority of these are benign, associated with dilatation of the aorta and fibrotic changes at the base of the aortic cusps. These murmurs are short, relatively quiet (<2/6), not associated with a thrill, usually peak early in systole and occur in the absence of the other signs and symptoms of aortic stenosis. When examining the venous pulse, compression of the left innominate vein by the unfolded aorta sometimes gives the erroneous impression that venous pressure is elevated, and the arterial pulse is normally more abrupt because of reduced compliance in the arterial system. Most authorities consider that a blood pressure greater than 160/95 mmHg is not normal for a patient of any age; raised pressure is associated with increased morbidity in old patients just as in younger age groups.

Electrocardiography and chest X-ray

The clinical examination of a patient over 60 years old should include a standard 12 lead electrocardiogram (ECG) and posteroanterior chest X-ray. At least 50% of patients aged over 65 years can be expected to have abnormalities in their ECG, and this proportion increases sharply with age. Table 3.4 lists the only changes which can be considered to be benign in old patients, as well as those which have a high correlation with clinical disease; all other changes and rhythm disturbances have the same implications as in younger people.

The chest X-ray can be expected to give important information

Table 3.4. Electrocardiographic changes in the old

Not associated with reduced life expectancy[1]
  Left axis deviation without left anterior hemiblock
  Counterclockwise rotation
  Minor clockwise rotation
  Incomplete right bundle branch block
  Possible left ventricular hypertrophy (voltage changes only)
  Occasional (<10%) ectopic beats
  First degree heart block[2]

Having a high correlation with clinical heart disease[3]
  Atrial fibrillation
  Left bundle branch block
  Intraventricular conduction defects
  ST segment and T wave changes

Reflecting structural damage to the heart[3]
  Myocardial infarction patterns
  Left anterior hemiblock
  Right bundle branch block

[1] Caird *et al.* (1974)
[2] Coodley & Coodley (1985)
[3] Fisch (1981)

about the size and shape of the heart, and is an invaluable tool in the diagnosis of pulmonary congestion. Although the presence of age-related pulmonary and skeletal changes slightly alter interpretation of the X-ray, it is broadly similar to that for other age groups (see Table 3.5).

Table 3.5. Examination of the heart: the chest X-ray in the aged patient

Normal changes without pathological significance
  (i) 'Unfolded aorta'
      Tortuous and prominent, projects to right
      Aortic knob higher, may reach clavicle, may be calcified
      Descending aorta more prominent (may mimic aneurysm)
      Widening of superior mediastinum (brachiocephalic vessels)

  (ii) Cardiothoracic (standard PA projection)
      May be increased; >50% (men) and >60% (women) usually pathological

Pathological changes
  (i) All abnormalities of pulmonary vasculature
  (ii) All calcification in heart, valves and pericardium
  (iii) All other changes considered pathological in younger patients

Strategy for further investigations

The results of the patient's history, clinical examination, chest X-ray and ECG can be used — in combination with knowledge of the proposed operative procedures — to plan any further investigation of the cardiovascular system. At least half the aged population will have evidence of heart disease, or limitation of cardiorespiratory function from these investigations (see Fig. 3.3), and this proportion will increase with age; those in certain groups, e.g. those presenting for vascular surgery, will have an even higher incidence. There will also be a proportion of patients in whom there is no evidence of heart disease but their medical condition precludes adequate provocation of symptoms, or the assessment of cardiorespiratory reserve, e.g. those severely restricted by arthritis. If the clinician considers it necessary, further tests can be selected to detect pathology (screening tests), to further elucidate heart disease which has been diagnosed, or to give information about functional ability. In Table 3.6, investigations have been classified according to the information which they are likely to provide, and also whether they are invasive or non-invasive.

If a *structural lesion* is suspected, the first investigation should almost always be an echoardiographic (ultrasound) examination. This is completely safe and non-invasive, and well tolerated by the patient. It can detect abnormalities in the size and wall thickness of the cardiac chambers, and the presence of valve lesions or septal defects. It is usually possible to detect dyskinetic segments (suggesting areas of fibrosis and infarction) and aneurysms. Flow can be detected and measured with ultrasonic Doppler techniques, so pressure gradients across a stenosed valve may be estimated. Echocardiography is extremely useful in discovering the cause of cardiomegaly, and is the method of choice for detecting pericardial effusions. However, because the technique involves 'sampling' a line (in M-mode) or a plane in two-dimensional echocardiography, it is possible to miss the presence of aneurysms or other dyskinetic lesions. Finally, ultrasound is becoming increasingly accurate in the measurement of EF and cardiac output, although at present the information derived from RNV is more reproducible.

Further information about structural lesions can be derived from radionuclide studies. RNV is particularly useful in demonstrating dyskinetic segments and aneurysms, while thallium scanning detects areas of low myocardial blood flow (ischaemia) or zero blood flow (infarcts). The latter is useful when an old person has left bundle branch block which precludes electrocardiographic diagnosis of an infarction; an acute infarct may be diagnosed by the uptake of technetium pyrophosphate.

Although other techniques such as computed tomography and nuclear magnetic resonance imaging may supercede it, at present the most specific way of delineating structural changes in the heart is by cardiac catheterization and angiography. This will give definitive information on the anatomical changes present, as well as being the only way to quantify coronary artery stenoses and measure intracardiac pressures. In the old patient, the extra structural information acquired may well not merit performing this investigation unless cardiac surgery is contemplated. On the other hand, the functional data (pressures, flow and shunts) may be invaluable.

If a patient has no limitation on physical exercise, it is unlikely that the *functional* state of their heart needs investigation (although they

Table 3.6. Further investigation of the heart

Investigation	Structural information	Functional information	Screening
Non-invasive			
Exercise electrocardiography		Can define exercise ability Provocation of dysrhythmias	Diagnosis of occult CAD Severity of CAD
Echocardiogram	Chamber size, shape Wall thickness Abnormal communications Valve abnormalities Abnormal wall motion (dyskinesia) Pericardial disease — effusion	Ejection fraction Cardiac output Flow direction (Doppler) Gradient across valves	Detects abnormalities mentioned
Nuclear angiography			
Ventriculography (RNV)	Chamber size Abnormal wall motion (dyskinesia)	Shunts Ejection fraction Cardiac output	Exercise RNV: occult IHD
Thallium scintigraphy	Ischaemic areas of myocardium Infarcted areas of myocardium		Screening for IHD
Technetium pyrophosphate imaging	Detects recent (<10 day) infarction		
Invasive			
Cardiac catheterization:			
Right-sided (pulmonary artery)		Right-sided pressures Cardiac output Physiological shunt	
Left-sided (angiography)	Chamber size, shape Abnormal connections Valve abnormalities Extent and site of CAD Abnormal wall motion (dyskinesia)	Shunts Ejection fraction Cardiac output Intracardiac pressures	
Intracardiac electrocardiography		Diagnosis of conduction defects Investigating rhythm disorders	

may have structural defects which are important). Unfortunately, most old patients are not in this position. A supervised exercise test will demonstrate the workload which a patient can achieve, and may also provoke symptoms or signs diagnostic of disease, but gives no direct information about cardiac output or ventricular function. In contrast, both of these can be measured with RNV, which is a non-invasive technique requiring only the injection of radioisotope labelled material, and detecting equipment; consequently it is very suitable for most old patients, causing the minimum of distress, although it is difficult to perform with a confused, restless or uncooperative individual. Although it is usually assumed that LV function is being studied, comparable results can be obtained for the right side of the heart. The EF at rest should not change with age in a healthy heart (see p. 32) and is approximately 65%; likewise, an increase in EF is normal during exercise (although this increase is reduced in old age). An EF which is less than 50% at rest is pathological, while an abrupt fall during the stress of exercise also implies poor left ventricular function, at any age. Systolic and diastolic volumes and the cardiac output can also be measured with RNV, at rest and during exercise, and quantify overall function.

Although RNV is an excellent tool for gaining an impression of patients' overall myocardial function, and is applicable even when they cannot exercise for non-cardiac reasons, it does not give direct information about intracardiac pressures. If this is required — possibly after RNV has demonstrated poor LV or RV function or for assessing and planning therapy — it is necessary to perform cardiac catheterization. The normal approach is via the right side of the heart with a pulmonary artery flotation catheter ('Swan-Ganz', PAC). It is then possible to make a physiological profile, with measurement of pulmonary capilliary wedge pressure, cardiac output, shunt, oxygen delivery, etc. Recently, various indices of RV function have also been derived from pulmonary artery catheterization (Kaplan, 1987). While the same sort of arguments can be advanced against this technique as against left-sided cardiac catheterization and angiography, the benefits may be greater, since the patient's status can be optimized by appropriate therapy; in addition, a PAC is useful for peroperative monitoring of the circulation. However, there is the danger that the information derived from a PAC may be misinterpreted, particularly in view of the normal increase in left ventricular compliance in the elderly (Kaplan, 1987). It is beyond the scope of this chapter to discuss the arguments and evidence for and against the use of invasive monitoring. However, it is the author's opinion that if a particular type of monitoring or investigation is indicated (in the view of the anaesthetist) for a young patient in order to provide optimal care peroperatively, then it is illogical to consider it inappropriate for an old patient undergoing the same operation.

Finally, it is possible that a *screening* test is required to discover occult disease in an apparently fit patient. Clearly any of the investigations above could be used for screening, but this would be relatively costly. Exercise electrocardiography is probably the easiest and cheapest test available. It is only applicable to patients who can perform the type of exercise involved, and usually provides evidence of the presence and severity of IHD, as well as defining exercise capacity. Similarly, exercise RNV gives evidence of (usually) ischaemic dysfunction. Coronary angiography has been used to screen younger patients (who would then be offered 'prophylactic' coronary bypass surgery) and the use of PAC for screening and assessing risk is discussed above.

References

Buskirk, E.R. & Hodgson, J.L. (1987) Age and aeobic power: the rate of change in men and women. *Fed. Proc.* **46**, 1824–1829.

Caird, F.I. *et al.* (1974) Significance of abnormalities of electrocardiogram in old people. *Br. Heart J.* **36**, 1012–1018.

Coodley E.L. & Coodley, G. (1985) Electrocardiographic changes associated with aging. In *Geriatric Heart Disease* (Ed. E.L. Coodley) PSG Publishing, Massachusetts, pp. 182–188.

Dehn, M. & Bruce, R.A. (1972) Longitudinal variations in maximal oxygen intake with age and activity. *J. Appl. Physiol.* **33**, 805–807.

Del Guercio, L.R.M. & Cohn, J.D. (1980) Monitoring operative risk in the elderly. *JAMA* **243**, 1350–1355.

Fisch, C. (1981) The electrocardiogram in the aged. In *Geriatric Cardiology* (Eds R.J. Noble & D.A. Rothbaum) F.A. Davis, Philadelphia, pp. 65–74.

Gerson, M.C. *et al.* (1985) Cardiac prognosis in noncardiac geriatric surgery *Ann. Intern. Med.* **103**, 832–837.

Goldman, L. *et al.* (1977) Multifactorial index of cardiac risk in noncardiac surgical procedures. *New Engl. J. Med.* **297**, 845–850.

Kaplan, J.A. (Ed) (1987) *Cardiac anesthesia*, 2nd Edn., Ch. 6. Grune-Stratton, New York.

Kennedy, R.D., Andrews, G.R. & Caird, F.I. (1977) Ischaemic heart disease in the elderly. *Br. Heart J.* **39**, 1121–1127.

Long, C.L. (1984) The energy and protein requirements of the critically ill patient. In *Nutritional Assessment*, (Eds R.A. Wright, S. Heymsfield & C. McManus). Blackwell Scientific Publications, Oxford, pp. 157–181.

Noble, R.J. & Rothbaum, D.A. (Eds) (1981) *Geriatric Cardiology*. F.A. Davis, Philadelphia.

Pomerance, A.R. (1981) Cardiac pathology in the elderly. In *Geriatric Cardiology* (Eds R.J. Noble & D.A. Rothbaum). F.A. Davis, Philadelphia, pp. 9–54.

Rao, T.L.K. *et al* (1983) Reinfarction following anesthesia in patients with myocardial infarction. *Anesthesiology* **59**, 499–505.

Rodeheffer, R.J. *et al.* (1984) Exercise cardiac output is maintained with advancing age in healthy human subjects. *Circulation* **69**, 203–213.

Shephard, R.J. (1978) *Physical Activity and Aging.* Croom Helm, London.

Shephard, R.J. (1985) Physical fitness: exercise and ageing. In *Principles and Practice of Geriatric Medicine* (Ed. M.S.J. Pathy). Wiley, Chichester, pp. 163–177.

Vasilomanolakis, E.C., Licht, J.R. & Ellestad, M.H. (1985) Exercise physiology, testing, and training in the geriatric population. In *Geriatric Heart Disease* (Ed. E.L. Coodley). PSG Publishing, Massachusetts, pp. 131–143.

Williams, B.O. (1985) The cardiovascular system. In *Principles and Practice of Geriatric Medicine* (Ed. M.S.J. Pathy). Wiley, Chichester, pp. 459–501.

Suggestions for further reading

Coodley, E.L. (Ed) (1985) *Geriatric Heart Disease*, PSG Publishing, Massachusetts. (Further details on the clinical side of geriatric cardiology, including investigations and ausculatory findings.)

Lakatta, G.L. (1987) Why cardiovascular function may decline with age. *Geriatrics* **42**, 84-94. (A recent review on the subject.)

4 | The aged pulmonary system

J.G. JONES

Introduction

In contrast to younger patients the old have a greater predisposition to pulmonary dysfunction during and after anaesthesia and this chapter explains some of the factors involved.

The pulmonary problems most likely to be encountered by anaesthetists who are caring for old patients are as follows:

(i) an impairment of gas exchange with more frequent and profound postoperative hypoxaemia due to prolonged basal atelectasis

(ii) a greater degree of airway obstruction, both of the upper and intrapulmonary airway

(iii) an impaired control of ventilation

(iv) respiratory muscle fatigue

(v) pulmonary oedema in multisystem failure.

None of these problems is easy to prevent and all are likely to create difficulties in patients, particularly in the postoperative period. Nevertheless, an awareness of the nature of pulmonary disorders in the old is important if the morbidity and mortality of postoperative pulmonary dysfunction in these patients is to be reduced.

One of the most important causes of respiratory dysfunction with increasing age is a change in the elastic properties of the lung parenchyma, the chest wall and in the walls of the airways. It is unclear whether some of these pulmonary changes are due simply to the effects of ageing or are the results of chronic exposure of the lungs to environmental or personal pollution (i.e. active or passive smoking).

The pulmonary impairment which precedes surgery may predispose the old patient to a greater degree of basal atelectasis when anaesthetic drugs are administered. Dependent atelectasis may not disappear with the elimination of anaesthetics from the body but may persist for days or weeks into the postoperative period. This causes a persistent background of impaired gas exchange and hypoxia which may be exacerbated by any other added abnormality of respiratory control.

Changes in the control of breathing with increasing age are easily demonstrated with standard tests but it is less clear whether or not there is also an increased sensitivity to the anaesthetic drugs which depress ventilation. The problems posed by patients with an aged pulmonary system predominate in the postoperative period rather than during anaesthesia itself. However, the increased use of oximetry during anaesthesia also demonstrates a greater degree of intraoperative impairment of gas exchange in the old than in young patients.

With a clear understanding of the changes that occur in pulmonary function with increasing age and the added effects of anaesthesia, surgery and postoperative medication, a reasonable prediction can be made of the likely postoperative respiratory state. Nevertheless, there is room for a considerable improvement in postoperative monitoring and management of respiratory dysfunction in the old.

Although the appearance of the patient in the postoperative period gives a useful guide to the development of respiratory problems, in practice clinical signs are missed and respiratory failure is often diagnosed only after many hours of severe hypoxia or when respiratory arrest supervenes. The sleeping patient is at risk of opioid-induced obstructive sleep apnoea with hypoxia, and this is a particular postoperative problem in old patients. It is unreasonable to devote costly resources and elaborate monitoring to the care of a patient during the operation and then leave the patient completely unmonitored for many hours in the critical postoperative stage when unrecognized, episodic, hypoxia may produce irreversible cardiac or cerebral damage.

Admission to a high dependency unit with continuous computerized monitoring of oxygen saturation, particularly during sleep, is the present ideal standard of postoperative management after major operative procedures in the aged.

Lung parenchyma, chest wall and gas exchange

Elastic properties and ageing

It is unusual for clinicians to think in terms of the elastic properties of the lungs, chest wall and airways. Nevertheless, a grasp of the basic ideas about lung and chest wall elasticity is important to obtain a good understanding of how the lungs work and how the processes of ageing and disease might alter normal function. The term tissue elasticity refers to a tendency of a tissue to recover to an original form if deformed by some stress. The stiffer, or more elastic, the tissue the more readily it returns to its original form. In the case of the lungs it is a common observation at post-mortem that the normal lung removed from the chest cavity collapses to a small volume. What is less obvious is that the thoracic cavity from which the lungs are removed is larger than it would normally have been in life. Both the lungs and chest wall have elastic properties which act in opposite directions, tending to make lung volume smaller and the thoracic cavity larger. The two surfaces of the pleura couple together these opposing forces and the pleural pressure between them is a measure of the elasticity of the opposing tissues. If the tissues become inelastic, they will be easily deformed and will not readily return to their original form. The ageing process tends to have opposite effects on the chest wall and the lung — the chest wall becomes *more elastic* and the lung *less elastic* so that there is an age-related increase in functional residual capacity. In an extreme form this results in the barrel shaped chest, the consequences of this which are (i) the diaphragm becomes flatter and (ii) airways become narrower (Fig. 4.1).

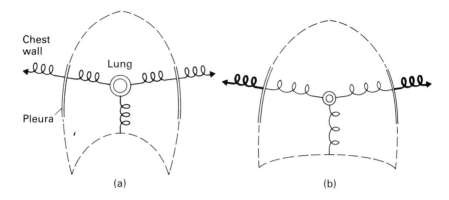

Fig. 4.1. (a) The elastic properties of the chest wall and lung help to maintain the patency of the airways and curvature of the diaphragm. (b) Ageing leads to an increased chest wall elasticity, but the loss of lung elasticity is more important and leads to airway narrowing, enlargement of the thorax and flattening of the diaphragm.

Diaphragm shape and lung elasticity

Flattening of the diaphragm is a well known phenomenon, particularly in emphysema where lung elasticity is considerably reduced. However, its functional significance is not well recognized in the context of breathing difficulties in older patients following surgery. On the basis of the Laplace equation where $P = 2T/r$, it can be seen (Fig. 4.2) that for the same diaphragm tension (T) produced by muscle contracture, a 10-fold increase in diaphragm radius (r) leads to a 10-fold reduction in maximum diaphragmatic pressure (P). Thus, a patient with a flat diaphragm is using more energy in diaphragm muscle for the same work of breathing and is more liable to fatigue, especially in the presence of hypoxia. The flat diaphragm will therefore fatigue more readily if there is (i) an increase in airway resistence (mucus) or (ii) increased loading on the diaphragm (abdominal distension), (iii) reduced ability of the respiratory muscles to contract (muscle relaxants or metabolic disturbance), (iv) increased stiffness of the lungs (atelectasis), (v) hypoxia.

If a preoperative X-ray film of the chest shows flattening of the diaphragm, this may predict a reduced ability of the patient to resist muscle fatigue postoperatively. The clinician responsible for the postoperative respiratory management must then be on the look-out for any signs of respiratory difficulty and hypoventilation.

The aged pulmonary system

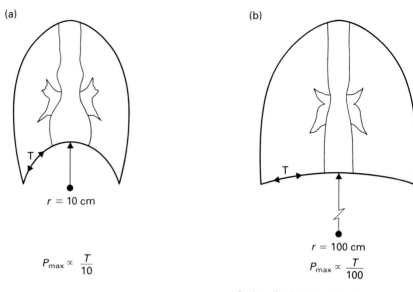

(a) (b)

$$P_{max} \propto \frac{T}{10}$$

$$P_{max} \propto \frac{T}{100}$$

$$\text{Maximum diaphragm pressure} \propto \frac{\text{Active diaphragm tension}}{\text{Diaphragm radius}}$$

Fig. 4.2. Application of the Laplace equation to diaphragm contraction in (a) the normal and (b) the aged lung. For the same degree of diaphragm muscle contraction there is less pressure generated by the flat diaphragm in the aged patient.

Lung elasticity and airway calibre

A change in lung volume caused by the action of the respiratory muscles produces the well known elastic recoil or compliance curve of the lung (Fig. 4.3a). This relates changes in lung volume to changes in pleural pressure; an index of the latter is obtained using a small balloon lying in the oesophagus. Ageing and emphysema cause a loss of elastic recoil and shift the curve to the left, whereas pulmonary fibrosis; atelectasis or adult respiratory distress syndrome (ARDS) shift the curve to the right (Fig. 4.3b). More pulmonary function laboratories should produce lung compliance curves in patients. A clue to a loss of elastic recoil pressure is obtained from a low carbon monoxide transfer combined with expiratory rather than inspiratory airflow obstruction. The latter is demonstrated using the maximum flow–volume curve. The elastic recoil pressure is not only a measure of the stiffness of the lung but it is also the distending force on intrapulmonary airways. From Fig. 4.3b, it can be seen that the factors causing *airway narrowing* are a reduction in lung volume or ageing/emphysema. In contrast, *airway dilatation* is promoted by an increase in lung volume or pulmonary fibrosis.

It would appear from Fig. 4.3b that at any lung volume V_L, the elastic recoil pressure for the whole lung is either P_1, P_2 or P_3 depending on which curve is relevant to the lung in question. Thus at the same lung volume airways are narrower in the aged/emphysematous lung than in the lung of fit, young subjects or those with pulmonary fibrosis.

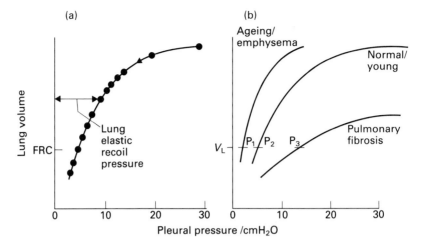

Fig. 4.3. (a & b) Elastic recoil curves in normal and abnormal lungs.

Furthermore, because of the effect of gravity, the airways in the dependent part of the lung are much less distended than the upper part because the elastic recoil becomes progressively smaller with vertical distance down the lung (Fig. 4.4). This means that the elastic force holding the airways open at the bottom of the lung is very much smaller

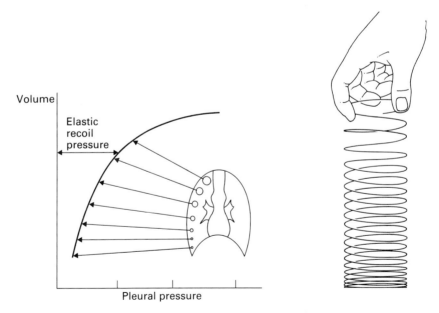

Fig. 4.4. (Left) Gravitational force causes a gradient of recoil pressure, and therefore of airway size, from the top to the bottom of the lung; consequently the airways are very narrow in the dependent part of the lung, and the top of the lung has a lower compliance than the bottom. J. Mead (personal communication) suggests that this effect of gravity on the lung can be illustrated using a 'slinky' spring (right); the top is more distended than the dependent part but the dependent part moves more than the top.

The aged pulmonary system

than the force distending airways at the top of the lung. The direction of this gradient of elasticity is determined by the direction of the force of gravity and extends from the upper to the lower lung, regardless of posture.

Loss of lung elasticity with increasing age will shift the elastic recoil curve to the left and airways will now close at a critical closing pressure which is achieved at a higher lung volume (V_2) than in young subjects (V_1) (Fig. 4.5). This age-dependent shift in the point of airway closure to progressively higher lung volumes may be the explanation for the progressive deterioration of gas exchange with increasing age. This is because a much larger proportion of the lung volume is poorly ventilated in relation to its perfusion. Although the relationship between age and closing volume is well known, the effect of increasing age on closing volume may be considerably less than is generally believed. Holtz et al. (1976) showed that taking a vital capacity breath prior to the closing volume manoeuvre exaggerated the size of the closing volume in aged subjects. Their study showed that during tidal breathing in older subjects, airway closure occurred at a substantially *lower* lung volume than was previously considered. On the basis of their study, airway closure is likely during the tidal breathing in sitting subjects at about 85 rather than 65 years of age, and in supine subjects at about 60 rather than 45 years of age. Thus, the effect of age on airway closure is less severe than was previously believed.

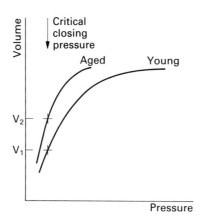

Fig. 4.5. This shows the effect of age on the elastic recoil and closing volume of the lung. The critical closing pressure of dependent airways is achieved at a higher volume (V_2) than in the younger lung (V_1) and may exceed functional residual capacity.

Impaired gas exchange: anaesthesia and afterwards

One of the most consistent changes in pulmonary function following induction of general anaesthesia is a 20% reduction in functional residual capacity (FRC) which is closely correlated with an increase in alveolar-arterial Po_2 gradient. It was originally thought that this correlation could be explained by a reduction in lung volume, e.g. from V_2 to V_1 in the right-hand curve in Fig. 4.5, to the point when basal airways began to close. If this was in fact the mechanism it would be expected that an increase in lung volume, e.g. by positive end expiratory pressure (PEEP), back to V_2 would open the airways and improve gas exchange. Unfortunately, this does not normalize gas exchange (Heneghan *et al.*, 1984) and the closing volume hypothesis no longer attracts wide support as the explanation for the increased impairment of gas exchange during anaesthesia. Brismar *et al.* (1985) and Hedenstierna *et al.* (1986), using computerized tomography, have now shown that following the induction of general anaesthesia there occurs widespread extensive atelectasis in the dependent part of the lung (Fig. 4.6), and the magnitude of the atelectasis is correlated with the magnitude of shunt and to the impairment in arterial oxygenation.

Not only does this elucidate the mechanism of impaired gas exchange during anaesthesia but it also explains why gas exchange abnormalities persist, sometimes for many days, into the postoperative period. Basal atelectasis does not re-expand immediately postoperatively, nor is it completely re-expanded by large inflations during the operative procedure. This is because the atelectatic and the non-atelectatic lung units have quite different elastic recoil curves, the former having much higher recoil and more hysteresis than the latter and even with a high distending pressure the degree of expansion of the atelectatic dependent parts of the lung is very much less than the non-atelectatic lung. This is why sighs and transient higher inflation are of little or no value in reversing this effect. A much more useful procedure for expanding atelectasis is frequent turning of the patient, even including the prone position, to allow gravity to open up these units.

The implications of the findings for older patients are as follows:

(i) atelectasis of the dependent parts of the lungs is a common feature during anaesthesia, and is detected with computerized tomography but not with conventional radiography

(ii) the lower the elastic recoil pressure of the lung the easier it is for dependent airways to close and the more difficult it is to re-expand them by periodic inflation

(iii) the more extensive and persistent the atelectasis, the more severe and prolonged is the impairment of gas exchange postoperatively

(iv) persistent postoperative atelectasis may lead to secondary infections because of impaired ciliary clearance of secretions, a particular feature in old patients (Pavia, 1984).

Thus, the problems in the aged lung with loss of elastic recoil pressure are (i) flattening of the diaphragm with impaired efficiency and greater susceptibility of fatigue, and (ii) basal atelectasis induced at the time of anaesthesia and persisting for several days postoperatively, with a predisposition to postoperative hypoxaemia. The latter sets the scene for episodes of even more profound hypoxia during obstructive sleep apnoea, which is commonly induced by the administration of opioids postoperatively.

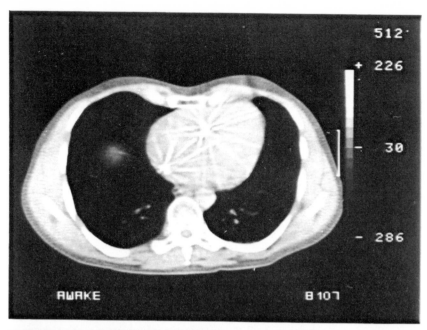

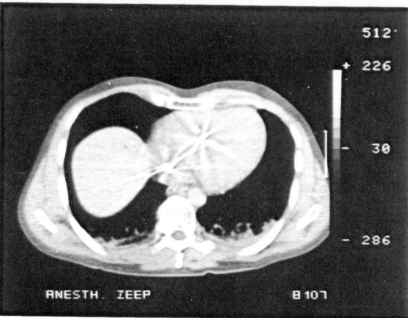

Fig. 4.6. Computerized tomograph of the chest before and after induction of anaesthesia, to show development of atelectasis in the dependent lung. Note that the dome of the diaphragm has also moved into the field of view. (Kindly supplied to the author by Dr Hedenstierna.)

Airways dysfunction in the aged

Abnormalities of airway function are conveniently divided into those of (i) the *lower* and (ii) the *upper airway*.

The lower airways

Effect of lung elastic recoil on airway resistance   As mentioned above, a major determinant of intrapulmonary airway calibre is the elasticity of the lung parenchyma. Because age reduces lung elasticity the basal airways narrow, in a passive fashion, at a higher lung volume than in younger patients. This relationship between airway calibre, or resistance, and lung volume can be measured in anaesthetized patients using forced airflow oscillation (Jones *et al.*, 1987) and is shown in Fig. 4.7 for a young and an old subject. This shows that lung volume is a major determinant of airway resistance. During anaesthesia the FRC may be considerably reduced due to the reduced tone of the muscles of the chest wall. Consequently the FRC may be only a little larger than residual volume and the airway resistance at end expiration may be very large. This is particularly likely in the obese patient when FRC is reduced to a greater extent during anaesthesia than in thin patients. In the older subject the whole airway resistance curve lies above that of the young subject. This may be due to changes in the elastic properties of the airways and of the lung parenchyma as well as to increased airway mucus.

A number of points therefore arise:

(i) airway resistance rises steeply with diminishing lung volume

(ii) if FRC is reduced (supine posture, abdominal distension, obesity) there is an increase in airway resistance

(iii) the increased airway resistance in aged subjects (and in emphysema) may, in part, be due to loss of lung elastic properties

(iv) the low elastic recoil and high airway resistance in the lung base predispose to atelectasis.

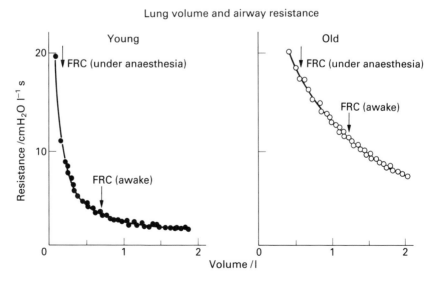

Fig. 4.7. Airway resistance versus lung volume in a young subject (left) and in an old subject (right). Note that during general anaesthesia the FRC may be considerably reduced.

55 | *The aged pulmonary system*

Particular attention must be directed to reversing basal atelectasis by instructing the nurses and physiotherapists to produce frequent large changes in posture in these patients.

Elastic properties of the walls of larger airways   A major, but fortunately not too common, problem in the aged is an increased tendency of the large airways to collapse because of the change in the elastic properties of the airway wall. This change may occur quite independently of changes in lung elastic recoil pressure and leads to an increase in airway obstruction quite refractory to bronchodilators and is quite difficult to diagnose without bronchoscopy or dynamic bronchographic studies of the large airways.

To understand something of the effect of increased airway collapsibility a brief outline is needed of the factors which determine maximum expiratory flow. The principal methods of quantifying the degree of airway obstruction are the forced expiratory volume in one second (FEV$_{1.0}$), peak expiratory flow rate (PEFR), or the flow–volume curve. Once a certain expiratory effort has been exceeded, the maximum expiratory flow rate is determined by three factors: (i) lung elastic recoil pressure, (ii) small airway resistance, and (iii) elastic properties (collapsibility) of the large airways (Fig. 4.8a). In the aged all three of these may change so as to reduce expiratory flow but the effect of changes in the elastic properties of the large airway is not widely known. To simulate the effect of ageing on the elastic properties of the trachea and large bronchi the large airway of post-mortem lungs can be exposed to the proteolytic enzyme, pronase. After a few hours these airways become very much less inelastic (i.e. more easily collapsible) than normal (Jones *et al.* 1975).

Fig. 4.8b shows that the normal trachea requires a pressure of

(a)   (b)

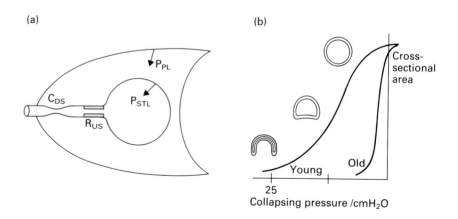

Fig. 4.8. (a) The determinants of maximum expiratory flow. These are the lung elastic recoil pressure (P$_{STL}$), upstream resistance of small airways (R$_{US}$), downstream compliance (C$_{DS}$). P$_{PL}$ is pleural pressure. (b) The increased collapsibility (compliance) of the large airways in some old patients.

25 cmH$_2$O to produce complete closure, wheareas after pronase only a few cmH$_2$O are needed to produce major airway closure. The effect on expiratory flow is very dramatic so that with no change either in the elastic properties of the lung parenchyma or in small airway resistance there is a profound fall in expiratory flow. The only clinical clue to the existence of this phenomenon is the incidental finding at bronchoscopy of very compliant large airways (De Kock, 1977) which may present as a postoperative problem because of a considerable difficulty in clearing bronchial secretions. Not only is there a problem in clearing secretions but there is a large increase in the work of breathing because major airway collapse will occur during relaxed tidal breathing. Assisted ventilation and vigorous humidification will be necessary until the secretion of viscid bronchial mucus decreases.

Two-phase gas liquid flow in airways   Another important factor that produces a considerable increase in airway resistance is a layer of mucus on the walls of the airways. It might be supposed that this effect is fairly obvious and is produced simply by narrowing the lumen of the airway. However, in a detailed analysis of the effects of mucus-like liquids in airways (Clarke *et al.*, 1970) it was found that the increase in airway resistance might be as much as 10 times greater than expected by narrowing alone because of a complex interaction between gas flow and the liquid layer on the wall of the tube. This interaction is called two phase gas liquid flow. The increased resistance to flow in this system is very sensitive both to gas flow rate as well as the the thickness and visco-elastic properties of the mucus layer. To clear fluid from the wall the gas flow rate has to be very high (with a Reynolds number > 5000) If this flow rate is not achieved there is a very high airway resistance but no expulsion of airway mucus. An increase in bronchial secretions may be a feature of chronic exposure to polluted atmospheres or tobacco smoke and is also caused by anaesthesia and intubation. The problem of clearing secretions from the lungs of the postoperative patient has not been solved but lowering the viscosity of mucus using aqueous aerosols may considerably reduce the flow rate needed to achieve critical two phase flow with expulsion of mucus.

Removal of viscid secretions from the airways of aged patients may be particularly difficult for the following reasons:

(i) there are more secretions

(ii) impaired humidification causes an increase in the visco-elastic properties of mucus

(iii) the airways are more collapsible

(iv) expiratory flow rate may be considerably reduced.

The upper airway

One of the commonest problems during and after anaesthesia is obstruction of the upper airway and it is paradoxical that anaesthetists have largely failed to investigate the underlying mechanisms of this problem. However, sleep apnoea has been extensively investigated (Strohl *et al.*, 1980) and the findings are relevant to postoperative apnoea and hypoxia which are common in the older patient.

Obstructive apnoea is caused by closure of the upper airway which may remain closed despite increasing breathing effort (Remmers *et al.*, 1978). The oropharynx is the only collapsible segment of the extra thoracic airway because its walls are very compliant and cannot resist the effects of a negative transmural pressure (Rodenstein & Stanescu, 1986). Reduced airway patency is promoted by four factors: (i) negative pressure in the airway lumen, (ii) neck flexion, (iii) mucosal adhesion once the airway has closed, and (iv) abnormal anatomy.

In normal, awake man a large pressure, as much as 80 cmH$_2$O, is needed to close the upper airway, whereas only a few cmH$_2$O pressure are needed to close the airway in some stages of sleep and under general anaesthesia (Brouillete & Thach, 1979). The large force opposing airway collapse when awake is due to the tonic and phasic activity induced in the upper airway wall muscles by neural activity. This activity dilates the airway, decreases its compliance and increases its resistance to collapse. During inspiration the muscles of the upper airway are activated just prior to activation of the intercostals and diaphragm. In this way the upper airway can resist the collapse pressure produced on inspiration. When the neural control of the upper airway is impaired or abolished, as in *old patients*, in *REM sleep*, after *alcohol consumption* or *anaesthesia*, the phasic activation of the upper airway may be reduced or abolished with a considerably increased tendency to episodic closure of the oropharynx. Flexion of the neck has a marked closing effect on the oropharnyx and there are well known anatomical factors, such as short thick neck, small jaw and obesity, which predispose to upper airway obstruction during sleep or anaesthesia.

That this may be a particular problem postoperatively has been emphasized by Catley *et al.* (1985) who showed that in the 24 h following surgery older subjects were particularly liable to show periodic apnoea if given morphine analgesia but not if regional analgesia was used for postoperative pain relief. It is clear that in old patients following surgery, particularly on the hip, upper abdomen or chest, there is an interaction between the effects of anaesthesia, analgesia, surgery and sleep to give episodes of quite severe arterial oxygen desaturation. These factors are indicated in Fig. 4.9. The impairment of gas exchange caused by atelectasis induced by anaesthesia persisting into the postoperative period has already been noted. This produces a background of hypoxia against which episodes of sleep apnoea exacerbate oxygen desaturation, particularly in older patients given morphine infusions. Although central apnoea was a common phenomenon, it was never associated with hypoxia, whereas obstructive apnoea or partial upper airway obstruction was always associated with hypoxia.

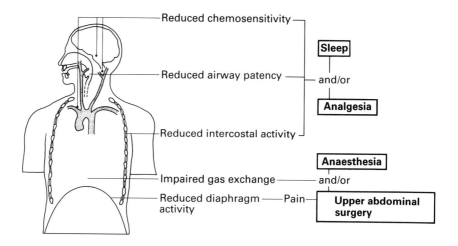

Fig. 4.9. The relationship between the effects of anaesthesia, surgery, analgesia and sleep on oxygenation in the postoperative period. (Reproduced with permission of authors and publishers of *International Anesthesiology Clinics.*)

The problem of obstructive apnoea and hypoxia occurs during sleep only in patients given morphine infusions, and it becomes more frequent with increasing age (Fig. 4.10). This is an important clinical point because, in contrast to young patients, more frequent and more profound episodes of hypoxia occurred in the older age group over long periods of time in the postoperative period. It would seem likely that patients in this age group would be less tolerant of hypoxia than younger patients, both for cerebral as well as cardiac reasons. Those patients with a recent history of cerebrovascular insufficiency or myocardial infarction are particularly at risk if hypoxia is associated either with a fall in cardiac output or an increased tissue demand for oxygen.

In view of these findings some change in practice is required with these patients. In particular, (i) the high risk group of patients and operative procedures should be identified, (ii) regional analgesia used as postoperative pain relief would rarely be associated with hypoxia, (iii) if opioids are used for postoperative pain relief the administration of oxygen will be needed for much longer periods than had been previously considered to be necessary (Jones *et al.*, 1985). This is because the danger of hypoxia with sleep apnoea may last for several days after an operation. A factor that may prolong this effect is that surgery and anaesthesia abolish REM sleep for several days postoperatively. When REM sleep returns, these hypoxic episodes may become even more frequent and prolonged and associated with a greater degree of hypoxia. Thus, the most dangerous time for postoperative hypoxia may be during the second or third night following the operation, a time when patients are rarely given extra oxygen to breathe (Moote *et al.*, 1986).

The continuous measurement of oxygen saturation may be an advance in patient safety in the postoperative period. Nevertheless,

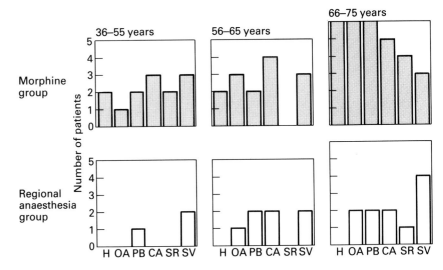

Fig. 4.10. The effect of age on respiratory abnormalities during sleep in the postoperative period in two groups of patients having morphine or regional anaesthesia for postoperative pain relief. H — hypoxia ($SaO_2 < 80\%$); OA — obstructive apnoea; PB — paradoxical breathing; CA — central apnoea; SR — slow respiratory rate; SV — small tidal volume. Total numbers of patients in the three age ranges were 5, 5 and 6 respectively. (Reproduced with permission of authors and publishers of *Anesthesiology*.)

fairly simple computer processing of this information will give a clearer picture of the proportion of time a patient may spend at any particular oxygen saturation. This will be discussed further in the next section.

Control of breathing in the aged

Control of breathing in the aged has been reviewed by Pack & Millman (1986) and the salient features, together with studies of the effects of anaesthetic drugs, are presented below.

Ageing and ventilatory control

The automatic control of the ventilatory system depends upon a number of different signals which originate from two groups of receptors: (i) the peripheral mechanoreceptors in lungs, chest wall and joints, and (ii) central and peripheral chemoreceptors. In awake subjects the former feedback predominates in the fine control of ventilation, particularly in the response to mechanical loading, whereas during sleep the chemoreceptor input predominates in the control process.

Mechanical loading

In conscious man a sudden increase in the airflow resistance of a breathing circuit is usually well compensated for without a change in PCO_2 or PO_2. This is because of the abrupt change in afferent information from the various mechanoreceptors. There is evidence that the aged have a reduced compensatory response to such mechanical loading and it was at one time postulated that this was due to a reduced perception of the abnormal sensations arising in the chest wall during loading. However, it has been shown by Tack *et al.* (1982) that the aged do not have a reduced perception of loads and some other mechanism may underly this undoubted effect of ageing on impairing load compensation.

Chemoreceptor activity

More information is available on the effects of ageing on chemoreceptor activity. The standard challenge techniques for evaluating respiratory control include quantifying the ventilatory response to either an increased carbon dioxide or a decreased oxygen concentration in inspired gas. Kronenberg & Drage (1973) showed that in a group of men aged 64–73 years the hypoxic responses were 50% of a control group of younger subjects, and in the case of the hypercapnic response there was a 40% reduction in response. One explanation for these results is that the chemoreceptor response to stimulation is quite normal but, because of the effect of ageing on the lung and chest wall, ventilation cannot increase appropriately. If ventilation cannot respond to the increased drive, e.g. because the lungs and chest wall are abnormally stiff, there is an alternative technique that can be employed to evaluate chemoreceptor response. If, just at the beginning of inspiration, the airway is rapidly occluded there is an abrupt fall in pressure within the occluded airway which is proportional to inspiratory muscle activity. The fall in airway pressure 100 ms after the initiation of inspiration, the $P_{0.1}$, is a measure of respiratory muscle activation unimpeded by the mechanical resistance of lung and chest wall and is a closer correlate of ventilatory drive than change in ventilation *per se*. Nevertheless, Peterson *et al.* (1981), using the occlusion pressure technique, showed that the reduction in ventilation was not due to mechanical factors in lung and chest wall, and that there was a real reduction in central chemoreceptor response in the old.

Effect of anaesthetic drugs on the control of breathing

It has long been customary to reduce the dose of opiate preoperative medication in aged subjects in the belief that the old are more susceptible to respiratory depression than the young. The effect of intravenous morphine 10 mg per 70 kg body weight on ventilation in two groups of subjects, young (aged 28–37 years) and old (aged 65–82 years) was studied by Arunasalam *et al.* (1983). They studied minute ventilation, end tidal CO_2 and ventilatory frequency and showed that, whereas morphine produced a significant degree of respiratory depression as measured by these three variables, there was no difference between the magnitude of the effect in the two groups. However, 7 of the 13 old subjects and only 3 of 13 young subjects showed frequent periods of sleep apnoea following morphine.

Pack & Millman (1986) pointed out that young (19–29) and old (67–88 years) subjects showed no significant difference in the fall in ventilation and rise in end tidal P_{CO_2} during sleep. However, the pattern of ventilation was more irregular in the old subjects with both central and obstructive apnoea, particularly in male subjects during stage 1 and 2 sleep. Catley et al. (1985) found that respiratory disturbances were particularly pronounced in patients age 66–77 years who had received postoperative morphine infusions for pain relief (Fig. 4.10). In contrast, patients of a similar age having regional anaesthesia had fewer apnoeic episodes with no occasions where Sa_{O_2} fell below 85%.

In an analysis of the factors causing respiratory irregularity Khoo et al. (1982) predicted that respiratory irregularity would be enhanced by hypoxia. However, we had noticed that hypoxia (Sa_{O_2} below 80%) caused arousal, an increased ventilation and a rise in Sa_{O_2}. To examine the effect of oxygen administration on postoperative sleep apnoea and hypoxia, we (Jones et al., 1985) administered 28% oxygen to patients recovering from anaesthesia. Oxygen saturation was measured continuously and, with the aid of computer analysis, plots were produced to show the percentage of time spent at any particular Sa_{O_2} during the period of the study (Fig. 4.11). This study gave the following results:

(i) oxygen therapy always produced an *improvement in oxygenation*
(ii) there was a *gradual improvement* in oxygenation throughout the night
(iii) oxygen administration did not influence the number or duration of *hypoxic* episodes.

Effects of general anaesthesia on ventilatory control

There is no information on the different susceptibilities of young and old patients to the effects of volatile or intravenous anaesthetics on ventilation. However, it is well known that volatile anaesthetics reduce tone and phasic movement of the upper airway and rib cage musculature to a greater extent than that of the diaphragm (Jones, 1977). Because of this, the depressant effect of volatile agents on the hypercapnic response can be explained almost entirely by the depressant effect on rib cage movement. Since the effect of anaesthetics in reducing rib cage movement is so potent it is doubtful that there would be a significant difference between young and old patients.

Similarly the effect of volatile anaesthetics in reducing hypoxic chemoreceptor responses is very potent. Even 0.1 MAC (minimum alveolar concentration) is sufficient to produce a 90% reduction in the hypoxic response. Although there is an age-related reduction in hypercapnia and hypoxic ventilatory responses, the effects of conventional

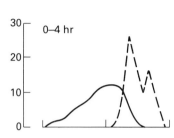

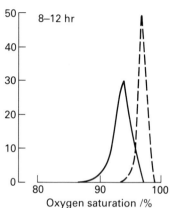

Fig. 4.11. Method for quantifying saturation versus time during a 12 h period while recovering from surgery. The patient was breathing air or 28% O_2 as shown. Note the gradual improvement in oxygenation with time. (Reproduced with permission of authors and publishers of *Journal of the Royal Society of Medicine.*)

doses of volatile anaesthetics in reducing ventilatory responses are considerably more potent but it is possible that the effects are additive. Thus, the older patient may show a greater degree of respiratory depression during anaesthesia than the younger patient.

The rapid elimination of volatile anaesthetics in the postoperative period is an important factor in reducing this cause of postoperative respiratory depression. Nevertheless, as discussed above, the effects of opioids may persist for many hours and their elimination from the body may be compromised in the aged.

Respiratory muscle fatigue and weaning

It has been pointed out that 20% of patients who undergo mechanical ventilation in intensive care units are unable to continue spontaneous ventilation when it is discontinued. There is a clinical impression that this may be a greater problem in the old than in the young. In patients with malnutrition and/or chronic obstructive lung disease it is established that there are particular difficulties in weaning after several days of mechanical ventilation. Weaning may also be a problem in old patients with these disorders after mechanical ventilation for anaesthesia and surgery. The factors contributing to the difficult transition to spontaneous ventilation are the inefficient flat diaphragm, increased airway secretions, hypoxia and persistent muscle weakness. Furthermore, the effects of neuromuscular blocking drugs on muscle power are not immediately reversed by the administration of neostigmine. Generally the factors that must be considered in evaluating the patient prior to weaning can be divided into non-pulmonary and pulmonary.

Non-pulmonary factors favouring weaning are near normal mental and nutritional state (calories, muscle mass, phosphate and potassium) and a normal circulation. Pulmonary factors include a vital capacity of 10–15 ml per kg body weight, normal acid base status, and a right-to-left shunt of less than 20%.

Two other important factors are *ventilatory drive* and *respiratory muscle fatigue*. Both are difficult to evaluate in this situation but because of the reduction in muscle power with increasing age, muscle fatigue may be a more important factor in old patients. In order to make a distinction between muscle fatigue and reduced ventilatory drive the airway occlusion pressure technique mentioned above has been employed (Sassoon *et al.*, 1987). This technique measures ventilatory drive during the first 100 ms of airway occlusion, the $P_{0.1}$. The range of normal values of $P_{0.1}$ is up to 6 cmH$_2$O but if ventilation is impaired without any obvious cause, such as stiff lungs or abnormal chest wall, the $P_{0.1}$ is considerably greater than 6 cmH$_2$O, the implication being that ventilatory drive is *increased* to compensate for *weakness* of the respiratory muscles. Under these conditions of increased ventilatory drive the respiratory muscles are too fatigued to sustain contractions sufficient to maintain normal ventilation.

A maximum inspiratory pressure greater than 30 cmH$_2$O may be a useful guide to easy weaning but this does not take into account the relationship between the maximum pressure that can be generated and the pressure needed to maintain ventilation. If the pressure needed for normal ventilation is greater than 40% of the maximum inspiratory pressure then the muscles will fatigue (Fig. 4.12). Thus, in a patient who can just achieve a maximum inspiratory pressure of 30 cmH$_2$O, a high resistive or elastic load (because of airway obstruction or interstitial lung disease) may cause the pressure required to maintain ventilation to exceed 15 cmH$_2$O and the respiratory muscles will quickly fatigue.

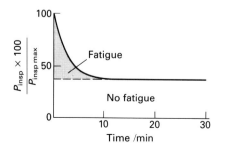

Fig. 4.12. The time to fatigue at different inspiratory loads (P_{insp}) measured as a function of maximum attainable inspiratory pressure ($P_{insp\,max}$). In this example fatigue occurs in 10 min at 40% of ($P_{insp\,max}$).

The electromyograph pattern of respiratory muscle may be a useful indicator of fatigue by showing the ratio of muscle force produced at a high (50 Hz) versus a low (20 Hz) stimulating frequency (Moxham, 1984). However, this approach has been of limited clinical value in predicting respiratory muscle fatigue.

Pulmonary oedema

Adult Respiratory Distress Syndrome (ARDS)

Pulmonary oedema is a complication which may occur more frequently in the aged because of the greater risk of (i) left-sided heart failure due to myocardial ischaemia or infarction and (ii) hypoproteinaemia because of liver or renal disease. Nevertheless, it would be quite wrong to assume that all pulmonary oedema in the aged is due to these causes. There is an increased risk of the ARDS because many of the disorders which predispose to ARDS are more common in old patients. For example, acid aspiration may occur in an unconscious patient with laryngeal incompetence and sepsis may occur more commonly following major bowel surgery for carcinoma. The fundamental defect in the lung in the pulmonary oedema of ARDS is quite different from that in left ventricular failure, although in the aged the two conditions may coexist, giving rise to considerable diagnostic confusion.

To obtain a clear understanding of the mechanism of pulmonary oedema and their management in old patients with multisystem disease, an outline is needed of the structure and function of the alveolar wall. Details of the structure of the alveolar wall, together with new studies of its solute permeability (Barrowcliffe & Jones, 1987) and the factors which influence the net fluid flux across the barrier, are summarized in Fig. 4.13. Starling's original concept of these factors oversimplifies these forces in a number of ways. The osmotic pressure gradient ($\Delta\Pi$) must be modified to take into account the efficacy of the barrier as a semipermeable membrane. This is described by the reflection coefficient (σ)

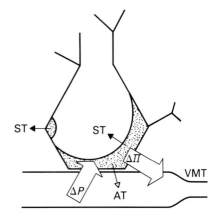

Fig. 4.13. Summary of the forces, active and passive, which influence fluid balance across the alveolar wall. ST — surface tension; AT — active transport; VMT — venomotor tone; ΔP — hydrostatic pressure gradient; $\Delta\Pi$ — osmotic pressure gradient.

The aged pulmonary system

which for a perfect semipermeable membrane is unity and for a very leaky membrane falls to zero. In this way, $\sigma \times \Delta\Pi$ describes the effective gradient of osmotic pressure.

In ARDS there is a leaky barrier where the reflection coefficient σ for protein in many alveoli may be near zero; as a consequence there is no effective colloid osmotic pressure gradient in these alveoli. In these circumstances the hydrostatic pressure gradient across the capillary wall is no longer opposed by an osmotic pressure gradient. This is a very important concept in that it emphasizes the basic principle in the management of ARDS which is to reduce the hydrostatic pressure in the pulmonary capillaries to less than 10 mmHg. This contrasts with the situation in left-sided heart failure, when the hydrostatic pressure must be reduced only below a critical value of about 25 mmHg, i.e. the magnitude of the normal colloid osmotic pressure gradient.

Other factors which maintain a fluid-free alveolus are active transport of solute, both crystalloid and colloid, and the effects of surface forces. Surfactant reduces the surface tension which would otherwise exert a considerable force, tending to pull liquid into the alveolar space. However, Hills (1987) suggests that because the surfactant acts as a water repellant it promotes alveolar dryness by the formation of convex droplets and these act as pumps which remove fluid from the alveolar lumen. Surfactant deficiency promotes alveolar collapse by increasing the forces tending to close the alveoli; it causes alveolar flooding by abolishing the action of corner pumps and also causes a considerable increase in solute permeability of the alveolar barrier.

Active transport is an important factor in maintaining the large concentration gradient of solute across the barrier which, if the reflection coefficient is near unity, results in a highly protective gradient of osmotic pressure which keeps the alveoli free of fluid. Thus, from the physiological point of view, ARDS causes a breakdown in the integrity of the barrier, particularly of the epithelium, a reduction in the reflection coefficient (σ) of both the epithelial and endothelial components, and an increased flux of protein into the alveolar space which denatures surfactant and promotes further flooding and alveolar collapse.

The most common causes of ARDS are aspiration of gastric contents (roughly one-third of reliably witnessed aspirations may develop the syndrome) and serious infections including pneumonias and gram-negative septicaemia. The source of such infection is frequently intra-abdominal, and positive blood cultures do not have to be obtained to make the diagnosis. ARDS is reported to occur in 25–60% of such cases.

Diagnosis and management of ARDS

The basic criteria in the diagnosis of ARDS are radiological evidence of pulmonary oedema, hypoxaemia due to a mismatch of pulmonary ventilation to perfusion, and a reduced lung compliance. Other tests are

Table 4.1. Tests of pulmonary function following lung injury

1 Gas exchange (P(A-a)o_2 difference, V/Q distributions)
2 Radiography (CXR, angiography)
3 Mechanics (compliance)
4 Alveolar liquid analysis (pulmonary oedema protein, alveolar lavage)
5 Pulmonary artery pressures (wedge pressure)
6 Lung permeability (^{99m}Tc-DTPA, labelled protein)
7 Lung metabolism
8 Lung water (thermodilution, CT scan)
9 Lung inflammation (labelled neutrophils, gallium, biopsy)

outlined in Table 4.1. Some workers advocate a measurement of pulmonary wedge pressure using the Swan-Ganz catheter. They insist that it is important to distinguish between a high microvascular pressure oedema and a low pressure oedema. Their point is that ARDS is a low pressure pulmonary oedema because of reduced σ and a low effective colloid osmotic pressure. However, in aged patients left-sided heart failure may coexist with ARDS and a raised pulmonary wedge pressure does not exclude ARDS. Many aged patients show evidence of incipient left ventricular failure by a rise in pulmonary wedge pressure on exercise despite a normal pressure at rest (Ehrsam *et al.*, 1983).

A marked increase in pulmonary venous resistance, and hence pulmonary capillary pressure, can cause a haemodynamic form of pulmonary oedema with a normal wedge pressure. This may be a particular problem in ARDS because many mediators of lung injury promote an increase in pulmonary venomotor tone.

Thus, a 'low' wedge pressure in an ARDS patient may seriously underestimate the actual, unbalanced pressure in the pulmonary micro-circulation. There are techniques available (Collee *et al.*, 1987) with which the actual pulmonary capillary pressure may be measured.

The mainstay of the treatment is threefold:
 (i) reduce pulmonary capillary pressure
(ii) avoid overdistension of the lung
(iii) treat the underlying cause.

Fluid restriction and the maintenance for days or weeks of a careful fluid balance are of paramount importance. Vasodilators (isosorbide, nitro-prusside or prostaglandin E1) may be needed to reduce pulmonary venoconstriction. Plateau pressures greater than 40 cmH$_2$O are likely to produce overdistension of unaffected lung units and exacerbate lung injury. A high PEEP obviously promotes a high plateau pressure. A pulsed oximeter may be of value in facilitating adjustments of ventilator settings in that it gives an indication of change in Sao_2 if peripheral circulation is satisfactory. There are no specific treatments for ARDS but the elimination of septic foci is of supreme importance.

The only factor that may necessitate modifications of this regimen is the need to maintain an adequate oxygen delivery to the brain and heart.

Otherwise, the maintenance of a low pulmonary capillary pressure must be paramount.

Although the mortality of ARDS is high, Rinaldo & Rogers (1986) suggest that most patients, especially those where trauma is implicated, can be treated succesfully and survive. If sepsis can be treated by surgical drainage, then this may not preclude clinical recovery if the vigorous regimen advocated above is conscientiously applied.

Conclusion

Respiratory dysfunction in the old patient is common because of reduced elasticity of the lungs leading to airway closure and impaired gas exchange. There is impaired control of breathing and upper airway patency during sleep. These two factors lead to severe episodes of sleep-related apnoea and hypoxia, particularly following the administration of morphine in the postoperative period. Respiratory muscle fatigue may be precipitated by malnutrition in patients with increased work of breathing due to obstructive airway disease. Finally, pulmonary oedema must be regarded as a multifactorial disorder and care must be taken not to misdiagnose the increased permeability type of oedema. The use of more prolonged non-invasive monitoring of arterial oxygen saturation in high dependency units will increase patient safety following major surgery. Oxygen therapy and vigorous mobilization may be needed for much longer periods in the aged than in younger patients.

References

Arunasalem, K., Davenport, H.T., Painter, P. & Jones, J.G. (1983) Ventilatory response to morphine in young and old subjects. *Anaesthesia* **38**, 529–533.

Barrowcliffe, M.P. & Jones, J.G. (1987) Solute permeability of the alveolar capillary barrier. *Thorax,* **42**, 1–10.

Brismar, B., Hedenstierna, G., Lundquist, H., Strandberg, A., Svensson, L. & Tokics, L. (1985) Pulmonary densities during anesthesia with muscular relaxation — a proposal of atelectasis. *Anesthesiology* **62**, 422–428.

Brouillette, R.T. & Thach, B.T. (1979) A neuromuscular mechanism maintaining extrathoracic airway patency. *J. Appl. Physiol.* **46**, 772–779.

Catley, D.M., Thornton, C., Jordan, C., Lehane, J.R., Royston, D. & Jones, J.G. (1985) Pronounced, episodic oxygen desaturation in the postoperative period: its association with ventilatory pattern and analgesic regimen. *Anesthesiology* **63**, 20–28.

Clarke, S.W., Jones, J.G. & Oliver, D.R. (1970) Resistance to two-phase gas-liquid flow in airways. *J. Appl. Physiol.* **29**, 464–471.

Collee, G.G., Lynch, K.E., Hill, R.D. & Zapol, W.M. (1987) Bedside management of pulmonary capillary pressure in patients with acute respiratory failure. *Anesthesiology* **66**, 614–620.

De Kock, M.A. (1977) *Dynamic Bronchoscopy.* Springer-Verlag, Berlin, Heidelberg, New York.

Ehrsam, R.E., Perruchoud, A., Oberholzer, M., Burkart, F. & Herzog, H. (1983) Influence of age on pulmonary haemodynamicals at rest and during exercise. *Clin. Sci.* **65**, 653–660.

Hedenstierna, G., Tokics, L., Strandberg, A., Lundquist, H. & Brismar, B. (1986) Correlation of gas exchange impairment to development of atelectasis during anaesthesia and muscle paralysis. *Acta Anaesth. Scand.* **30**, 183-191.

Heneghan, C.P.H, Bergman, N.A. & Jones, J.G. (1984) Changes in lung volume and (PAO_2-PaO_2) during anaesthesia. *Br. J. Anaesth.* **56**, 437-445.

Hills, B.A. (1987) Bursting the alveolar bubble. *Anaesthesia* **42**, 467-469.

Holtz, B., Bake, B. & Oxhoj, H. (1976) Effect of inspired volume on closing volume. *J. Appl. Physiol.* **41**, 623-630.

Jones, J.G. (1977) The chest wall — tone and movement. *Anesthesiology* **47**, 325-326.

Jones, J.G., Fraser, R.B. & Nadel, J.A. (1975) Prediction of maximum expiratory flow rate from the area-transmural pressure curve of compressed airway. *J. Appl. Physiol.* **38**, 1002-1011.

Jones, J.G., Jordan, C., Scudder, C., Rocke, D.A. & Barrowcliffe, M. (1985) Episodic postoperative oxygen desaturation: the value of added oxygen *J. Roy. Soc. Med.* **78**, 1019-1022.

Jones, J.G., Jordan, C., Slavin, B. & Lehane, J.R. (1987) Prophylactic effect of aminophylline and salbutamol on histamine-induced bronchoconstriction. *Br. J. Anaesth.* **59**, 498-502.

Khoo, M., Kronauer, R.E., Strohl, K.P. & Slutsky, A.S. (1982) Factors including periodic breathing in humans: a general model. *J. Appl. Physiol.* **53**, 644-659.

Kroneberg, R.S. & Drage, G.W. (1973) Attenuation of the ventilatory and heart rate responses to hypoxia and hypercapnia with aging in normal man. *J. Clin. Invest,* **52**, 1812-1819.

Moote, C.A., Skinner, M.I., Grace, D.M. & Knill, R.L. (1986) Severe sleep related hypoxaemia after abdominal surgery in the morbidly obese. *Can. Anaesth. Soc. J.* **33**, S105.

Moxham, J. (1984) Failure of the respiratory muscle pump. In *Effects of Anaesthesia and Surgery on Pulmonary Mechanisms and Gas Exchange* (Ed. J.G. Jones). International Anesthesiology Clinics, Vol.22, No.4. Little Brown, Boston, pp. 165-181.

Pack, A.I. & Millman, R.P. (1986) Changes in control of ventilation, awake and asleep, in the elderly. *J. Am. Geriatr. Soc.* **34**, 533-544.

Pavia, D. (1984) Lung mucociliary clearance. In *Aerosols and the Lung: Clinical and Experimental Aspects* (Eds S.W. Clarke & D. Pavia). Butterworths, London.

Peterson, D.D., Pack, A.I., Silage, D.A. & Fishman, A.P. (1981) Effect of aging on ventilatory and occlusion pressure responses to hypoxia and hypercapnia. *Am. Rev. Respir. Dis.* **124**, 387-391.

Remmers, J.E., deGroot, W.J., Sauerland, E.K. & Anch, A.M. (1978) Pathogenesis of upper airway occlusion during sleep *J. Appl. Physiol.* **44**, 931-938.

Rinaldo, J.E. & Rogers, R.M. (1986) Adult respiratory distress syndrome. *New Engl. J. Med.* **315**, 578-580.

Rodenstein, D.O. & Stanescu, D.C. (1986) The soft palate and breathing. *Am. Rev. Respir. Dis.* **134**, 311-325.

Sassoon, C.S.H., Te, T.T., Mahutte, C.K. & Light, R.W. (1987) Airway occlusion pressure: an important indicator for successful weaning in patients with chronic obstructive pulmonary disease. *Am. J. Respir. Dis.* **135**, 107-113.

Strohl, K.P., Hensley, M.J., Hallett, M., Saunders, N.A. & Ingram, R.H.Jr (1980) Activation of upper airway muscles before onset of inspiration in normal humans. *J. Appl. Physiol.* **49**, 638-642.

Tack, M., Altose, M. & Cherniack, N.S. (1982) Effect of aging on the perception of resistive ventilatory loads. *Am. Rev. Respir. Dis.* **126**, 463-467.

5 | The aged nervous system

M. HILDICK-SMITH

Introduction

The changes which occur in the nervous system with ageing make it difficult to interpret the elderly patient's signs and symptoms. For example, it is hard to distinguish clearly between the benign forgetfulness of ageing and the forgetfulness of early dementia. There may be confusion between the gait changes of old age and those of Parkinson's disease. There may be false clues, such as absent vibration sense below the knees and absent ankle jerks, which do not have the same significance in the elderly as they would have in a young patient. Disease in systems other than the nervous system are very likely to be present and to complicate the picture. For example, painful arthritis in a shoulder may make it difficult to assess tone in the arm, while cataracts and small pupils may make it difficult to see the fundi.

Despite the many difficulties, it is essential that those who prepare elderly patients for necessary surgery or for intensive care treatment have a clear grasp of the ways in which ageing and disease of the nervous system and elsewhere will influence the outcome. The balance between risks and likely benefit can then be clearly weighed for each individual elderly patient. If it is decided to proceed, suitable modifications, e.g. in surgical technique, in anaesthetic or in drug dosages, can be made to take account of the patient's condition.

Neuropathology and neurochemistry of ageing and disease

Before certain changes in the ageing brain can be accepted as due to normal ageing, we must be confident that pathological processes have been excluded. As this subject is more thoroughly explored, some degree of consistency is emerging in the findings of different workers, suggesting that these findings do now reflect the changes of normal ageing. As age increases there seems to be some decrease in brain weight and flattening of cerebral gyri, and Davis & Wright (1977) have shown that the majority of normal people aged 70 or more have a considerable degree of cerebral atrophy. Reduction in the volume of white matter has been shown, and neocortical cell loss has been estimated at about 1% per year in persons aged 69–95. The hypothesis that the remaining neocortical cells can undergo growth of dendrites is supported by the relative proportions of the changes in the white and grey matter with ageing.

The brains of some elderly normal people show a few neurofibrillary tangles and senile plaques (which are present in much larger numbers in those with Alzheimer's disease). Deposition of lipofucsin in the cells of the medulla and hippocampus with increasing age is well documented, though the function of the material is unclear.

There has been much interest in the subcortical nuclei. The basal nucleus of Meynert shows no cell loss in normal ageing, and is responsible for the majority of the cholinergic input to the cortex. The locus coeruleus controls the majority of the noradrenergic input to the cortex and shows cell loss with age, as does the substantia nigra.

Just as there is variation in cell loss from one region to another, so there is variation in neurochemical disturbance, and some of the contradictions in the literature on this subject may be due to different areas being studied. The cholinergic system is known to be relevant to memory disturbance, and local decrease in choline acetyl transferase (CAT) has been shown in normal ageing. The cell loss in the locus ceruleus is mirrored by a loss in noradrenergic activity with age, while the loss of cells in the substantia nigra is reflected in an age-related decline in the activity of dopamine in elderly people without clinical Parkinson's disease. Localized changes in activity of serotonin (5HT) with age may be responsible for the characteristic sleep disturbances in the elderly.

In Alzheimer's disease the presence of neurofibrillary tangles in the cortex is probably the most reliable indicator of the disease. Other characteristic changes include argyrophilic (senile) plaques consisting of a central amyloid-like core and abnormal surrounding nerve processes and glial processes (Tomlinson *et al.*, 1970). Granulovacuolar degeneration is present, with nerve cell loss and Hirano body formation, while new formation of dendrites is impaired. There is cell loss in the nucleus of Meynert together with decrease in CAT (Rossor *et al.*, 1982). The intellectual deficit has been shown to correlate with the decrease in CAT, and particularly with the number of tangles in the cortex (Wilcock *et al.*, 1982). There are some deficiencies in other neurotransmitters, but these are less significant than the loss of CAT. The suggestion that the neuropathological changes in Alzheimer's disease may prove to be specific to certain pathways has not, disappointingly, opened the way to any treatment aimed at boosting acetylcholine.

In Parkinson's disease, the characteristic pathological changes are of degeneration in the pigmented nuclei of the substantia nigra and locus ceruleus, with characteristic Lewy bodies, and there is corresponding decrease in dopaminergic activity. There is correlation between the decrease in dopamine and the degree of cell loss, with atrophy and glial scarring in the zona compacta of the substantia nigra. There needs to be a loss of 80% of dopamine below normal before clinical Parkinson's disease appears, and before this stage there are compensatory mechanisms including increased turnover of dopamine in the remaining cells and increased sensitivity to dopamine in the striatum. The cholinergic system is normal in most areas of the brain in early and middle Parkinson's disease, but cortical CAT decrease has been shown in parkinsonian patients with dementia. A lesser decline in noradrenaline and 5HT has been shown in the brain in Parkinson's disease, but the fact that the primary deficit is in the dopamine system has opened the way to effective treatment.

Normals of neurology in old age

Macdonald Critchley in his classical lectures on the neurology of old age (Critchley, 1931) implied that the problems of diagnosis and treatment of neurological conditions were neglected in the old. It is still true that potentially treatable conditions such as spinal cord compression or subdural haematoma may be disregarded in old patients who might benefit from surgery, while other elderly patients may be subjected unnecessarily to procedures because the extent of their mental and physical incapacity has not been appreciated.

An estimate of the degree of neurological abnormality present in non-neurological patients admitted to hospital was attempted by Prakash & Stern (1973). They examined 100 patients, of average age 81 years, admitted to a geriatric unit: 30 patients were mildly confused; the fundi were visible in only 44; 33 patients had sluggish or irregular pupils; more than 60 had some muscle wasting in the hands; only 14 had a stride length greater than the length of their own feet; tone seemed increased in the legs in 45; and vibration sense in the legs was decreased in 33.

Similar widespread minor neurological abnormalities have been described in two American studies (Klawans et al., 1971; Kokmen et al., 1977) using elderly volunteers living at home. Particular attention was drawn to the progressive limitation of upward gaze with age, and to some loss of muscular strength, speed and dexterity in completing a task.

These findings highlight the difficulties in deciding which abnormalities should be given most weight in reaching a diagnosis. In clinical practice those which form a recognizable pattern or which relate to a functional disability will be considered most, while isolated findings may have to be disregarded.

Investigation of the aged patient with neurological abnormalities

Despite the difficulties much of the essential information for assessment and diagnosis in the elderly patient can be obtained — if not from the patient (because of deafness, confusion, speech disorder, etc.) then from a relative or carer. Instantaneous onset of the illness suggests a vascular or ictal cause (as in the young) while a slowly progessive problem is more likely to be due to a degenerative or malignant process. It is essential to get details from an observer of any 'turns', including whether the patient was unconscious, and to obtain a full list of the patient's medication, as drug-induced problems are more frequently encountered in the elderly (see Chapter 7).

After getting a reliable history, the first priority is to get an assessment of the patient's mental capability, using a questionnaire, such as that in Table 5.1, which tests orientation, short-term memory loss and simple calculation (by serial reversals), and takes 2.5 min to administer. Though there are disadvantages to all mental tests, it is more important to do one and repeat it later (using the patient as his own control) than to rely on the phrases 'somewhat confused' or 'rational' which can be subjective and inaccurate. If a patient has a low score, his confusion may be due to an acute illness and will improve with treatment, whereas a low score due to dementia will persist with minor variations. It is important to ensure the patient is not too deaf nor oversedated to hear the questions, or that a speech disorder does not invalidate the results. A depressed patient may also have a low score, and this may be difficult to distinguish — if suspected it is best to ask if the patient feels depressed, as this will often be readily admitted.

One advantage of administering the mental test first is that it shows what reliance can be placed on further details of history and physical examination (especially sensory aspects), and warns the examiner to proceed straight to the vital points in examination before the patient's attention span is over.

Examination of the fundi needs co-operation, but rarely reveals papilloedema even in the presence of raised intracranial pressure in the old. It is worth testing for hemianopia and for rough reading ability and possible visual neglect (reading only one half of a line of print) if

---

Table 5.1. Abbreviated mental test

Explain to the patient that memory, not mentality, is being tested
1 How old are you?
2 What time is it? (to nearest hour)
3 Address for recall at end of test — this should be repeated by the patient to ensure it has been heard correctly:
   42, West Street
4 What year is it?
5 What place is this? (name of institution or address)
6 Recognition of two people (doctor, nurse, etc.)
7 Day and month of birth
8 Year of start of the Second World War
9 Name of present monarch
10 Count backwards, from 20 down to 1

What was the address I asked you to remember?

Total number of correct answers = mental score
Scores: 8–10 normal
          4–7   moderate confusion
          1–3   severe confusion

Check patent is not deaf, depressed, dysphasic, drugged, severely ill (unable to co-operate) or struggling with a language difficulty

---

suspected, e.g. by the presence of a hemiplegia. In the ill elderly patient in whom meningitis or subarachnoid haemorrhage is suspected, cervical osteoarthritis may cause confusing decreased neck movement. However, in meningeal irritation lateral neck movements are usually significantly freer than those in the sagittal plane.

Examination for tone in arms and legs must take account of painful or restricting arthritis, but convincingly increased tone or sustained clonus or an unequivocally upgoing plantar reflex will be reliable, as will clear difference in strength or co-ordination between the sides of the body, or unequivocal small muscle fasciculation in hand or tongue. Unreliable signs include sluggish irregular pupil(s), wasting of the interossei, the glabellar tap, absent abdominal or ankle reflexes or absent vibration sense below the knee and sensory testing in general.

Relevant other examination may include checking for arrhythmia, postural hypotension (allowing 2 min after standing before measurement), checking for the murmur of aortic stenosis or the presence of carotid bruits, together with checking an ECG (for silent myocardial infarct), or a chest X-ray (for unsuspected bronchial carcinoma). The cervical spine X-ray is seldom helpful, as there is some abnormality in all patients over 60 and only gross changes may be relevant.

It is vital to assess function, which can conveniently be done by getting patients to take off their own pyjama jackets at the beginning of an examination, later asking them to stand from the bed and walk a few steps, as this will give quicker and more valuable information about their capabilities than detailed testing. It is important to know whether or not they can manage alone in the toilet.

There are a few 'short-cuts' which can be valuable. Any elderly patients who can walk 10 steps heel-to-toe on a line have nothing wrong with their nervous systems. Those who can easily 'find' their hemiplegic limb with their eyes shut have no serious body image problem. Those who can respond to the command 'Please rub your nose', delivered without gesture or explanation have no severe receptive dysphasia.

Investigation of elderly patients with primary or intercurrent neurological disorder will lean heavily on non-invasive tests. There is little indication now for lumbar puncture except in suspected meningitis, and sometimes subarachnoid haemorrhage, and other invasive tests such as carotid angiography will be performed only when clearly indicated (see later).

The electroencephalogram (EEG) is a useful non-invasive test. It shows age changes, particularly a decrease in the frequency of the dominant alpha rhythm with age, though the frequency still remains above the lower limit of normality (8 Hz) Some totally normal EEG tracings can be seen in centenarians. In many elderly individuals the EEG may show localized irregular slow waves in theta (4–7 Hz) and delta (0–3 Hz) bands in the temporal lobes, particularly on the left. If this abnormality is isolated it needs no investigation but its significance needs to be determined in each patient as it cannot be assumed to be due to ageing. The EEG is valuable as a tool of investigation in patients who have episodes of uncertain origin (?epileptic) or who have neurological or neuropsychiatric problems, and is particularly valuable if it shows a clear focal abnormality, e.g. in epilepsy.

The brain scan ('scintiscan') is a widely available non-invasive investigation which can demonstrate any lesion causing increased uptake, whether a bruise over the scalp, a cerebral infarct, or Paget's disease of the skull. It is useful to demonstrate large supratentorial lesions such as tumours, multiple metastases or infarcts, or subdural haematomas but is less accurate at showing lesions less than 2.5 cm in diameter or larger ones if they are in the posterior fossa. The computerized tomography (CT) scan, which is less widely available, is more accurate and can distinguish clearly cerebral infarcts from haemorrhages and tumours; it can delineate a subdural haematoma and demonstrate cerebral atrophy and normal pressure hydrocephalus. The place of this expensive investigation in the elderly is still being assessed. Its value probably lies in helping with diagnosis (stroke vs. neoplasm) in a slowly developing stroke, or where there is suspicion of subdural haematoma or of cerebral metastases. It may help when the preponderance of ataxia and incontinence over lesser mental impairment in a particular patient suggests normal pressure hydrocephalus. In general, it should be used only when the information it provides will affect patient management or enable a clearer prognosis to be given to relatives.

Other non-invasive tests used in the elderly include the visual evoked response (VER) and auditory evoked response (AER), both of whose latencies are increased with ageing, though not to a clinical extent. There is current work on the value of AER changes in dementia, and the VER can be used to demonstrate an old (forgotten) visual lesion. This can be valuable, for example, in an elderly patient with paraplegia as it suggests a diagnosis of multiple sclerosis rather than a spinal compressive lesion, and may save the patient an unrewarding and hazardous spinal operation.

Other non-invasive research tools include the positron emission tomography (PET) studies of local cerebral blood flow and metabolism, which may be useful in studies on dementia and stroke, and the nuclear magnetic resonance (NMR) studies which can demonstrate cortical thickness, and differentiate white from grey matter in dementias.

The electromyograph (EMG) is useful in distinguishing motor neurone disease from cord compression or cervical radiculopathy as a cause of wasting of the small muscles of the hand. It can be used to show the site of nerve entrapment, e.g. of the median nerve in the carpal tunnel, or of the lateral popliteal nerve (sometimes due to pressure from bad positioning of the leg during anaesthesia).

Cerebral blood flow (CBF)

The brain has a very high demand for oxygen and glucose and can function properly only if adequately perfused. There are delicate homeostatic mechanisms whereby the brain adapts to variations in systemic blood pressure by altering the calibre of cerebral arterioles. If the blood pressure falls the cerebral arterioles dilate and CBF is maintained. This poorly understood mechanism appears to adapt to persistent hypertension and, if the blood pressure is then too rapidly lowered, ischaemic brain damage may occur. CBF is also controlled by chemical and metabolic means, e.g. the most powerful dilator of cerebral arterioles is CO_2, the main product of cerebral metabolism.

Total CBF is uniform through the day, with no overall reduction during sleep (though it increases during REM sleep) and with no differences between the perfusion of the right and left hemispheres. There are, however, regional differences and the flow to the frontal and temporal lobes is greater than that to the parietal lobes, while grey matter is better perfused than white matter. There is a gradual decline in CBF from the age of about 30 onwards, but whether this is related to decreased brain weight and metabolism or due to degenerative arterial disease is not clear. Regional changes in perfusion occur (as in the young) when old people do physical or mental work. For example, speaking promotes bilateral activation (not only in Broca's and Wernicke's areas), whilst thinking about moving a limb gives increased perfusion in a different area from that involved when the limb is actually moved. CBF is increased in the early stages of anaesthesia (Lassen & Christensen 1976) as well as during epileptic seizures and in hyperthyroidism. Under all forms of general anaesthesia changes in P_{CO_2} continue to produce major changes in CBF, while there is lesser sensitivity of CBF to P_{O_2}. In multi-infarct dementia total CBF is reduced, whereas in Alzheimer's disease overall CBF is unchanged but perfusion of the grey matter (cortex, basal ganglia and thalamus) is reduced.

After a stroke, not only is CBF reduced to the affected side of the brain, but also the perfusion of the contralateral side is decreased for a period up to a month. In a transient stroke CBF on the affected side returns to normal after a few weeks, whereas those who are unconscious at the onset of the stroke usually have low CBF for some months — hence the CBF does correlate with the degree of recovery. In the acute stroke the normal relationship between CBF and brain metabolism is disrupted. There may be areas round the cerebral infarct where blood supply is more than adequate (luxury perfusion), as shown in PET studies, and in these areas reduced extraction of oxygen occurs. Other areas have 'critical perfusion' with inadequate blood supply, but higher oxygen extraction. Hence the overall picture after stroke is complex, but the perfusion of the brain depends on the systemic blood pressure, which should not be rapidly reduced as this may worsen the patient's condition.

Polycythaemia is associated with increased risk of stroke, as is a raised haematocrit (packed cell volume (PCV) over 0.46). If 250 ml of blood is removed and the haematocrit reduced the CBF can increase by up to 50% and this treatment is being assessed to see whether a reduction in further strokes can be obtained.

Epidemiology of strokes

The mortality of stroke increases with age, as does the incidence of stroke (average age at onset being 75 years). The incidence varies slightly from country to country but is roughly 200/100 000 of the population per year (Kurtzke, 1976). In the USA the prevalence of stroke varies from 0.35/1000 aged under 35 to 116/1000 aged over 85. As far as transient ischaemic attacks (TIA) are concerned, comprehensive recording of their incidence is inherently difficult. The symptoms, by definition, last for less than 24 h, and the patient may not report them. However, a Rochester study shows an average incidence of 31/100 000 population, rising with age to 220 at 65–74 years and 293 at 75 years or over. It is estimated that about one-third of TIA sufferers have a stroke in the following five years.

In developed countries such as the UK or America cerebrovascular disease has long been the third commonest cause of death (exceeded only by heart disease and cancer). There has, however, been a falling incidence of strokes and a declining mortality over the last 30 years or so. This tendency began before modern control of hypertension was established. It may owe something to declining salt intake (as freezing replaced salt curing in food preservation), though there is much salt in some processed foods. Other environmental risk factors related to stroke are cold temperatures, soft water, and low socio-economic class. Personal risk factors include male sex, age, history of TIAs, hypertension (even isolated systolic hypertension), heart disease, glucose intolerance, obesity, smoking and a raised PCV or serum cholesterol.

Stroke

In an emergency, the anaesthetist may need to prepare for operation a patient already disabled by a stroke, so it is important to be aware of the problems whether the patient has motor, cognitive or perceptual deficit.

Stroke can affect any part of the body, but Marquardsen (1969) found that 92% of stroke patients have some degree of weakness of one or more limbs. The arm is nearly always affected (suggesting a middle cerebral artery lesion), though in 3% of patients the paralysis affects the leg only (anterior cerebral artery lesion). About 90% of patients have flaccidity of the affected limbs immediately after the onset, but persistent hypotonia leads to a bad functional outcome. The classical pattern in hemiplegia is of increased tone in arm flexors and leg extensors, and undue reinforcement of this pattern can be prevented by careful positioning of limbs in the early weeks, as taught in the Bobath method and other physiotherapy techniques. The anaesthetist may be involved at this stage if a patient has unfortunately developed a stroke during anaesthesia. It is important to avoid pulling on the paralysed arm when lifting or moving such patients as this will worsen any subluxation of the humerus which has occurred and lead to later difficulties with a stiff and painful shoulder. (Many geriatric wards use a belt round the patient's waist when lifting or transferring new or old stroke patients to avoid the risk of pulling on the hemiplegic arm.)

Sensory aspects of stroke can occur at numerous levels. At the thalamic level sensation is reduced, but once the sensory threshold is reached the patient experiences extremely unpleasant sensations (often of swelling) on the affected side and will try to protect the affected limbs from any contact which may set off this sensation. At the level of the sensory cortex (where the face, lips and thumbs are disproportionately represented) a deficit will prevent patients identifying an object in the hand unless they can see it. This disability leads to difficulties, e.g. in finding keys in a pocket or in finding objects in the dark. If the stroke affects the parietal sensory cortex (an association area for sensory information) patients may totally forget a limb unless they look at it, or may deny there is any problem of sensation — and these aspects suggest a poor prognosis for recovery.

Visual disturbance may take the form of hemianopia (when patients will turn their heads in order to compensate for the visual loss) and visual neglect (when they will be unaware of one half of space and unable to compensate). Such patients may eat only the food on one half of a plate. An intermediate difficulty is visual inattention when patients can 'see' into the affected area only if there is no competition from the opposite side. Such patients have great difficulties feeding or dressing as they must see objects on both sides. One practical consequence of awareness of a patient's visual problem is in giving advice to relatives or nurses not to stand or help the patient from the neglected side, as the patient will not be visually aware of them there. All the above-mentioned perceptual problems carry the risk of high mortality or poor recovery.

Speech disorders complicate stroke, particularly when the receptive cortex or Wernicke's area is involved, leading to inability to understand (receptive dysphasia), or when the main motor area (Broca's area) is involved, leading to inability to speak or name objects (expressive dysphasia). Other problems include difficulty in initiating voluntary control of speech muscles (dyspraxia) in a patient who may be able to respond with clear automatic speech. Other patients have difficulties with facial and lip movements leading to dysarthric slurring of speech, while others with brainstem strokes have laryngeal muscle weakness and dysphonia. The more severe speech disorders have poor prognosis for recovery, and the question of whether a right or left hemiplegia has the better prognosis depends on the degree of perceptual or communication disorder present in each case, as these will be more important than the degree of motor loss.

One in four stroke patients has a significant degree of depression, but this usually arises about 6 months after the event, when the level of remaining disability is becoming clearer. Emotional control may be lost, especially in patients with multiple 'lacunar' strokes. These patients may suffer from emotional lability (or emotional incontinence), i.e. paroxysmal outbursts usually of crying when addressed, and this abnormality may persist for years.

If the anaesthetist is required to assess a patient, who has had an old stroke, for necessary or pain-relieving surgery, e.g. for abdominal or genitourinary disorder, only the briefest examination will be possible. This should include assessment of communication and mental ability, motor power in elbow extensors, wrist extensors, dorsiflexors of feet, brief assessment for loss of body image, ability to roll over in bed, stand and balance. He should try to see the patient undress if possible as a means of assessing function. All possible means of help need to be given to complement the patient's capabilities, e.g. it is important to have hearing-aid, spectacles, dentures, etc. available.

Recovery staff need to be aware of communication problems (if any) and for all care to be given in positioning, skin care, etc. especially for the hemiplegic side during the recovery period.

Parkinson's disease

This condition is the commonest disabling neurological condition after stroke. Its prevalence increases with age, being 14/1000 among those aged 70–84 and 26/1000 among those aged 85 or over. Since the advent of levodopa, patients are surviving longer and some studies suggest that the life-expectancy for patients who respond to levodopa is now nearly normal. Parkinson's disease is now largely a condition of the elderly, and 58% of British sufferers are aged 70 or over. The aetiology is still unknown, though twin studies have excluded a genetic component and the condition is not related to generalized vascular disease. The cause may be multi-factorial and may include contributions from a slow virus, and from individual variation (e.g. cigarette smokers are less likely to develope this disease) together with an environmental component. This may be related to MPTP (1-methyl-4-phenyl-1,2,5,6-tetrahydropyridine) a substance which has caused rapid onset of Parkinson's disease in young heroin addicts. Much research is now going on in this field of causation. In the elderly the increasing importance of drug-induced Parkinson's disease (in patients exposed to phenothiazines such as chlorpromazine and prochlorperazine) is being recognized.

The signs and symptoms of Parkinson's disease are a caricature of those of normal ageing including slowness in writing, cutting up food, dressing, rolling over in bed and getting in and out of chair or bed.

Problems of gait and balance dominate the picture in the elderly and the anaesthetist will frequently encounter these patients when they have fallen and sustained a fracture, e.g. of the femoral neck. Occasionally the condition will be undiagnosed; it should be looked for in any elderly patient having falls. Diagnosis, though difficult in the elderly, is made as in younger patients by thinking of the possibility of Parkinson's disease and confirming it by checking for tremor, muscle rigidity in trunk and limbs and assessing for bradykinesia by watching patients undo buttons or timing the writing of their names and addresses. Up to one in three aged parkinsonian patients may have dementia and the mental score (see earlier) is very valuable, as is an assessment of depression (Table 5.2). Many patients will have bladder problems — these may be a mixture of autonomic and detrusor hyper-reflexia with low bladder capacity, perhaps complicated by some degree of prostatism and worsened by anticholinergic drugs. Constipation occurs in 75% of sufferers and may be similarly related to autonomic dysfunction and/or anticholinergic drugs, compounded by the prolonged bowel transit time and the general immobility of the aged. These patients may be better taken off their anticholinergic drugs (which cause confusion in many aged parkinsonian patients) and will need attentive bladder and bowel care perioperatively. It is important to check whether there is significant postural hypotension (if the patient can stand) as this may recur under operative conditions. Periods of bedrest cause great reduction in mobility in parkinsonian patients, so it is important that they be kept as active as possible with breathing exercises, leg exercises, etc. before operation and as soon afterwards as possible with physiotherapy help.

Table 5.2. Short Zung interviewer-assisted depression rating scale

	Seldom or never	Some of the time	Good part of the time	Most of the time	Score
1 I feel down-hearted and blue	(1)	(2)	(3)	(4)	
2 I have trouble sleeping at night	(1)	(2)	(3)	(4)	
3 Morning is when I feel best	(4)	(3)	(2)	(1)	
4 I can eat as much as I used to	(4)	(3)	(2)	(1)	
5 I get tired for no reason	(1)	(2)	(3)	(4)	
6 I find it difficult to make decisions	(1)	(2)	(3)	(4)	
7 I feel hopeful about the future	(4)	(3)	(2)	(1)	
8 I feel that I am useful and needed	(4)	(3)	(2)	(1)	
9 My life is somewhat empty	(1)	(2)	(3)	(4)	
10 I still enjoy the things I used to do	(4)	(3)	(2)	(1)	

Total

$$\text{Short Zung LDS Index} = \frac{\text{Total}}{40} \times 100$$

Depression = >70
Score one response only for each question
Scoring numbers 1–4 not included on assessment sheet in routine use

(From Tucker *et al.*, 1987, with kind permission.)

The correct height of bed, chair, commode, etc. will aid independence, as will provision of a wheeled walking-aid such as the Delta-Aid for the postoperative period.

In early or moderate Parkinson's disease the drug regime will be simple, e.g. Sinemet Plus or Madopar 125, one tablet three to five times a day, and the early doses in the day can be omitted preoperatively without ill-effect. For nausea and vomiting it is best not to use a phenothiazine, and domperidone 10–20 mg up to three times daily is effective. The parkinsonian patient has an increased risk of aspiration pneumonia as the disease is associated with problems of swallowing and of oesophageal motility.

Patients with more advanced Parkinson's disease may be on more complex drug regimens, and many will carry a card on which the timings and names of their drugs are identified. Some will be on selegiline (a once a day MAOB inhibitor) which often smoothes out the end-of-dose deterioration which supervenes after some years of levodopa treatment. This drug can be omitted perioperatively. Bromocriptine, a dopamine agonist used for the same purpose as selegiline, has a shorter action and should be restarted as soon as food is permitted, as should antidepressants (such as dothiepin, lactulose or other bowel agents, etc). It is important that the anti-parkinsonian medication be kept under review each day; otherwise, an inadvertent 'drug holiday' may result in the patient becoming rigid, immobile, unable to swallow and very frightened. Even if no physical problem (such as deep vein thrombosis or pneumonia or pressure-sores) supervenes, such a patient's morale may require weeks of treatment before recovery.

Epilepsy

The incidence of epilepsy increases with age — the annual incidence for new seizures varies from 40/100 000 for those aged 60 to 80/100 000 for those aged over 75 (Hauser & Kurland, 1975). The incidence of primary epilepsy decreases with age but the increase in secondary epilepsy due to cerebrovascular disease more than compensates for this. Petit mal is almost unknown in the old, but grand mal and all variants of partial seizures occur. The cause of very late onset epilepsy may not be clear in up to 50% of cases, but cerebrovascular disease is the largest single cause (Hildick-Smith, 1974). About 5–8% of patients with hemiplegia go on to develop epilepsy. Fits in association with cerebral atrophy are likely to present an increasingly frequent problem as the population ages, but the present incidence is not known.

The extent of investigation of a patient aged 60 or more presenting with epilepsy is a matter for clinical judgement. In the minority of patients who are fit and alert and who have increasing focal neurological signs, CT scanning should be arranged. The patient should be fit to proceed to craniotomy if, for example, a benign tumour is discovered.

The majority of patients will present quite differently, as the epilepsy may appear against a background of old hemiplegia, or long-standing dementia, or tumours elsewhere in the body and may be only part of the disease picture. In these patients it seems right to concentrate investigations into potentially reversible causes of fits. These include changes in blood glucose, urea or calcium, alcohol or drug dosages or withdrawals, and cardiovascular causes such as arrhythmias or postural hypotension. Similar guidelines would seem reasonable for the anaesthetist if an elderly patient should develop 'turns' for the first time in the perioperative period.

It is now known that epilepsy can be satisfactorily controlled on one drug alone using carefully monitored dosage. Previous treatment was by combinations of drugs on the grounds that their therapeutic effects were additive while their individual toxicity was reduced. There was no evidence for this, and in fact phenobarbitone induced an enzyme which reduced the blood levels of the phenytoin with which it was frequently prescribed. Phenytoin once nightly at a dose of 300 mg frequently gives satisfactory fit control. The serum level can be monitored after about three weeks, and the dosage adjusted using a nomogram (Fig. 5.1). Small dosage increments above a critical level can lead to toxicity, as the enzyme concerned in the metabolism of the phenytoin in the liver can become saturated. Small dosage tablets (50 mg, 25 mg) of the same preparation should be used for this 'fine tuning', as other preparations have different bioavailability. The most important toxic effects in the elderly are drowsiness, slurred speech, nystagmus and ataxia, accompanied by confusion and perhaps an increased liability to fits. This clinical picture must be distinguished from stroke leading to cerebellar dysfunction. In practice, such symptoms are unlikely to occur below serum phenytoin levels of 120 μmol l^{-1} (30 mg ml^{-1}). In the steady state the half-life of phenytoin can be as long as 140 h, so omission of a dose in the perioperative period is not critical.

The alternative anticonvulsant for old people, carbamazepine, has been less extensively studied, but the drug is known to be effective in partial seizures. It is more expensive than phenytoin and has a shorter half-life, needing to be given at least twice a day. There is less good correlation of toxicity with serum levels than with phenytoin. The suggestion that carbamazepine may be associated with less cognitive side-effects than phenytoin needs to be confirmed in long-term, single-drug regimens.

There are so many interactions between anticonvulsants and other groups of drugs that it is not possible for the individual physician to remember them all. However, there are numerous wall-charts or pocket-discs which can be used as *aides-mémoires*. Examples of interactions which seem likely to affect the anaesthetist include the following: phenytoin decreases the effectiveness of benzadiazepines; anticholinergic drugs increase the serum phenytoin level (by allowing increased time

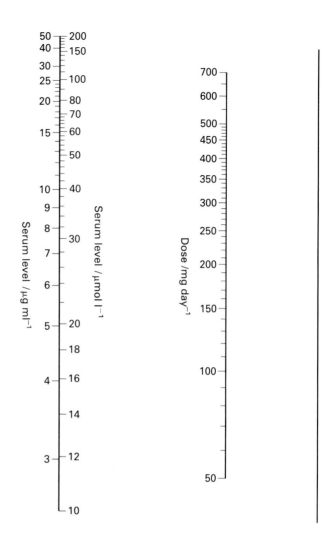

Fig. 5.1. Using the nomogram: a line is drawn connecting the observed serum phenytoin level (left scale) with the dose administered (centre scale) and extended to intersect the right vertical line. From this point of intersection, another line is drawn back to the desired serum level (left scale). The dose to produce the desired level can be read off on the centre scale. (Devised by A. Richens and B. Rambeck and reproduced with kind permission.)

for gut absorption); cimetidine increases the plasma phenytoin levels.

Patients on long-term anticonvulsants are at risk of folate deficiency and osteomalacia so the serum folate, calcium and alkaline phosphatase should be checked prior to operation.

Acute confusional states

The anaesthetist will very frequently come across elderly patients suffering from acute confusional states, as many of the illnesses which cause the patient to be confused, disorientated or hallucinated can occur in the perioperative period. Examples include chest and urinary tract infections and septicaemias, cardiac failure or 'silent' myocardial infarction, dehydration or electrolyte disturbances, anaemia or blood loss, disturbance of diabetic control or hypothermia. One of the reasons why it is valuable to check the mental score before operation is because a low score can alert the anaesthetist to the likelihood of postoperative disturbed behaviour. If the patient becomes disturbed and there is no adequate assessment of preoperative mental state (or if it was normal), careful checks need to be made for any episodes of hypotension or arrhythmia during anaesthesia, or for any other disturbance which would lead to temporary cerebral hypoperfusion, or predispose to a stroke. Drug reactions (e.g. to anticholinergic drugs, or barbiturates) or the effects of withdrawal (e.g. of tranquillizers or of alcohol) must also be considered.

The patient will exhibit behaviour which varies throughout 24 h, being alternately restless or slow, irritable or apathetic, and may suffer visual hallucinations, especially in a darkened ward. Calm and reassurance are essential, with repeated explanation to the patient whenever necessary. Sedatives may be needed, and drugs like haloperidol or thioridazine or chlormethiazole can be used, preferably in moderate dosages. Sometimes, if the confusional state is due to remediable cause, a non-urgent operation can be postponed until the patient is in a better state to benefit.

Dementia (see also Chapter 6)

It has been estimated (Kay, Beamish & Roth, 1964) that over 20% of those aged 80 years or more show evidence of dementia, so the likelihood of aged demented patients presenting for operation is fairly high. It is surprising how often supporting relatives are not aware of the degree of mental impairment suffered by the patient. They may be surprised to find the patient unable to answer the questions in the mental test and looking to them for the answers to simple questions. Later they may recall that the patient has not had to deal with financial or domestic matters for years, as the carers have gradually taken over any decision-making. Once the true state of affairs is realized a balanced judgment can be made about how urgent or necessary the operation is, and preparations made to help the patient and relatives afterwards if it is decided to proceed.

Balance and falls

There is an underlying decrease in balance with age, together with an increase in postural sway (Overstall et al., 1977). The old who are not fit and active have shorter and more variable step-length, and walk more slowly than their active counterparts. There is an increasing tendency to fall as age advances. In surveys of normal old people at home 20% of men and 40% of women had fallen in the last year, but only 3% needed medical treatment. The tendency to fall is compounded by difficulties in sight and vestibular function, and bent posture of head and neck with decreased proprioceptive information.

It is important to distinguish between an accidental fall, or 'trip', and falls which are not due to environmental factors. The former group of falls occur largely in mobile people under 75 years old, fit enough to risk climbing ladders or walking on icy pavements, and usually the prognosis for recovery after the resultant injury is good. Non-accidental falls have no clear cause — 'my legs just gave way' — and occur in older and frailer patients, often when changing position or when moving about indoors. These falls are often associated with underlying illness (infection, postural hypotension, Parkinson's disease, dementia, past strokes, arthritis of hips and knees). These illnesses affect the already impaired balance and gait mechanisms and worsen the prognosis.

Prolonged bedrest will impair an elderly patient's ability to return to his previous mobility, so this period should be as short as possible after operation, and physiotherapy and positive encouragement to become mobile and independent again must be given.

Bladder and bowel problems

The complex mechanisms involved in control of bladder and bowel are being increasingly studied in elderly patients, and have implications for pre- and postoperative care. One common disorder of micturition in the old is detrusor instability, associated with frequency and urgency, urge incontinence and nocturnal enuresis. When the balance between detrusor and sphincter mechanisms is disturbed the patient will suffer from hesitancy, poor stream and incomplete emptying. These and other disturbances of bladder function can be assessed by urodynamic studies and these may be important, e.g. in assessing whether a patient's symptoms are likely to be improved by prostatectomy.

Measures can be taken to help the aged patient retain continence during the operative period. It will help if the patient is as well and mobile as possible, and if urinals and commodes are readily available and the patient's bed or chair not too far from the toilets. Any urinary infection or faecal impaction should be promptly treated. A bladder record chart will often help to identify a pattern of incontinence which can be helped by regular toileting and training, and any drugs (e.g. diuretics) which may worsen the problem should be withdrawn if possible. Imipramine 10–25 mg may be helpful, as its anticholinergic effects can improve bladder capacity in suitable patients.

The majority of bowel problems in the elderly are due to constipation and faecal impaction, compounded in the aged surgical patient by lack of fluids and stool-bulking agents, by immobility, which increases colon transit time, by drugs and by the psychosocial factors of anxiety and strange surroundings. Attention to those factors before and after operation will prevent distress.

Autonomic disorders

There is an aged-related decline in the performance of the autonomic nervous system, both in the cardiovascular and the thermoregulatory responses.

In the cardiovascular reflexes, the changes in heart rate on standing after lying down are less in the elderly than the young. The response of blood pressure to the Valsalva manoeuvre is often abnormal in old age. The incidence of orthostatic hypotension increases with age (from about 16% aged 65–74 years to 30% aged over 75 years). It is usually due to a combination of autonomic impairment together with other clinical factors, such as other neurological disease (Parkinson's disease, strokes), or iatrogenic causes (diuretic or hypotensive drugs) or general medical causes (e.g. diabetes). Treatment will consist of stopping unnecessary drugs, and attempting to retrain the baroceptors by progressively elevating the head of the bed. Full-length elastic stockings may be of limited help, as may fludrocortisone, while the effect of flurbiprofen or of pindolol is being evaluated.

There is decline in the thermoregulatory responses with age, as shown by the decrease in core temperature with age demonstrated in large-scale population studies (Fox et al.,1973). There is a decreased vasoconstrictor response to cooling in up to 50% of elderly people, making them less able to maintain core temperature.

Accidental hypothermia is defined as the presence of a deep body temperature of <35 °C measured by rectal thermometer. Treatment of this condition, together with that of any contributory illness or injury, is often required in elderly patients 'found on the floor' having lain for some hours in a cool temperature. In winter 1975 some 3.6% of patients over 65 admitted to two London hospitals were hypothermic. Multiple factors are usually involved of which the first is cold exposure, complicated by impaired thermoregulation and lack of ability to warm up by shivering. Old people also have impaired thermal perception, and will take longer to act to change the room temperature when they are at risk. Finally, old people are liable to neurological diseases which cause autonomic damage either centrally as in Parkinson's disease, Shy-Drager syndrome and cerebrovascular disease, or peripherally as in diabetes and alcoholism. They also suffer from other non-neurological contributory causes such as hypothyroidism or hypopituitarism and are liable to be given drugs like phenothiazines which enhance the risk of hypothermia.

Clinical features of hypothermia include grey cool skin, e.g. on the abdominal wall, confusion or coma, and hypertonus with decreased reflexes. The ECG may show sinus bradycardia and delayed PR interval and there may be characteristic J waves (Fig. 5.2). A fall in blood pressure is an ominous sign. Respirations are slow and shallow with a low Po_2 and there is risk of bronchopneumonia and of aspiration of

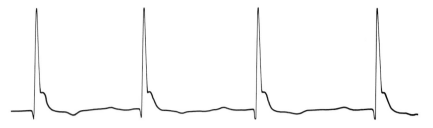

Fig. 5.2. ECG in hypothermia, showing J waves.

stomach contents. The serum amylase is often raised, sometimes the blood glucose and haematocrit are raised, and there may be oliguria. The prognosis depends on the degree and duration of the hypothermia and the reversibility of the underlying condition.

Too rapid rewarming of the patient can produce circulatory collapse with 'afterdrop' of core temperature leading to dysrhythmias. For a patient whose core temperature is 32–35 °C, providing a light covering and a room temperature of 25–30 °C will allow the core temperature to rise at about 0.5 °C h^{-1}. The patient should be given an antibiotic and O$_2$ should be provided via a Venturi mask. The patient should be on a ripple mattress, barrier-nursed, and pulse and blood pressure must be monitored. For otherwise recoverable patients with core temperature less than 32 °C, intensive care treatment and positive pressure ventilation may be appropriate, together with administration of warm fluids via a central venous line, and treatment with intravenous antibiotics and fluids to correct electrolyte disturbances, especially hyperkalaemia. Core temperature and ECG monitoring will be needed, but the prognosis is poor.

Syncopal attacks in the elderly are not usually a manifestation of autonomic dysfunction (being more often due to arrhythmias, TIAs, etc.) but carotid sinus syncope (due to a hypersensitive carotid body) or vasovagal syncope or the syncope associated with cough, micturition or defecation have a basis in impaired autonomic control.

Neurosurgical decisions

In many cases, examination of the nervous system in an elderly patient presenting for surgery will be a minor part of the assessment of risk factors. However, in patients for whom neurosurgery is contemplated the balance between operative risk and potential benefit must be clearly evaluated. Knowing the natural history of the untreated condition, and the likelihood of successful outcome are important factors, as are informed and realistic expectations on the part of the patient. Removal of a meningioma over the cortex may be justified if there is increasing neurological deficit. Slowly developing tumours such as acoustic neuroma or spinal meningioma will offer good chance of removal with benefit if surrounding blood vessels are not too distorted. Evacuation of chronic subdural haematoma (suspected in a patient with a two to three month history of fluctuating responsiveness and intellect) may give dramatic results even in the old. On the other hand, treatment of TIAs with carotid angioplasty will be a rare event in the aged, as the patient should be free of vascular disease elsewhere and be biologically young and alert.

With the advances that are occurring in anaesthetic and surgical techniques the benefits of surgery on the brain and elsewhere are being made available to many older patients who, 10–20 years ago, would have been regarded as too old or unfit for surgery. Evaluating which aged patient can or cannot benefit from a particular procedure will be more often required of surgeons and anaesthetists.

References

Critchley, M. (1931) The neurology of old age (Goulstonian Lecture) *Lancet* **i**, 1119–1127, 1221–1230, 1331–1336.

Davis, P.M.J. & Wright, E.A. (1977) A new method for measuring cranial cavity volume and its application to the assessment of cerebral atrophy at autopsy. *Neuropathol. Appl. Neurobiol.* **3**, 341–358.

Fox, R.H., Woodward, P.M. *et al* (1973) Body temperatures in the elderly: a national study of physiological, social and environmental conditions. *Br. Med. J.* **i**, 200–206.

Hauser, W.A. & Kurland, L.T. (1975) The epidemiology of epilepsy in Rochester, Minnesota 1935 through 1967. *Epilepsia* **16**, 1–66.

Hildick-Smith, M. (1974) Epilepsy in the elderly. *Age Ageing* **3**, 203–208.

Kay, D.W.K., Beamish, P. & Roth, M. (1964) Old age mental disorders in Newcastle-upon-Tyne. 1. A study of prevalence. *Br. J. Psychiatry* **110**, 146–158.

Klawans, H.L., Tufo H.M. *et al* (1971) Neurologic examination in an elderly population. *Dis. Nerv. Sys.* **32**, 274–279.

Kokmen, E., Bossemeyer, R.W. *et al* (1977) Neurological manifestations of ageing. *J. Gerontol.* **32**, 411–419.

Kurtzke, J.F. (1976) The distribution of cerebrovascular disease. In *Stroke* (Eds F.J. Gillingham, C. Mawdsley & A.E. Williams). Churchill Livingstone, Edinburgh, pp. 5–20.

Lassen, N.A. & Christensen, M.S. (1976) Physiology of cerebral blood flow. *Br. J. Anaesth.* **48**, 719–734.

Marquardsen, J. (1969) The natural history of acute cerebrovascular disease. *Acta Neurol. Scand.* **45** (Suppl. 38).

Overstall, P.W., Exton-Smith, A.N. *et al* (1977) Falls in the elderly related to postural imbalance. *Br. Med. J.* **1**, 261–264.

Prakash, C. & Stern, G. (1973) Neurological signs in the elderly. *Age Ageing* **2**, 24–27.

Rossor, M.N., Svendsen, C. *et al* (1982). The substantia innominata in Alzheimer's disease: an histochemical and biochemical study of cholinergic marker enzymes. *Neurosci. Lett.* **28**, 217–222.

Tomlinson, B.E., Blessed, C. & Roth, M. (1970) Observations on the brains of demented old people. *J. Neurol. Sci.* **11**, 205–242.

Tucker, M.A. *et al* (1987) Validation of a brief screening list for depression in the elderly. *Age Ageing* **16**, 139–144.

Wilcock, G.K., Esiri, M.M. *et al* (1982) Alzheimer's disease: correlation of cortical choline acetyltransferase activity with the severity of dementia and histological abnormalities. *J. Neurol. Sci.* **57**, 407–417.

Suggested further reading

Hildick-Smith, M. (Ed) (1985) *Neurological Problems in the Elderly*. Bailliere Tindall, London. (An up-to-date account, most chapters written by British consultant geriatricians with a particular interest in neurological disorders.)

Katzman, R. & Terry, R. (Eds) (1983) *The Neurology of Ageing*. F.A. Davis, Philadelphia. (A wide-ranging review of the field, most chapters written by American neurologists, psychiatrists and pathologists.)

6 | Psychological changes with ageing

C. TWINING

Normal ageing

For those of us fortunate enough to remain in good health, continuity rather than change will be the essence of ageing. However, as practitioners we are concerned primarily with how best to help those who need our skill in helping to overcome disease or disability. The problems that they face and indeed the treatments which we may offer make exceptional demands which can emphasize the effects of ageing. It is important therefore to make adjustments to our practice for the effects of ageing. To this extent we must pay special attention to the changes of ageing even if they are small compared with the many things that do not change.

Changes in psychological function may be important both in terms of the direct effects of anaesthetic agents on the older central nervous system and in respect of the way age affects people more generally. Examples of the former might include the possibility that any 'normal' age changes in intellectual function could put older patients at risk of more severe or prolonged postoperative confusion or other mental impairment. Examples of the latter would include the ways in which older people differ in their presentation for, and recovery from, surgery.

It is possible to draw some useful guidance in these matters from the now quite extensive research into the changes in intellect and personality which are to be found with age. This is a complex area especially as many of the findings depend on the method used. In particular, because successive generations show different backgrounds and patterns of psychological development, what we find from comparing today's young and old generations does not always hold true for those who will be old tomorrow. However, this difficulty, namely the relative merits of cross-sectional and longitudinal studies, need not concern us greatly here. We are seeking to know what are the relevant psychological differences between those who are older now and those who are younger now. It is enough to know *what* are the relevant differences between those born in the 1900s and those born in the 1940s. We do not need to ask *why* those differences occur.

Ageing and cognition

It is generally assumed that there are real and inevitable changes in cognitive function with age. This is seemingly an amalgam of inherited wisdom, such as Shakespearian notions of senility, and imperfect understanding of research findings. This is nowhere better illustrated than in the complexities of ageing and intelligence. The simplest summary of how we think of ageing is seen in the data relating to intelligence test scores. In the derivation of intelligence quotients (IQs) the effect of age is taken out in that each person's scores are compared with others in the same age band. However, it is also possible to compare the average raw scores of those at different ages and this yields data such as that shown in Fig. 6.1.

There is a steady rise in intelligence score until young adulthood and then a reversal. It is important to note, however, that the differences associated with age are mostly small compared with the differences between people of the same age. Thus, the spread of individual's scores at age 65 years is such that those scoring one standard deviation above the mean for this age are still doing better than the average 25 year old.

Moreover, the picture is more complicated than this because of different patterns of change both between different individuals and between different skills. Intelligence itself is simply the ability to solve a number of different types of intellectual problem. Thus, a typical intelligence test like the Wechsler Adult Intelligence Scale (WAIS) contains items which cover a variety of areas. There are tests of vocabulary, comprehension, information, simple memory, visual perception and spatial skill, etc., and looked at separately there are consistent differences in the way skills change with age. It is therefore not enough to say what happens to 'intelligence' with age. We must consider different skills separately.

In general, those skills which depend on language and especially those involving accumulated 'wisdom' show very little change until well

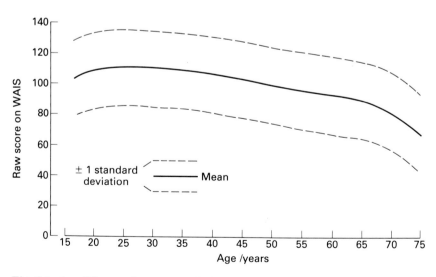

Fig. 6.1. Age differences in scores on the Wechsler Adult Intelligence Scale (from data in Wechsler, 1955).

into late life. Other skills, such as those involving spatial perception and thinking, tend to show earlier decline. One general finding is the reduction in speed of intellectual processing with age. This is seen not only in simple reaction time but in the speed of more complex visuo-spatial tasks and even in verbal fluency. The decline, however, is not a problem for most people, even those who are very elderly, in everyday life. Few of us operate at maximum mental capacity most of the time and in any case we can use our 'wisdom' and experience to compensate. However, if we have to carry out an unfamiliar task quickly then age differences are much more apparent.

Similarly there is an important difference between the practice of a well learned skill and the learning of that same skill for the first time. If we have learned to drive a car when young then there is no problem, pro-vided we are healthy, in continuing to do so at least into our 70s. Indeed, the advantage of greater experience is reflected by the insurance companies who offer special discounts to those over 50 years of age. However, the elderly or even middle-aged person who has never learned to drive finds it hard to develop the skills so ably practised by cohorts who have driven for years. Thus, speed of new learning is certainly impaired although this should not be taken as confirming that 'you can't teach an old dog new tricks'. The slope of the learning curve may be less but the end-point may be the same. The old need not be told that they can never learn to drive, just that it will take rather longer.

Rigidity of thinking is often cited as one reason for older people being less able to learn quickly. Certainly there is evidence that older people will tend to try to solve a new problem using tried and tested solutions. If these do not work then they are likely to persist with these rather than try some new approach. Thus, instruction in strategy may be particu-larly helpful to older people.

Memory

There is almost universal agreement that memory changes with age. Although there is some evidence to support this, at least in terms of small changes, the idea has had a disproportionately powerful influence on our image of ageing. For example, it may lie behind the erroneous notion that senile dementia is nothing more than an exaggeration of normal ageing. Thus, older people are often said to have poor recent memories (e.g. for what happened yesterday) but good remote memories (for what happened 30 years ago). Psychological studies do not, however, support this. Indeed, they suggest that such a model of the different types of memory is wrong for people of any age.

In terms of different mechanisms of memory, research suggests that it is appropriate to distinguish between three types. These are iconic, primary and secondary memory. The first of these relates to time-spans of less than one second and is more a part of what we usually think of as perception. Primary memory is the mechanism which enables us to remember a few things for up to about a minute. Anything longer than this requires repeated use of either primary memory or secondary memory. This secondary memory mechanism appears to be the same whether we are remembering things for 40 min or for 40 years. The quantity of memory will change over these times but the mechanism remains the same. It is primary and secondary memory which are of importance in our everyday notion of memory.

There is a slight but consistent age change in primary memory. For younger people the limit of this memory is about seven items. One everyday example is our ability to register the digits in a telephone number. Anything over about seven items and we have to adopt special strategies like dividing it into chunks (the area code first and then the number) or writing it down. For those aged over 70 this immediate memory store has slightly less capacity, namely about six items. For most purposes this is more than sufficient but the difference is apparent if maximum capacity is required.

Secondary memory covers both what we usually refer to as recent memory and what is called remote memory. Here too there are real age differences, though these are more apparent under some circumstances than others. In particular, the way in which information is presented (e.g. whether it is spoken or written), the instructions that are given and the way in which retention of the information is assessed all make a difference.

The most obvious way to test memory of this type is to present a set amount of information and then ask the subject to repeat back as much as he or she is able. If we present lots of information at a steady rate then only the most recent few items can be retrieved from primary memory, and the rest must rely on secondary memory. Indeed, if we get the subject to do some other mental task like counting backwards for a couple of minutes immediately after presentation, all the memory is from the secondary store.

This simple paradigm tends to show the greatest difference between young and old subjects. For example, in one experiment where people had to remember lists of words, those in their 20s could remember about 14 out of 24 words, whereas those over 60 could only recall about eight. There seems little doubt that memory is linked with age.

However, this particular experiment is of interest because some attempt was made to look at things in more detail. It also included an assessment of memory using recognition rather than recall. If the subjects were asked to pick the words that had been presented from a second, longer list the age difference was less pronounced. Thus, the younger subjects could recognize an average of 20 words out of 24 and the older group did just as well. Age differences are much less apparent for recognition than for recall.

One reason for this may be that it is the retrieval rather than the storage of information that is at fault. Having some organized strategy for getting back what has been stored is just as important as being able to store it in the first place. This is the difference between the well indexed library and the chaotic warehouse. There are also other reasons to think that changes in strategy are important in the impact of ageing.

First, there is the expectation of failure. If an older person is presented with a memory task he or she often reacts by saying something like 'I shall be no good at this, my memory is hopeless'. This preoccupation with failure may itself be enough to disrupt performance.

We know from many experiments that it is 'depth of processing' which matters in determining memory performance. Information which has been given a good deal of deep thought will be better remembered than that which has been given only superficial attention. Indeed, it would seem that this level of processing is more important than an explicit instruction to remember something. It may be that such instruction alerts us to the fact that we must 'pay attention' but no more than this. Thus, if we by some other means ensure deep processing then we will also facilitate memory. In the case of older subjects, finding some other way of ensuring that material is well processed has the advantage of not raising expectations of failure.

The second way that strategy has been shown to be important is by varying the instructions given to young and old subjects. For example, if we are given a list of items to remember, this will be more successful if we can organize the material into some sort of structure. This might be that the items are all 'things to eat' or 'the names of muscle groups', for example. Comparisons between young and old subjects show that older people are less likely spontaneously to adopt effective strategies of this sort. Giving instructions as to how to analyse material helps the older subjects more, and age differences are then less apparent.

Of course, most of the time we do not have to remember lists of items. We may more likely wish to remember some sort of narrative, e.g. the plot of a book or what happened at church on Sunday. In this case it seems that older people are more likely to remember the theme or moral of the tale rather than the specific factual detail. It is often ability to recall facts that is used, both experimentally and in everyday life, to judge whether someone has a good or bad memory. Again this favours the young rather than the old.

Likewise, the way in which material is presented makes a difference to our ability to remember. We may, for example, distinguish between spoken and written material. The best sort of presentation is a combination of both. Using only oral is, however, better than written presentation alone. Again, older people benefit more from using the best strategy.

One final point in relation to memory must unfortunately be to dispel one of the few positive myths of ageing. This is the notion that older people are especially good at recalling distant memories. There may be several reasons why this misconception is so popular. With senility, the striking difference is between recent and remote memory. The former is so obviously impaired compared with the latter. Moreover, many elderly people are happy to reminisce and some of the memories can seem prodigious. However, it is often impossible to tell whether they are correct or not.

One attempt to look at this involved getting old and young people to try and recall famous events of past years and even the names of their schoolteachers. This simple method yields answers that can actually be verified. Where direct comparisons were possible the younger subjects could remember more than the older ones. Nonetheless, the subjects in their 70s could recall correctly 45% of their schoolteachers by name. This is impressive, especially as those in their 20s, i.e. 50 years nearer to the original event, were only correct in 67% of cases. Memory over these sorts of periods is remarkable but we must conclude that the main reason older people remember further back is just because they have been alive longer!

Emotions and personality

Changes in emotions and personality are if anything rather less than those in cognitive function. Continuity is the key in normal ageing and those who are happy and stable are those who tend always to have been so. It has been said that as we grow older we become more like ourselves, that is to say our existing personality characteristics become exaggerated. This implies no particular shift in *direction* with age, rather that individuals become more distinct from one another. Certainly the differences between generations are more noticeable than the effects of ageing itself although it is possible to draw some useful general conclusions.

The two most commonly described personality dimensions are those of Emotionality (sometimes call Neuroticism) and Socialization (also known as Introversion-Extraversion). Both of these show slight changes with age.

There tends to be an increase in Emotionality, that is to say in the tendency to worry and to get upset easily. This has been termed Neuroticism because of its relation to predisposition to neurotic disorders. Certainly some workers have described very high rates for such disorders, including as high as 45% if mild disorders are included. However, there are problems of definition and the figures for those who need active help, let alone psychiatric treatment, are much less.

There is also some evidence of a consistent shift towards increased Introversion. This tendency to withdraw from social contact may be related to the phenomenon of disengagement which, it has been suggested, is a normal process in ageing. However, not only is this hypothesis much disputed but the causal chain is by no means clear.

Personality is often assessed by means of a questionnaire or interview. The aim is to enquire about a range of different behaviours and the individual's personality is inferred from the trends seen across various settings and occasions. Specific behaviours may, however, change for a number of different reasons. If an older person reports that he or she goes out to see friends less this may be due to arthritis or poverty rather than a personality change. The danger is that we may attribute such changes to some mysterious, and by implication unalterable, process of personality rather than the more practical and obvious reasons.

Conversely it may be easy to see someone as isolated and withdrawn because of their circumstances when in fact they have always been so inclined. We can only accurately interpret someone's behaviour in the light of their present condition and past performance. The best guide to an older person's *personality* is how that person has been during adult life.

Abnormal ageing

So far, the concentration on the differences in psychological function can reasonably be judged to part of 'normal ageing'. These changes are found at least to some degree in all older people. They are generally not as large as most people imagine. Perhaps more important from a clinical point of view are the disturbances of cognition and affect which beset many older people. These never afflict the majority but the minority is large enough to mean that these matters must be taken into account in everyday clinical practice with older people. Indeed, the sample of older people who make use of health services is biased towards those who have problems and therefore includes a disproportionately high number of those with psychological, as well as physical problems.

Some form of dementia (chronic progressive deterioration in cortical function) affects about 10% of those over 65 and about 20% of those aged over 80 (see Chapter 5). It is therefore important to recognize these conditions, to distinguish them from normal ageing and to change clinical management where appropriate. The fact that these conditions afflict one in five of those over 80 should not lead us to dismiss the problem as being due to old age. Similarly the fact that we are unable to ameliorate the underlying condition for the great majority of the dementias should not deflect us from considering what may be done to avoid making things worse.

Similar principles must apply to our understanding of emotional distress. The fact that multiple loss is so common in later life may be the reason why depression is the commonest psychiatric disorder in older people at least until the age of 75 and why the rate for successful suicide is highest in this age group (Post, 1982). However, it is not enough simply to catalogue the painful events and to conclude that 'if all that had happened anyone would be depressed'. There are many older people who are not distressed despite multiple problems. There is more to successful adjustment than being appropriately unhappy. To describe distress as 'understandable in the circumstances' is to devalue it and to make it easy to do nothing to help. To give one example: rates for depression following stroke are high, treatment is often not given but can be shown to be effective. The recognition and management of emotional disorders following physical illness in older people is an important and neglected component of 'whole patient' care.

In order to give the best care to each individual patient it is important to have at least some idea both whether there are problems of psychological dysfunction and whether that individual is showing a greater or lesser degree of 'normal' age changes. This demands at least some sort of assessment.

The assessment of mental function

It is nonsense to suggest that every older person being considered for anaesthesia should have a formal psychological assessment, and obviously they cannot all be seen by a clinical psychologist. However, we do all make some sort of judgement, albeit implicitly, about cognitive function and/or personality in assessing patients. As the likelihood of 'abnormality' is relatively higher in older people it is as well to think a little about how to make good assessments rather than bad ones. It is often said in case presentations that an older patient 'looks demented'; if we can go beyond this by using some form of systematic method then we are likely to be more accurate.

The assessment of mental function relies on three sources of information: the patient's self-report, the report(s) of those who know the patient and formal testing and observation. It is necessary to consider each of these in relation to both cognitive function and emotional behaviour.

Cognition

It is hardly surprising that self-report is not the most reliable source of information for assessing an individual's memory and intellect. There are of course many patients who complain of difficulties in memory or concentration but this is not a good guide to what is wrong. It is a useful indicator that *something* is wrong but not *what* is wrong. Several studies have shown that self-report of memory difficulties in older people are most often associated with anxiety or depression, not with dementia. So it is worth asking the question 'Do you have any trouble with your memory?', provided the answer is interpreted correctly.

Much more important for the evaluation of cognitive function is the report of those who know the patient well. If the spouse, daughter or other carer says that he or she 'is very forgetful' this should certainly be followed up. This sort of information may not be easy to obtain in the presence of the patient if he or she does not think there are problems. The relative may have been reprimanded repeatedly by the patient for suggesting any decline in mental function. It is often necessary to ask the patient whether there are such problems and look at the relative as the patient answers. It is still better to have a chance to ask the relative separately if forgetfulness is a problem.

It is also important to get specific examples of problems if any are reported. Sometimes normal lapses of memory or uncertainty due to anxiety are reported as signs of senility. Persons who complain that they often find that they have gone to fetch something from another room and then forgotten why they went there are not necessarily in the early stages of Alzheimer's disease.

It may seem that the obvious answer is to use some formal brief, psychometric assessment. There are several examples of this, notably the Abbreviated Mental Test (AMT) (Hodkinson, 1972) the Mini-Mental State (MMS) questionnaire (Folstein *et al.*, 1975) and the Clifton Assessment Procedures for the Elderly (CAPE) (Pattie & Gilleard, 1979). These procedures are quick and easy to administer but, particularly in the case of the AMT and MMS, yield only very rough measurements.

The AMT consists of 10 questions (Chapter 5) and is designed primarily to screen for signs of disorientation and other signs of memory loss in hospital in-patients. Because it is easy to use it has been included in many studies of elderly people including those undergoing anaesthetic procedures. It has been used to assess both the presence of dementia and, by repeated testing, the incidence of acute confusion. Its use is largely confined to Britain. There are virtually no published studies of its validity as a screening measure for dementia, though some reports have shown that it may relate to clinical outcome. It is a shortened version of a test which has been shown to correlate with post-mortem histopathology in dementia. There are no normative data as such, although several people have suggested cut-off points for 'abnormal' function.

The MMS is North American in origin and has been used to test thousands of aged US citizens. It covers more than orientation, having some items of language and visuospatial function. It has been widely used and studies have included its application to several thousand 'normal' old Americans. The results suggest that those able to complete the test without errors are very unlikely to be suffering from dementia. However, those scoring many errors include many who do *not* suffer from dementia. It seems that there may be many reasons for making errors on the test, of which cognitive impairment is but one. In particular, it appears that those of lower educational level are likely to make errors whilst not suffering from dementia. Its use in screening can therefore be said to be limited to the exclusion of 'normals' rather than the positive identification of those with specific difficulties.

The CAPE combines brief formal tests of cognitive function with a rating scale of behaviour. It was developed for, and is best suited to, the evaluation of elderly people's dependency levels and their likely needs for supportive care. It has been tested for both reliability and validity and there are normative data for elderly people with a variety of diagnoses and from a variety of care settings. It is not, however, particularly sensitive to small changes in individual function.

Many other procedures have been used for the evaluation of cognitive function in older people, including almost all possible combinations of the sub-tests of the WAIS (Wechsler, 1955). The WAIS has been widely used but it has to be administered by a trained tester, usually a psychologist. The full battery takes at least an hour and for these reasons its clinical use is restricted to the most selected cases and fatigue is a real problem for frail elderly subjects. There is also some uncertainty about how much the various skills needed to do the WAIS are affected by dementia or other impairment. It can be difficult to judge accurately the level of premorbid intellectual function and consequently the present level of impairment.

Of more general interest in the measurement of such premorbid function is the suggestion that this can be estimated from word reading ability. The National Adult Reading Test (Nelson, 1982) consists of a set of 50 irregular words which the subject is asked to read out aloud. The number of words read out correctly is reported to correlate with premorbid intelligence even in those with moderate dementia. The potential for combining this with some of the existing procedures seems worth further exploration.

There has also been a move towards developing assessments of more direct relevance to the activities of daily living. Of course if we are interested in abilities to cope day by day then the obvious answer would seem to be to do this directly. The only problem is the time and skill necessary to do this. There is still a good deal of scope for collaboration between psychologists and occupational therapists to develop reliable standardized measures of this type.

In short there is a wide variety of procedures which have been devised for the assessment of cognitive function in older people. The priority now is not to devise new tests but to carry out proper evaluations using the techniques already developed.

Emotions

There are relatively few techniques specifically designed for the measurement of emotions in elderly subjects. Mostly it is assumed that those developed for younger groups will give similar results. Thus, studies of depression in older people rely on the ubiquitous Hamilton Rating scale for the measurement of severity of depression (Hamilton, 1960).

In some cases there are real problems of validity in applying even well developed methods such as this to older people. For example, the first factor on the General Health Questionnaire (Goldberg, 1978), which has been widely used as an indicator of psychological dysfunction, focuses on somatic complaints. However, in the elderly the results are confounded by the frequency of chronic physical disease. For example, reports of aches, pains and fatigue are as likely to be due to arthritis as to depression or anxiety. Similar problems apply to the use of the Beck Depression Inventory. Using this scale on one sample of 70 year olds suggested that 48.3% of them might be depressed (Stenback, 1980). The use of such self-report measures in elderly subjects has been reviewed (Gilleard *et al.*, 1981).

Of course things are further complicated because it has been demonstrated that for older people chronic poor health is a risk factor for depression (Murphy, 1982). This has not been found to be the case for younger people. It is difficult to discern therefore how much a particular symptom is related to physical disorder and how much to emotional distress.

There have been some attempts to produce measures specific to older people, including a Geriatric Depression Screening scale (Yesavage *et al.*, 1983; Lesher, 1986). Such approaches deserve to be more widely applied. The previously mentioned danger of dismissing distress as 'normal in the circumstances' might be prevented by a more structured assessment of emotional state, just as formal cognitive assessment does in the case of dementia.

There is relatively little consideration given to the ways in which emotional distress rather than, for example, frank depressive illness may present in older people. A number of studies of physical disorders show that presentation in older people tends to be in terms of signs rather than symptoms. This is known to have implications for how early older people present for surgery.

Similarly it does seem that older subjects tend to present emotional disorder with somatic rather than the psychological symptoms. There are almost certainly 'cultural' differences in the use of terms such as anxiety so that it is not at all clear whether older subjects even interpret the questions on emotional behaviour in the same way as younger subjects.

Fortunately this is more of a problem for those engaged in formal research than for those in clinical practice. In the latter case the issue is whether we can detect those in sufficient distress to warrant special help. This depends on interpersonal sensitivity rather than formal questionnaires, though we can all think of some practitioners who might be better *replaced by* a questionnaire! The value of a questionnaire may be that it structures the clinician's thinking and approach to the patient. Any 'score' that is produced is likely to be of use in describing a group of patients but not in giving the particular answers to an individual's problems. It is fair to say that questionnaires and rating scales help us to ask questions of individuals rather than answer them.

In the case of emotions, for example, the questionnaires or rating scale may suggest that this person is very upset but does not tell us why.

The implications for anaesthetic practice

The central question must surely be: 'How does what we know of the psychology of ageing help us to help older people?' It is not enough simply to express some pious hope that this sort of knowledge will somehow make us 'understand old people better'. This sounds splendid but must be translated into some specific changes in our own behaviour if it is to mean anything in reality.

Patient selection

There is little evidence of any change in mental function in older people which might exclude them from anaesthesia on the grounds of age alone. Certainly there may be cases where there should be careful thought given but this is due to other factors — abnormal rather than normal ageing. The most obvious example would seem to be the case of those older people with some degree of dementia. It has been suggested that there might be risk of exacerbation or acceleration of the decline in such patients. There is certainly very good evidence that impairment of cognitive function is associated with poor outcome for conditions such as fractured neck of femur. However, the reasons for this are not clear and it may prove to be some underlying debilitation that causes this association. This is something that requires further research but we can already enhance our prognosis by taking cognitive function into account.

What we do not yet know is precisely which procedures are of specific benefit to older people in terms of mental function. It is quite possible that age and mental function interact in some way so that no one procedure can be said to be 'best for older people'. This is of practical importance in view of the wide range of techniques now available, including regional anaesthesia (see Chapter 13). However, there is still need to carry out studies which control adequately for other variables, notably the type of surgery (Chapter 10). Only in this way can the effects of the anaesthetic procedure itself be determined. Preliminary research has suggested that in older subjects undergoing elective orthopaedic surgery those having general anaesthesia are more likely to have detectably impaired memory function after surgery than those having regional anaesthesia (Hole *et al.*, 1980). However, much more work is needed to confirm this and to look at whether any sub-groups of those at special risk can be identified.

Patient preparation

It is perhaps here that we can most usefully use our knowledge of *normal* ageing. There is no doubt from both clinical observation and a number of studies that good patient preparation in terms of information and re-assurance speeds postoperative recovery. This applies to older patients as to younger but we can enhance the impact of such intervention considerably. For example, we know that how we present material to older people makes a big difference. Having both spoken and written material helps. Similarly, if we are wishing to help someone to make use of previously presented material, cues to aid recall will be helpful (e.g. not 'try to remember what I told you yesterday' but 'I want you to remember the things I told you about the breathing exercises which were written on the yellow card').

The speed of presentation of information will need to be slightly less to allow for the slight but real reduction in processing speed. This does of course mean taking into account individual differences and does *not* mean treating every older person as if they are mentally handicapped.

It may be especially helpful to find out what experience, personal or second-hand, the older person has of surgery. If they have not been in a hospital since they had their appendix out 50 years ago, they could have some incorrect images of what to expect. Indeed it may be fascinating to hear what it was like being in hospital before the last war.

Recovery and rehabilitation

One of the things that is most likely to have changed during an older person's lifetime is the length of time someone spends in bed after an operation. The pattern of recovery will take longer for many older people but this does not mean that it need be incomplete. However, it is important to recognize that it can be discouraging to see younger people making more rapid progress, especially if taking longer means that one has to move from one ward or hospital to another. There is good evidence to show that how well older people are prepared for moves of this sort can determine whether the move enhances recovery or speeds decline.

It is generally accepted that the risk of postoperative delirium is increased where there is pre-existing cognitive impairment. There is a widespread suspicion than the problems of postoperative delirium may be worse in older people irrespective of any evidence of abnormality preoperatively. This seems a reasonable hypothesis since we know that there is some decrease in maximum cortical function with age and it seems likely that the stress of anaesthesia might reveal this. The current state of knowledge of postoperative delirium in the elderly has recently been reviewed (Seymour, 1986). Studies carried out to date have indicated that age is certainly a risk factor but there is less evidence with respect to impaired preoperative psychological function. In part this may be because most studies have used only the crudest measures of such function. Often there is no more than a clinician's or relative's rating of the presence or absence of 'abnormal mental status' (e.g. Hole *et al.*, 1980; Millar, 1981). Even where formal measures have been used these are confined to brief screening instruments such as the AMT. This leads to problems of ceiling effects since the great majority of patients get all the items correct. Such tests may simply not be sensitive enough to pick up changes, especially if these are in functions other than memory and orientation.

Seymour also referred to the problem of postoperative fatigue. This appears to be more common than delirium but there is even less research on this topic. Similarly there is little work using formal measures of daily living activity to assess outcome and few if any attempts have been made to look carefully at the reports of relatives on whom the burden of longer term practical problems usually falls.

In short, there are some intriguing pointers to suggest areas for investigation. To date, however, there is little in the way of good descriptive work let alone any controlled trials which may enable us to draw conclusions on the specific effects of anaesthesia. Closer collaborative efforts between anaesthetists and clinical psychologists would help to secure the most effective progress.

References

Folstein, J., Folstein, S. & McHugh, P. (1975) Mini-mental state. *J. Psychiatr. Res.* **12**, 189.

Gilleard, C.J., Willmott, M. & Vaddadi, K.S. (1981) Self-report measures of mood and morale in elderly depressives. *Br. J. Psychiatry.* **138**, 230–235.

Goldberg, D. (1978) *Manual of the General Health Questionnaire.* NFER-Nelson, Windsor.

Hamilton, M. (1960) A rating scale for depression. *J. Neurol. Neurosurg. Psychiatry.* **23**, 56–62.

Hodkinson, H.M. (1972) Evaluation of a mental test score assessment of mental impairment in the elderly. *Age Ageing* **1**, 233–238.

Hole, A., Terjesen, T. & Breivik, H. (1980) Epidural versus general anaesthesia for total hip arthroplasty in elderly patients. *Acta Anaesth. Scand.* **24**, 279–287.

Lesher, E.L. (1986) Validation of the geriatric depression scale among nursing home residents. *Clin. Gerontol.* **4(4)**, 21–28.

Millar, H.R. (1981) Psychiatric morbidity in elderly surgical patients. *Br. J. Psychiatry.* **140**, 426–35.

Murphy, E. (1982) The social origins of depression in old age. *Br. J. Psychiatry.* **141**, 135–142.

Nelson, H.E. (1982) *National Adult Reading Test: Test Manual.* NFER-Nelson, Windsor.

Pattie, A.H. & Gilleard, C.J. (1979) *The Clifton Procedures for the Elderly.* Hodder & Stoughton, London.

Post, F. (1982) Functional Disorders. In *The Psychiatry of Late Life* (Eds R. Levy & F. Post). Blackwell Scientific Publications, Oxford.

Seymour, G. (1986) *Medical Assessment of the Elderly Surgical Patient.* Croom Helm, London.

Stenback, A. (1980) Depression and suicide behaviour in old age. In *Handbook of Mental Health and Ageing* (Eds J.E. Birren & R.B. Sloane). Prentice-Hall, Englewood Cliffs, New Jersey.

Wechsler, D. (1955) *The Manual for the Wechsler Adult Intelligence Scale*. The Psychological Corporation, New York.

Yesavage, J.A., Brink, T.L., Rose, T.L., Lum, O., Huang, V., Adey, M. & Leiver, V.D. (1983) Development and validation of a geriatric depression screening scale: a preliminary report. *J. Psychiatr. Res.* **17**, 37–49.

Suggested further reading

Woods, R.T. & Britton, P.G. (1985) *Clinical Psychology with the Elderly*. Croom Helm, London. (This book describes the wide range of contributions which clinical psychologists have been developing for helping older people. It is the current standard text for British work in this specialty.)

Hanley, I. & Hodge J. (Eds) (1984) *Psychological Approaches to the Care of the Elderly*. Croom Helm, London. (A collection of papers covering a variety of approaches to assessment and psychological treatments.)

Stott, M. (1981) *Ageing for Beginners*. Basil Blackwell, Oxford. (One of a series of short texts on 'Understanding Everyday Experience'. The author, a journalist and broadcaster, gives a very readable, personal view of the pros and cons of growing older and advice on making the best of later life.)

7 | The extent, character and patterns of disease in the aged

M.R.P. HALL

Introduction

'The importance of a special study of the diseases of old age would not be contested at the present time. It is agreed, in fact, that if the pathology of childhood requires clinical consideration of a special kind and with which it is indispensable to be practically acquainted, senile pathology too has its difficulties which can only be surmounted by long experience and profound knowledge of its peculiar characters'. This quotation was not was not written recently, or even during the last 30 years, a time during which the discipline of geriatric medicine has taken root and flowered, but 106 years ago in 1881 by the great French Physician, J.M. Charcot in his *Clinical Lectures on Senile and Chronic Diseases*.

Senile pathology, the basis underlying 'disease in the aged', does have 'its difficulties', for the features of a specific disease may not be easy to detect. As an example, a request was received to see an old man aged 83 years because every time he got out of bed he fell over and his son and daughter-in-law were finding it difficult to care for him, for they were frequently having to lift him up from the floor. His general practitioner was puzzled for he could find no reason for his falls. When seen in consultation, the reason for his falling was soon discovered — his blood pressure (normal when lying in bed) fell dramatically when he sat up and became immeasureable when he began to stand. The problem was to find the cause of the postural (orthostatic) hypotension and decide which of the many alternatives was operative here (Table 7.1). He looked pale but was not clinically anaemic; he was afebrile and careful examination revealed nothing else apart from a respiratory rate of 32 per minute. Could this be the reason? He was admitted to hospital, where investigations including a chest X-ray were negative, but a blood culture grew *Streptococcus pneumoniae*, and over the course of the next 48 h he developed classical physical signs of a right lower lobe pneumonia with appropriate haematological and radiological changes. Antibiotic therapy cured him and with the return of his normal health his postural hypotension disappeared.

This case illustrates some of the typical problems posed by illness in an aged individual. The first of these relates to the presentation, which could hardly be described as typical or specific, although McFadden *et al.* (1982) have shown that elevation of the respiratory rate will precede the physical or radiological signs by as much as 48 h.

Following admission this man became very ill, his lying blood

Table 7.1. Causes of postural and exercise hypotension

Table 7.1. Causes of postural and exercise hypotension

1 Abnormal baroceptor reflexes
    Increased sensitivity of aortic and carotid sinus baroceptors
    Damage to central pathways in brain, e.g. after stroke
    Disease of spinal cord, e.g. ischaemic myelopathy
    Interference with sympathetic nerve supply, e.g. peripheral
        neuropathy, ganglion blocking drugs

2 Diminished cardiac output
    Myocardial infarction
    Bedrest
    Arrhythmias
    Febrile illness

3 Reduced blood volume
    Haemorrhage
    Dehydration

4 Abnormal sodium handling
    Alteration in renin-angiotensin II–aldosterone mechanism
    Endocrine disease, e.g hypopituitarism; hypoadrenalism
    Diuretics

5 Drugs (other than diuretics and ganglion blockers)
    Hypnotics, e.g. barbiturates
    Antidepressants — tricyclics and MAO inhibitors
    Tranquillizers, e.g. phenothiazines
    Levodopa

6 Severe varicose veins

pressure dropped and intravenous therapy and antibiotics were started before the blood culture result was known. Rapid deterioration of illness, if it is untreated, is another common occurrence.

There were two futher aspects of this case which are often part of the pattern of illness in the aged. Firstly, he took a long time to recover and it was almost six weeks before he was fully capable of self-care. The old take much longer to recover from illness than the young. Secondly, he lived alone and although his family were very supportive he was most anxious not to be a burden to them. Social, economic and environmental factors will often play a larger role. These need to be borne in mind when considering the overall management of each individual case.

The patient in this case was lucky in that he was reasonably fit prior to his illness, but multiple pathology is common and most aged patients will have other medical problems. Also, although this patient became very ill, he did not develop any secondary complications. With this sort of illness he could easily have become incontinent, faecally impacted, developed venous thrombosis, pulmonary embolism, heart failure, pressure-sores or mental confusion.

To summarize, illness in the old may be characterized, or affected by the following:
  (i) non-specific and/or atypical presentation
  (ii) rapid deterioration if not treated
  (iii) a longer recovery period

(iv) the effect of social, economic and environmental factors

(v) secondary complications

(vi) multiple pathology.

This old man also exhibited one of the 'Giants of Geriatrics' (Isaacs, 1982), namely instability (falls). The others are immobility, incontinence and intellectual impairment — common complications of illness and often the presenting features.

The extent of disease in the aged

The demographic changes in the age patterns show that while the total numbers of the elderly have reached a plateau, the number over 75 years and in particular those over 85 years, are increasing and the increase in the latter group will continue for another 25 years. This means that the number in the 65–74 age group is declining (Fig. 7.1). It is well known that the specific rates of hospital admissions per 1000 community population rises with age. Though this varies from condition to condition, the overall effect is of a 50% increase in the 75–84 age group as compared to the 65–74 age group, and of a further 50% increase in the 85+ age group compared to the 75–84 group. This, linked to the increasing numbers in both these older age groups, means that the demand on hospital services will continue to rise.

This is confirmed by examination of the data provided from the Hospital In-Patient Enquiry (HIPE). The data is based on approximately a 1 in 10 sample of all discharges and deaths. Unfortunately strictly comparable figures are not available as these relate to England and Wales in 1979, but only England in 1982 and 1984. Nevertheless, comparing 1979 England and Wales data, with regard to discharges and

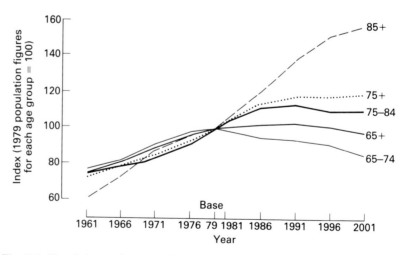

Fig. 7.1. Trends in population aged over 65 years (UK). (Indices are calculated from 1979 population figures.)

deaths, to the 1984 England data we find a 20% increase in the figures for the 65 years and over age group, against a 9% increase for all ages. Considering the two medical specialties, general medicine and geriatric medicine, one finds a 16% increase in the general medical discharges and deaths compared to a 35% increase for geriatric medicine for the same age group over the same period. This increase is mainly in the older age groups, i.e. 75–84 years and over 85 years, and this particularly relates to geriatric medicine. In spite of this, the mean duration of stay is steadily dropping, even in the oldest age group (86.2 days in 1979 to 60.7 days in 1984) which suggests that the increased number of patients are being treated more rapidly without necessarily an increase in the number of beds. In view of the potential complexity of illness in the aged already indicated, specialist knowledge of management becomes even more important if the hospital service is not to be overstretched. The following case history illustrates some of the problems facing the multi-disciplinary team in the management of illness in the very old.

A 90 year old widow, who had been diagnosed seven years previously as having diverticulosis coli, was admitted with central abdominal pain and vomiting. In addition she gave a three day history of central chest pain of a 'dull, crushing character'. There was no radiation of the pain and apart from swollen ankles, present for many years, there were no cardiovascular symptoms and her previous health had been good. Her only drugs were 'Moduretic' for her ankle swelling. She lived alone on the ground floor of the house and her daughter helped her with the cooking and shopping.

On examination she was found to be a small, thin woman whose blood pressure was 100/50 but whose heart was well compensated. She was tender in the epigastrium but otherwise had no abnormal physical signs apart from abnormal bowel sounds, bilateral cataracts, slight ankle oedema and erythema ab igne of both legs.

The clinical impression was of peptic ulceration or high bowel obstruction, but myocardial infarction had to be excluded. Investigations revealed an abnormal electrocardiogram (ECG) with sinus rhythm, a rate of 80 min^{-1}, Right bundle branch block, poor R wave progression, bifascicular block and atrial ectopics. Abominal X-ray revealed a dilated large bowel with a suggestion of a block at the splenic flexure and some fluid levels. Blood chemistry revealed a high blood urea of 19.9 mmol l^{-1}, a potassium of 6.9 mmol l^{-1}, T.protein 54 g l^{-1}, albumin 30 g l^{-1} and alkaline phosphatase 450 iu l^{-1} (due to Paget's disease). Her haemoglobin was 15.0 g dl^{-1} and her white count was raised, being 13.8 × 10^9 l^{-1} with a neutrophilia.

A nasogastric tube was inserted. She was given intravenous fluids and referred for a surgical opinion. The surgeons felt that her 'illness' was due to a combination of faecal impaction and hyperkalaemia but were puzzled as to the reason why her Potassium was so high in the presence of a moderately raised urea. We felt this was probably related to her 'Moduretic' (amiloride hydrochloride 5 mg and hydrochlorothiazide 50 mg) since hyperkalaemia is a well recognized complication of amiloride. It was also felt that the ECG changes were related to the hyperkalaemia.

However, after 10 days of i.v. fluids and aspiration no improvement in the bowel symptoms had occurred and the surgical team agreed to undertake a laparotomy. A small annular carcinoma at the junction of the sigmoid and descending colons was found and a sigmoid colectomy performed.

The postoperative course was complex, her blood pressure and urine output both being low. This responded to a dobutamine infusion but her respiratory rate then became slow (5 per minute) and irregular. This was felt to be due to opiate overdose, in spite of a total opiate dosage of only 50 mg Omnopon in 48 h. She was given naloxone, with immediate improvement.

During the first postoperative week she became increasingly oedematous, in spite of blood transfusion and diuretic therapy. Investigation showed her proteins had fallen further to 47 g l^{-1}. She transferred back to the geriatric medicine department on the ninth postoperative day and the oedema gradually resolved with diuretic therapy, i.v. albumin and blood transfusion, combined with a high protein diet which she had great difficulty in taking. Four months postoperatively she was still in hospital. Her blood chemistry was now within normal limits, with the exception of her proteins which were still low, total protein being 59 g l^{-1}, albumin 27 g l^{-1} and calcium 2.02 mmol l^{-1}. Her urea was 8.6 mmol l^{-1} and potassium 3.2 mmol l^{-1}. Her general condition was much improved but her colostomy closure failed and she had a faecal fistula. The smell of the faecal discharge revolted her and she was greatly distressed by this and the nursing staff felt that this contributed to her inability to eat and lack of further progress. After ensuring that the distal bowel was patent her colostomy was successfully closed. The improvement in her psychological state was dramatic and within a week her zest for life had returned.

The problem then was to increase her mobility and to return her to her own home.

There is no doubt that there are many lessons to be learned from this old lady's case, not least her own 'toughness' and tenacity to life for there is no doubt that many patients would have 'given up'. Maintenance of morale is, therefore, one factor which is very important. The case also illustrates many other important points and contains examples of all the characteristics described earlier. It is proposed, therefore, to develop these further in the rest of this chapter.

Morale

Maintenance of morale — the 'will to live' or the will and vigour to fight illness and overcome disability — is essential if the old are to make good recoveries from disease. This is a topic which has been studied relatively little in relation to disease in old age and its outcome, though all of us practising within the fields of geriatric medicine and psychiatry recognize that patients suffering from mental illness do less well when taken ill than those who have no mental disease. There is no doubt that depressive illness is associated with demoralization. There is a close association between loss and morale (Coleman, 1986). Ageing, regardless of social class or status, is frequently associated with loss. Retirement itself is a time of loss for many people. They lose status and work (occupation) and as a result interest and self-esteem. Unless they take action to counteract these losses they will neglect abilities and it is well known that disuse leads to atrophy. Consequently more loss of ability will occur. This can have clinical implications since muscle loss will be accentuated. It is perhaps no exaggeration to extend this line of reasoning so that decrease in muscle mass leads to increase of inactivity with reduction in ability to exercise, reduction in lung function, increase in osteoporosis and increase in body fat. Hence reduction in physical fitness, increased risk of fracture, reduced metabolic ability, altered metabolism of lipophilic drugs. These factors need to be taken into consideration when assessing the 'physical status' of an individual. Patients with low morale may need to be managed differently to those with high morale.

Special senses

Ageing itself will also contribute to loss in many patients. Deterioration of the special senses can lead to increasing isolation and it is seldom recognized that hearing loss may be an even greater disability than visual loss, for the hard of hearing are divorced from other people's minds and thoughts to a greater extent than the visually handicapped. Consequently communication becomes a barrier and with it understanding and knowledge. The elderly with hearing impairment, therefore, require just as much special consideration as the blind. Because of their disability they are often intensely suspicious of others and may become isolated or reclusive. They may suffer auditory hallucinations and believe people are making derogatory remarks about them and develop a true paraphrenic illness (schizophrenia of old age).

Similarly the visually handicapped may develop visual hallucinations, often associated with patterned bed curtains or wallpaper in conditions of low illumination. These can take the form of people's faces or of 'heads popping out of walls'. Such hallucinations often occur in the evening or at night when ward staffing levels are low, and when junior medical staff with limited experience are on duty. They can be frightening, even though the patient may recognize them as being imaginary, and lead to confusion. This may be exacerbated by drugs and occur both pre- and postoperatively. These patients can often be reassured and settled if time is taken to explain and allay their fear. A confusional episode (delirium) often appears to the patient as a bad dream occurring when they are awake. Given a warm drink and reassurance that they are safe and cared for will often enable the patient to settle. This is infinitely preferable, though much more time consuming, than giving a sedative drug, such as haloperidol. There is no doubt that the phenothiazine group of drugs are effective in the management of such cases but they often have to be given in too large a dose to produce their desired effect. The result is the patient tends to sleep the next day. Inversion of the sleep rhythm then becomes a real hazard. Should this happen then rehabilitation and recovery are put at risk.

The prevalence of disease increases with age and many old people lose functions because of this. However, in spite of this, many are able to compensate and may develop resilience that enables them to come to terms with, and even benefit from, their illness and disability. Many old people can adapt well to ageing and their physical state, and some have few deficits and life of excellent quality.

In the old lady's case, maintaining morale over a long time proved extremely difficult. The initial delay was not the best of starts for she was ill, uncomfortable and malnourished. Transfer to the surgical ward was disruptive but unavoidable, and she was transferred back to the acute admitting geriatric ward within 10 days though still very ill. She needed constant support and reassurance from both medical and nursing staff during this period and it was fortunate that the ward staff were in a stable state during this time so that she was managed by the same group of doctors and nurses who had made a clear management plan. They barely held their own, however, until the colostomy/faecal fistula was closed and her morale remained low until then.

Recognition of the need to maintain morale is essential, combined with careful assessment of the social circumstances, the sort of life the individual has led and his or her personal philosophy.

Assessment

The word 'assessment' is frequently used in geriatric medicine and its meaning is not always understood by other practitioners or professionals. Acute (admitting) geriatric medical wards are frequently called 'acute assessment wards' and as a result are sometimes thought not to be as 'acute' as acute surgical or general medical wards. They are, however, just as 'acute', perhaps more so, for as has already been said the aged patient deteriorates rapidly unless treated promptly. 'Assessment' means making an accurate physical, mental and social diagnosis, sometimes called triple assessment. The importance of maintaining morale has already been discussed, and faced with an acute, life threatening physical crisis it may seem inappropriate to consider the mental and social diagnosis. Yet unless some attempt is made to do this, disastrous mistakes can be made. Once a line of treatment is initiated it may be difficult to reverse and cause unnecessary suffering to the patient and distress to relatives, nursing staff and others involved in day to day care.

General aspects

The basic question which we all need to ask in assessing a patient is how will our treatment (management) affect the length and quality of his life. We need to perform what the economist calls a Cost Utility Analysis (CUA). If quality of life is bad there may be no point in prolonging life unless we can also improve the quality of life. This may well be possible for many old people and their relatives are ignorant of social benefits which could greatly improve their lot. It is not uncommon to find people leading happy lives four or five years after a hospital admission, prior to which they were a burden to themselves and their families (or carers).

It is comparatively rare to be unable to obtain information about the social state of an individual. The unconscious or confused old person admitted to the casualty department as the result of an accident, or having 'collapsed' in the street, will be an exception. In these cases the treatment of the critical condition will take precedence over other considerations. Usually, however, aged patients will be able to give an account of themselves and this can, and should, be confirmed with a relative or other person who may know them. Memory in old age can be untrustworthy and confabulation may occur.

Communication with the patient can be difficult. Almost one in three suffer from presbyacusis, the hearing loss of old age. If one speaks loudly, one is told, sharply, not to shout, they are not deaf. Yet the normal voice represents a jumble of sound which they find difficult to interpret. Shouting or speaking very loudly provokes the phenomenon of 'recruitment of sound' which is painful; hence their reaction. The use of an appliance to overcome hearing loss is, therefore, an advantage. The patient's own hearing-aid (if they have one) appropriately adjusted is often the most effective. It is a good idea, if the patient has a 'body worn aid' to hold this in your own hand and adjust the volume control yourself to suit the patient. If the patient does not possess an aid then the standard NHS speaking tube is probably the best amplification device available, since sound is not distorted. It is cheap and should be available on all geriatric wards, casualty departments and other places where the old are treated. In the case of the deaf, as opposed to those who are 'hard of hearing' greater amplification may be necessary and the 'Linco' speech trainer amplifier with headphones and a microphone may be needed. The alternative will be to resort to writing or using a communication card. This is obviously time consuming but one must always allow more time when dealing with an old person. Even when a communication problem is not present they can often be loquacious and difficult to keep to the point.

Social aspects

Today's old people have in most cases lived interesting lives. Though only a few now will have been old enough to have fought in the First World War, many will have been brought up during it. Others will remember the 1920s, the depression and most will have clear memories of the 1930s and the Second World War, in which some will have served overseas. They are people, therefore, with a considerable experience of life. Talking with them can be interesting and helpful in evaluating them. It is important to remember that they themselves will often not look on themselves as old though they may consider people younger than themselves as old. My own aunt in her 80s was active in providing entertainment for 'old people' in the village, who were 10 and 15 years younger than herself. For the benefit of medical students I ask those patients attending my clinic what age they look upon themselves as being. The answer is commonly 20 years below their real age.

A considerable literature now exists with regard to the physical, mental and social ability of the aged. Many of these assessment procedures are research tools which are much too long for everyday use. Nevertheless, in assessing patients it is important to consider their daily life and some of the headings one should explore are shown in Table 7.2. These are taken from the Nottingham Health Profile but are also included in many of the research questionnaires designed specifically for the aged. All are applicable to the aged and may be important for some individuals; they enable the doctor to obtain a much better mental picture of his patient. To these should be added knowledge of the patient's habits, particularly in relation to smoking and alcohol.

While it is helpful to build up a picture of the individual as a person, it is equally important to know about his domestic circumstances and support network. These are shown in Table 7.3. Knowledge of these is important since it may enable steps to be taken to plan discharge even before the recovery has taken place. It is also very reassuring to older patients to know that their doctors are so certain of his recovery that they are making preliminary plans for and consulting them about their discharge.

Looking after the house
Social life
Home life
Sex life
Hobbies
Interests
Holidays
Employment
  Past
  Present (full or part-time)

Table 7.2. Questions worth asking in regard to aspects of life style and ability

Table 7.3. Domestic circumstances and support network

Dwelling	House — own/council/rented	
	Flat	
	ground floor?	
	upper — lift? Yes/No	
	Bungalow — own/council	
	Sheltered housing — resident ward? Yes/No	
	Residential — local authority/private/voluntary	
Lives	With spouse/family member (specify)/other/ alone	
Daily support or services	Family member (specify)/neighbour/friend/ home help/meals on wheels/laundry service — other (voluntary)	
Finance	Supplementary benefit/additional pension/ attendance allowance	

Mental assessment

It is often stated that mental function deteriorates with ageing. Psychological tests have shown that the changes are variable and some functions are more likely to be affected than others. 'Vocabulary', for example, may actually improve until quite advanced age before beginning to diminish, while other functions may begin to change relatively early in life. One such function is the ability to make decisions. This is probably related to the fact that because the longeval individual has obtained so much experience with regard to 'pro' and 'con' factors, choosing a course of action proves difficult. This may affect 'informed consent', particularly if the inability of the aged to fully understand the advances in modern technology is also taken into consideration. Consequently the reply often received, after a long and careful explanation is 'Well, I'll do whatever you think is best, doctor'! This places considerable responsibility on the doctor and underlines the importance of knowing more about the 'medicine of old age'.

Depressive illness

It has already been said that loss is associated with demoralization. Many of the questions used in the assessment of morale are also used in the assessment of depression. Depression is common in the old; indeed, the prevalence is higher then than at any time in life. This is almost certainly due to relapses in people who have previously suffered depressive illness. The true incidence (i.e. occurring for the first time) in people over 75 years is low and the highest incidence is in the 40–65 age group (Post, 1981). Consequently in taking a history from an old person it is important to ask about previous depressive illness or the taking of antidepressant drugs. Like episodes occurring earlier in life, depression in old age will be triggered by environmental stresses such as a move from a family home, bereavement of spouse or siblings as well as physical illness resulting in loss of function. In addition, alteration in neuroendo-crine function undoubtedly plays a part and there is some evidence to suggest that depression is associated with mild intellectual deterioration (early dementia). Equally, depressive illness can be confused with dementia and this 'pseudodementia' will improve dramatically when the depression is treated.

Depression may also be marked by the patient's preoccupation with a real physical disability. During her illness, the 90 year old lady described earlier became undoubtedly depressed as a result of her preoccupation with the disability caused by her colostomy. Treatment with an anti-depressant might have helped her to tolerate the disability better until it was surgically relieved. Similarly hypochondriacal complaints may frequently mask mild depression which requires treatment. This is particularly common in patients who may have other disabilities or whose life style is poor, or whose supportive network is deficient. These problems will often coexist. Such patients will complain of loneliness, being a burden or having no one close to them. They complain of pain, or dry mouth, or swollen tongue, or nasty taste, to a greater degree than would seem justified by the clinical findings though the basis for the complaint may exist. Trial of an antidepressant drug may be more effective than attempting to improve life-style or increase supportive networks though these may also be justified.

A flat mood, gloomy appearance, lack of interest and activity, tearfulness associated with sleep disturbance such as early morning waking and poor appetite and weight loss, should always suggest the diagnosis of depression. Severely affected patients may become so apathetic as to become almost comatose or difficult to rouse.

Trial of antidepressant drugs with a good response (though this may take some time) will help to confirm the diagnosis. Remembering and suspecting that depression exists is, however, most important and psychogeriatric opinion should be sought if there is doubt. In severe cases electro-convulsive therapy may be indicated.

Anxiety states

Like depression, anxiety is common, particularly in old people who come into hospital for the first time to have an operation. It may be treated with a small dose of an anxiolytic. It does, however, need to be differ-entiated from hyperthyroidism (p. 120).

Delirium (acute confusional states)

Reversible mental confusion giving rise to outbursts of irrational behaviour, aggressiveness, refusal to accept therapy, visual halluci-nations and noisiness is more common in the aged. As has already been described, hallucinatory symptoms may be associated with deterioration in the special senses, sight and hearing. While this may be a symptom of an underlying paraphrenic illness and need long-term drug treatment, they and the other symptoms of confusion are much more likely to be due to a delirious state.

The onset is sudden, developing rapidly over minutes or hours. The pattern may vary with time with exacerbations of florid symptoms, often at night. Consciousness is clouded, disorientation of place, time and person is present and thinking disorganized. Sometimes the thoughts have themes from the past, which may be rational in themselves but not understood by hospital staff. The patient is often anxious and afraid, and speech may be incoherent. The episodes may be interspersed with lucid intervals. During these, patients may retain some insight of their condition and liken it to a 'bad dream'. Calm, friendly reassurance that they are not 'mad' and that their disturbed mental state is only temporary will often help a return to reality.

The causes of these states are legion and are listed in Table 7.4. They may frequently follow anaesthesia and surgery and can be anticipated if a careful psychiatric history has been taken, and mental assessment (see below) made. They may be associated with underlying cerebral cortical disease, which may not have been previously recognized by relatives, who later blame 'that operation' for their 'loved one's' continuing mental deterioration.

While delirious episodes usually recover when the cause is treated, they do need taking very seriously since they may provoke complications, e.g. rupture of suture lines, falls and fractures; some patients do not recover. Episodes may sometimes be provoked by moving a patient from a familiar ward to another, or even by altering the position of the bed in the ward. Management should be aimed at ensuring comfort, e.g. relieving pain, checking bladder, bowel and pressure areas; seeking a source of infection (blood culture, urine examination); ensuring adequate hydration and nutrition without provoking or worsening heart failure; checking drug therapy for a potential source (hypnotic, digitalis, etc.); checking electrolyte and metabolic state.

Apart from treating the cause (if possible) it may be necessary to use a tranquillizer to allay anxiety. Probably the simplest and easiest to use

Table 7.4. Causes of delirium (acute confusion)

Category	Example
Infections	Lung, urinary tract, gut, skin
Neurological	'Stroke', cerebral tumour, epilepsy, subdural haematoma, chronic brain disease (e.g. SDAT)
Cardiorespiratory	Myocardial infarction, pulmonary embolism, cardiac failure
Endocrine	Diabetes, hypothyroidism, hyperparathyroidism
Metabolic	Dehydration, vitamin deficiency (B_{12}, B_1)
Miscellaneous	Trauma, drugs (especially anticholinergic), anaesthetic agents, alcohol

is haloperidol which in elixir form is colourless and tasteless, so that it can be given in ordinary drinks and the risk of refusal to take a tablet (because it is thought to be a poison) is reduced. The dose should be tailored to the patient's need and response. While adequate dosage is essential, the minimum necessary should be used and the patient restored to normal ward life as soon as possible. Treatment of these patients is time consuming and can tax the patience and endurance of medical and nursing staff. Nevertheless, the temptation to 'flatten' the patient with a large dose of drug must be resisted and appropriate staff allocated to 'special' them. Oversedation carries an excessive risk of complications and must be avoided.

In cases where alcohol withdrawal is suspected, intravenous vitamins or chlormethiazole may be helpful and some will benefit from being given alcohol.

Dementia

The simplest definition of dementia is that of Marsden (1978): 'The syndrome of global disturbance of higher mental functions in an alert patient'.

The two common causes in old age are due to loss of brain tissue, as a result of either multiple infarcts — multi-infarct dementia (MID) — or diffuse brain changes producing a pathological picture similar to that seen in younger patients with Alzheimer's disease — senile dementia of the Alzheimer type (SDAT). In the case of MID, the history may indicate a stepwise deterioration in the mental state, each step being associated with an episode of deterioration which may then improve but not to the extent that the patient regains his previous level of competence. Elevation of the blood pressure is common and neurological signs, indicating a localized brain lesion, are found. The intellectual deterioration is often patchy and islands of preservation are found. In contrast, patients with SDAT may have no neurological signs but show signs of a gradual deterioration, particularly affecting memory. In the early stages of the disease it is sometimes difficult to distinguish from the memory disturbance which is sometimes seen in old people. This may be particularly so in the case of women over 80 years. SDAT affects many women of this age, yet some 'normal' memory loss is common. This particularly relates to short-term memory and the ability to recall things to order (Chapter 6). However, in SDAT the deterioration is more global. Disorientation in both space and time are present and as the disease progresses individuals become unable to recognize relatives or their current home, and many wander in search of a home vacated in early adult life. They may also suffer apraxia, agnosia and aphasia. Aimless wandering can become difficult to contain, and defecation and micturition become inappropriate so that care becomes a heavy burden.

Differentiation between MID and SDAT can be difficult and except

for research purposes is relatively unimportant. In series where pathological and clinical findings have been compared, approximately 50% of
cases had SDAT, 20% had MID and 20% had mixed SDAT and MID.
The remaining 10% had either normal histology or other causes.

Diagnosis of dementia is important since confusional episodes, depression and paranoid states can complicate the condition. A simple 10
question test can be helpful; even though it can give false positives . . .,
serial testing may help to differentiate conditions, e.g. patients with
confusion or depression will improve with treatment, while those with
dementia will not do so and may deteriorate.

Conclusion

Mental ill health is common in old age and should always be borne in
mind. Diagnosis can be difficult and the patient may not always be able
to give an accurate history. It is important, therefore, to interview
relatives and other carers who may be able to give a more accurate
picture of the mental state of the patient.

Physical assessment

General comments

Earlier in this chapter the importance of accurate diagnosis and early
treatment was stressed. It was also stated that multiple pathology was
common and that the presentation of illness was often non-specific or
atypical. In both the illustrative cases quoted the initial diagnosis was
not easy to make. In the second patient there was considerable delay before curative treatment was initiated. While this could be justified the
distinct possibility remains that in part the delay was due to the age of
the patient and the reluctance of both physicians and surgeons to be
more active until it became obvious that the only chance of survival was
via a surgical procedure. Yet here, at the time of admission, was a 90 year
old who was mentally well preserved and who until this illness had been
capable of living alone, albeit with support. Generally speaking nonagenarians are amongst the 'physiological elite' who recover well from illness,
unless they are in a terminal phase. Nevertheless, treatment needs to be
expeditious and once quality of life has been assessed, age by itself
should never be a barrier to treatment.

Cardiorespiratory system

In the second patient the diagnosis was in part obscured by a history of
chest pain. The diagnosis of myocardial infarction was possible and the
electrocardiograph was abnormal. The aged cardiopulmonary system
has been considered in Chapters 3 and 4 but two comments will be made

here. Firstly, electrolytic disturbance particularly relating to potassium, calcium and magnesium is common, especially in those who have been receiving diuretics with or without potassium supplements and potassium sparing agents. Hypomagnesaemia may be particularly important and *must* be remembered. Secondly, the possibility of temporary pacing should be considered, particularly if arrythmias are likely to occur during anaesthesia or surgery, or in the immediate post-operative period.

One further topic affecting the cardiopulmonary system, postural (orthostatic) hypotension, has already been mentioned and its causes outlined (Table 7.1). Autonomic disorders have been discussed in Chapter 5; an age-related decline in the autonomic nervous system activity undoubtedly occurs. It is likely that this is due to multifactoral changes within the nervous system and many of these may be disease related rather than true ageing changes, though it is likely that some slowing of conduction along nerve fibres occurs and neurotransmitter levels alter. There is no evidence, however, that either high or low pressure baroreceptors are affected by age.

Cardiopulmonary complications

Cardiopulmonary complications are common. Hypostatic pneumonia will complicate the bedfast state, hence the insistence of geriatricians that 'bed is bad'. Differentiation, in the postoperative phase, between lung infection and heart failure can be very difficult and it is probably wise to 'back both horses' and treat with diuretics and antibiotics. The smoker and ex-smoker are more prone to chronic airway disease and should be given pre- and postoperative chest physiotherapy. It has only recently been recognized that asthma is common; this must be remembered. As stated earlier, respiratory rate is an important measurement and must be monitored.

Pulmonary embolism is, of course, an obvious complication and steps are now routinely taken to avoid deep vein thrombosis. However, presentation in the elderly may be atypical and acute confusional episodes, apathy and a general 'failure to thrive' and progress as well as expected may indicate that small embolic episodes are occurring. A high index of suspicion is necessary to make the diagnosis, and special investigations should not be delayed. The presence of varicose veins is common and therefore may be unhelpful as a physical sign.

Nutrition

The Department of Health and Social Security (DHSS) nutritional survey (1979) of the elderly indicated that sub-nutrition was not common. Nevertheless, it was more common in people over 80 years old, where a prevalence of 14% was found. Other surveys have shown that there is a close link between illness and nutrient intake and that the longer the patient is ill the worse the nutritional state is likely to be. There is no doubt, in the case of our old lady, that she was considerably undernourished by the time she reached the operating theatre and indeed was suffering from sub-nutrition on admission. Surprisingly little is known about nutrition in the old, although more is gradually being discovered. Generally speaking the fit old are well nourished and in balance, though their intake of potassium and calcium may be on the low side. With illness, intake of nutrients — particularly protein, vitamins, essential elements and trace elements — all diminish. In hospital the situation may worsen and the modern habit of allowing patients to choose their own menu may compound matters. Studies on our own wards have shown that patients tend to choose diets deficient in iron and other vital components. When nurses are left to choose the diet it is of better quality. The importance of expert dietary advice cannot be over-emphasized and studies suggest that when nutrient intake is balanced, adequate recovery and discharge are speeded up.

Assessment of nutritional state in the old is difficult. Measurements such as skinfold thickness, mid-arm circumference, biochemical and haematological values are of doubtful worth unless they are very abnormal, in which case cachexia is usually obvious. Moreover, some patients on appalling dietary regimes are actually obese! A dietary history is worth taking, and if the individual can recall what they have eaten in the previous seven days a reliable guide to nutritional intake may be obtained. However, this should be checked by enquiry from a relative and should be recorded in the notes.

The most important aspect of nutrition lies in monitoring intake in hospital during the illness. Studies suggest that protein intake may need to be twice normal to counteract metabolic loss. There is no doubt that many patients are starved in hospital. The manner in which meals are served (all three courses arriving together) does not help the old, who may require much more time to eat than the young. Consequently a carefully drawn up supplementary feeding schedule needs to be prescribed and may even need to be supplemented by nasogastric drip through a fine tube during the night until recovery enables a normal diet to be taken.

Endocrine system

Diabetes mellitus: many old people have impaired glucose tolerance in response to a 50 g glucose load. In a study of women over the age of 85 years who all had normal fasting blood sugars, a third had abnormal 2 h sugar values. A random blood sugar measurement is probably as valuable a guide to the diagnosis of diabetes as more formal testing. Values over 11 mmol l^{-1} (198 mg per 100 ml) are indicative of diabetes and treatment depending on how high a level is found should be considered. Repetition of the blood sugar either as a random or fasting sample or measurement of HbAl (glycosylated haemoglobin) together with the absence or presence of symptoms, which may not be volunteered, will help to decide what treatment, if any is justified. Often simple dietary advice will enable the blood sugar to remain below 11 mmol l^{-1}. However, treatment with sulphonylureas may be indicated in some and insulin in a few. If oral therapy is indicated then a short-acting sulphonylurea should be used (e.g. tolbutamide) and biguanides should not be given.

Neurological complications of diabetes in the old are not uncommon and when present indicate that treatment is necessary.

Thyroid disease: both hypo- and hyperthyroidism are frequently found in the aged and hypothyroidism is the more common. In a recent survey of over 300 'normal elderly' living at home four were known to be hypothyroid and a further nine cases were discovered (Southampton Ageing Project).

The diagnosis of *hypothyroidism* can be difficult since the facies it presents is similar to that of ageing. A high index of suspicion is necessary in uncovering the condition. 'Failure to thrive' is suggestive, as is gruffness of the voice, bradycardia and slow relaxing reflexes. Thyroid function tests may be unreliable in the presence of acute illness and also affected by a wide variety of drugs. Direct measurement of free thyroxine concentration may help to make the diagnosis. Thyroid stimulating hormone (TSH) is also raised and levels over 10 u l^{-1} are diagnostic of primary hypothyroidism. It should be remembered that drug compliance is sometimes poor and patients supposedly on thyroxin may be under-replaced. Estimation of TSH may help to elucidate this problem.

Diagnosis of *hyperthyroidism* also may be difficult on clinical grounds. It should always be suspected in patients who have arrhythmias, particularly atrial fibrillation with or without evidence of heart failure. The classical symptoms of weight loss, palpitations and feeling the heat may all be present. Tremor should not be difficult to distinguish from the tremors seen in ageing, but sweating may be less prominent due to loss of sweat glands. Some patients are apathetic and appear slow and depressed, yet on biochemical testing they have levels of thyroxine consistent with hyperthyroidism. This group is obviously difficult to diagnose.

Hyperparathyroidism is not unusual and may be quite asymptomatic. It can account for hypercalcaemia and recent evidence suggests that in the absence of symptoms it is best left untreated.

Hypoparathyroidism is uncommon but may occur as a result of thyroid surgery.

Parathyroid hormone levels may well rise in disease, perhaps linked to reduction in vitamin D levels. Levels in normal, fit, healthy aged people seem to be lower than in the younger population.

Hypophysoadrenal axis: while both hypo- and hyperfunction of the pituitary and adrenal glands are seen in old age they are not common and the diagnosis has usually been made previously. Hypopituitarism (Simmonds Sheehan syndrome) may rarely present as hypotension complicating other disease in aged women. Past history of post-partum haemorrhage is usually obtainable and should be sought.

Phaeochromocytoma has been described over the age of 80 years but is very uncommon.

Skeletal system

Diseases of the bones and joints are common and frequently lead to the need for surgery. Bone and joint disease may also inhibit rehabilitation after surgery and attention should be paid to both conditions during periods of relative immobilization.

The three common *bone disorders* are osteoporosis, osteomalacia and Paget's disease.

Osteoporosis has been defined as a state of 'too little bone but what bone there is, is normal'. It is much commoner in women, may be associated with immobility and disuse, excess cortisol (natural or iatrogenic), thyrotoxicosis, and age itself. Evidence is accumulating that some women are more affected than others. While this may relate to calcium intake early in life and therefore total bone mass, it is more likely that some are 'fast calcium losers'. This can prevented by replacement of female sex hormone (hormone replacement therapy). Differentiation of these women is possible and it seems likely that many more women will be taking oestrogens than in the past. This can be justified on a cost-effective basis when one considers that the incidence of fractures of the upper femur in women is four times that of men. Currently no evidence exists for the value of giving hormones after the age of 70 years, but in view of the possible 'catch up' effect when they are stopped, it is possible to envisage some women remaining on 'the pill' for life.

Osteomalacia results from vitamin D deficiency. The clinical indications which may lead one to suspect the diagnosis are shown in Table 7.5. It may often complicate osteoporosis. Vitamin D levels are lower in the ill aged and a case can be made for supplementation in the housebound and institutionalized.

Table 7.5. Clinical indications of osteomalacia

Vague generalized pain
Back ache
Muscle weakness and stiffness
Waddling gait
Skeletal deformity
Bone tenderness
Long confinement indoors
Malabsorption states and malnutrition

Paget's disease causes disfiguration of bone and may give rise to bone pain and heart failure, as well as lead to immobility by involving joints or producing fractures. All these bone diseases increase the risk of fracture and consequent immobility. Severely osteoporotic people can easily sustain fractures as a result of minor trauma, e.g. being lifted carelessly in bed or by being stood up! Many suggest that treatment is of no avail though evidence does exist of increased cancellous bone deposition as a result of treatment with vitamin D, calcium and fluoride.

The two common *joint diseases* are rheumatoid arthritis and osteo-arthritis.

Rheumatoid arthritis may present for the first time in old age, although it is more common to see patients who have been long-term sufferers. New cases respond well to steroids and often have a relatively short, limited illness. The problem lies in the complications of immobi-lity, osteoporosis and the dangers of drug therapy, particularly when non-steroidal anti-inflammatory drugs are used.

Osteoarthritis gives rise to pain and immobility. The importance of the physiotherapist in maintaining mobility and function in both these conditions is great.

Prevention of complications

The importance of early mobilization, adequate diet and hydration have already been stressed, together with the risk of hypostatic pneumonia. Three other common complications are worth consideration.

Pressure-sores (decubitus ulcers)

The prevalence of pressure-sores increases with age and studies have shown an overall prevalence of almost 9%. Mean capillary pressure is about 20–30 mmHg so the degree of pressure needed to occlude the microcirculation is not great. The skin will recover when the pressure is released. However, if the pressure persists for too long, infarction of the skin and deeper tissues will occur. A pressure of approximately 40 mmHg maintained for one hour or so is sufficient to cause infarction of skin and deeper tissues. Ordinarily patients move when they feel uncomfortable but will not when unconscious or heavily sedated. Consequently attention must be paid to supporting surfaces such as mattresses, cushions, covers on operating tables, and trolleys on which patients may lie or be transported. Ward nurses are often incorrectly blamed for the development of a pressure-sore that may have been initiated elsewhere. Particular attention must therefore be paid to the vital pressure points — heels, sacrum, shoulders and hips — where breakdown is more likely to occur because pressure is greatest. Develop-ment of a sore can delay discharge by as much as four months. Cost in terms of suffering is great but so too is the cost in financial terms.

Incontinence of urine

True incontinence is the loss of the ability to control bladder emptying to order. Patients may also 'wet the bed' because they cannot wait for an appropriate receptacle to be provided. A colleague, recently in hospital, asked me if I knew that a nursing minute was three-quarters of an hour! Urinary incontinence is common in the old; prevalence of 18% for women and 7% for men has been quoted. The commonest form is 'urge' incontinence. In these cases the desire to micturate can only be suppressed for a relatively short time (approximately three minutes) before voiding becomes compulsory. It can be seen that maintaining continence even for the alert, active, ambulant patient can be difficult. Apart from its embarrassing and 'shameful' connotations, incontinence increases the risk of pressure sores. The maintenance of a continence chart can help nurses to promote continence by regular toileting. This must be encouraged and catheterization avoided unless absolutely necessary.

Constipation

Immobility, lack of fibre in the diet and dehydration are all predisposing factors for constipation. To these can be added drugs.

Symptoms include abdominal pain and mental confusion, and the condition may lead to faecal impaction with spurious diarrhoea and urinary incontinence, often with retention and overflow, even in women. Patients may, in their confused state, attempt to disimpact themselves, with resultant smearing of faeces over themselves, bed clothes and furniture. The condition is insiduous and often difficult to spot if the impaction is high, when the rectum may be empty.

Laboratory results

Haematological findings

Anaemia is diagnosed if the haemoglobin level is less than 12 g dl^{-1}, and further investigation is necessary. Hypochromia — a low mean corpuscular haemoglobin concentration (MCHC) — suggests iron deficiency, which is the commonest form of anaemia found. It may be associated with blood loss, most frequently from the gastrointestinal tract. A high mean corpuscular volume (MCV) with anaemia and macrocytosis indicates vitamin B_{12} or folic acid deficiency. Red cell folate levels are more reliable than serum folate levels. A bone marrow examination is sometimes necessary to confirm anaemia. Absence of iron staining particles in the marrow confirms iron deficiency, while serum iron can be unreliable and even iron binding saturation can mislead.

A high MCV with macrocytosis in the absence of anaemia may relate to a high alcohol intake and be particuarly useful evidence for the anaesthetist. The white cell count tends to fall with age and a white count about 9×10^9 1^{-1} may indicate infection or abnormality. Leukaemias are common and high lymphocyte counts above $5 \times 10^9 1^{-1}$ are not uncommon. However, a marrow examination is necessary to make firm diagnosis. The peripheral blood film may, however, indicate leucoerythroblastic processes and thrombocytosis may also occur. Low white cell counts down to $3 \times 10^9 1^{-1}$ are not abnormal.

The erythrocyte sedimentation rate (ESR) tends to rise with increasing age and levels up to 30 mm h^{-1} (Westergren) can be considered within normal limits. Very high levels are not uncommon and should be investigated. Sometimes, however, no cause can be found, in which case they should not be treated but the patient followed up. A raised ESR in excess of 100 mm h^{-1} may persist without treatment for years and settle spontaneously.

Biochemical tests

In the healthy aged, the ranges of the common biochemical parameters measured are identical to those found in younger age groups. Abnormal findings indicate disease or else result from drugs (e.g. diuretics) given to treat disease. The significance of some abnormalities, however, is of less importance in the old. This particularly applies to blood urea and creatinine. The upper limit of normal for blood urea concentration is 10 mmol 1^{-1}. Higher levels are not infrequently found and may indicate heart failure or dehydration rather than severe renal failure. Indeed, it is not uncommon to find levels of over 20 mmol 1^{-1} returning to normal levels with recovery of health. Creatinine levels may also be higher. They are, however, a poor indication of renal failure since creatinine levels may be low in thin, ill old people who have a raised blood urea concentration. With the exception of calcium and uric acid, the remainder of biochemical findings usually indicate disease in the same way as they do in the young.

Calcium levels may often be in the high normal range without indicating active disease, though as previously mentioned hyperparathyroidism does occur. Metastatic bone disease, particularly of breast, is another cause.

Uric acid levels tend to follow the blood urea and acute gout is not uncommon in patient on diuretics, even in women.

Serum cholesterol tends to rise with age but is often found to be lower in older age groups, perhaps a cohort effect, those with higher levels having died.

Total proteins may be above 80 g 1^{-1} in myeloma and liver disease while hypoalbuminaemia less than 35 g 1^{-1} may indicate sub-nutrition, chronic infection, malignancy, diffuse liver disease or chronic renal disease. Associated with a low albumin is a low calcium; this was the finding in the 90 year old lady described earlier in this chapter. In her case this was certainly associated with sub-nutrition since values returned gradually to normal as her appetite and nutrient intake improved.

Alkaline phosphatase is commonly high and may indicate Paget's disease of bone. Estimation of isoenzymes to differentiate liver from bone as a cause may well be indicated when doubt exists. Usually, however, if liver is the cause, other liver function tests are abnormal.

Conclusions

While in many cases the findings and the presentation and character of disease are similar in the aged and the young, it is important to remember that the findings can be different. Because of age more factors can influence the character and pattern of illness. The medical notes should be read carefully for indications which will help the anaesthetist to better assess the older patient. The social history and previous life-style of the patient is particularly important since low social class or poverty may indicate poor nutrition and low morale. This is recognized by doctors working on geriatric wards but may be absent from notes on surgical wards. The anaesthetist may need to ensure that such information is available to him. Often the nursing staff will know but if they do not then information may need to be obtained from relatives to confirm or supplement the history given by the patient.

References and further reading

Brocklehurst, J.C. (Ed.) (1985) *Textbook of Geriatric Medicine and Gerontology*. Churchill Livingstone, Edinburgh.

Bromley, D.B. (1966) *The Psychology of Human Ageing*, Penguin Books Ltd, Harmondsworth.

Charcot, J.M. (1881) *Clinical Lectures on Senile and Chronic Diseases*. The New Sydenham Society, London.

Coleman, P.G. (1986) *Ageing and Reminiscence Processes. Social and Clinial Implications*. Wiley, Chichester, p. 23.

DHSS (1979) *Nutrition and Health in Old Age. Report on Health and Social Subjects No. 16*. HMSO, London.

Hodkinson, M. (Ed.) (1984) *Clinical Biochemistry of the Elderly*. Churchill Livingstone, Edinburgh.

Isaacs, B. (Ed.) (1982) Introduction to geriatric medicine: the state of the nation. In *Recent Advances in Geriatric Medicine*. Churchill Livingstone, Edinburgh, p. 4.

McFadden, J.P, Price, R.C, Eastwood, H.D, *et al.* (1982) Raised respiratory rate in elderly patients: a valuable physical sign. *Br. Med. J.* **284**, 626–627.

Marsden, C.D. (Ed.) (1978) The diagnosis of dementia. In *Studies of Geriatric Psychiatry*. Wiley, Chichester, pp. 99–118.

Pathy, M.S.J. (Ed.) (1985) *Principles and Practice of Geriatric Medicine*. Wiley, Chichester.

Post, F. (1981) Affective illnesses. In *Health Care of the Elderly*, (Ed. T. Arie). Croom Helm, London, pp. 89–103.

8 | Mechanisms of altered drug effects in the aged

G.T. TUCKER

Introduction

A need for lower dosage of many drugs and an increased risk of toxicity in the aged has long been part of clinical experience. However, scientific interest in the effects of ageing on pharmacokinetics ('what the body does to drugs') and pharmacodynamics ('what drugs do to the body') is relatively recent. In turn, this has also stimulated regulatory concern, accentuated by the recognition of the implications of the 'Opren affair' for the evaluation of new drugs.

Altered dosage requirements of anaesthetic agents and adjuvants in the aged are based largely on anecdote, but some objective data are available, examples of which now follow.

(i) Decreased dosage of thiopentone (Dundee, 1954; Christensen & Andreasen, 1978) and propofol (Hilton et al., 1986; Dundee et al., (1986) is particularly well documented.

(ii) The minimum alveolar concentrations (MAC values) of inhalation agents decline by about 20% between the ages of 20 and 80 years (Krechel, 1984).

(iii) Although in fit patients dose–response relationships of non-depolarizing neuromuscular blocking agents are independent of age, onset time and recovery may be prolonged in the old (Donati & Bevan, 1986; Duvaldestin et al., 1982; Matteo et al., 1985).

(iv) A lowered dosage of benzodiazepines is indicated both by epidemiological evidence (Boston Collaborative Drug Surveillance Program, 1973; Greenblatt & Allen, 1978) and by the results of controlled studies (Swift et al., 1985).

(v) Atropine is more sedative in the old (Smith et al., 1979), but produces a diminished cardiovascular response (Virtanen et al., (1982).

(vi) A direct inverse relationship between the epidural dose of local anaesthetic required to block each spinal segment in adults and patient age was established by Bromage (1978). Although more recent studies (e.g. Park et al., 1980), using fixed volume injections, suggest weaker and more complex correlations, higher levels of blockade should be anticipated in the old.

(vii) *Acute* respiratory depression 10 min after a single i.v. injection of morphine was found to be similar in fit old and young subjects (Daykin et al., 1986). Nevertheless, the old are generally more sensitive to morphine (Bellville et al., 1971) and it remains 'wise to use minimal doses and exercise extra care in monitoring older patients given opiates'

(Arunsalem *et al.*, 1983). Evidence that this applies also to the epidural and intrathecal injection of these drugs has also been reported (Gustaffson *et al.*, 1982).

In considering possible mechanisms of altered drug response and dose requirements in the elderly, this review will concentrate primarily on pharmacokinetic changes, since these have been studied more extensively than pharmacodynamic changes. The latter are more difficult to investigate and generally require the prior exclusion of kinetic mechanisms.

Many factors complicate the design and interpretation of pharmacokinetic studies in the aged. For example, considerable difficulties arise from inequalities in biological and chronological age. Thus, older individuals become more diverse with advancing age and the consequences of the natural process of senescence must be delineated from the confounding effects of disease, poor nutrition and drug interactions, all of which are more prevalent in the aged. Studies are invariably cross-sectional rather than longitudinal, and therefore more is known about age differences in drug action than changes of drug action with age. Other problems are more avoidable and relate to the use of inadequate numbers of subjects and samples in each decade, leading to low statistical power. Failure to allow for all of the relevant pharmacokinetic factors, especially plasma binding, is common. Conclusions about alterations in drug absorption are often made from data obtained after extravascular administration only, without the use of intravenous controls.

Such experimental deficiencies tend therefore to give rise to a confused literature with many instances of conflicting conclusions from different studies of the same drug. The literature on the kinetics of anaesthetic drugs and adjuvants is no exception to this. Nevertheless, an objective can be to see whether or not some generalizations can be made as guidelines for the choice of drug and dosage. Instances where there is good evidence that altered pharmacodynamics contribute significantly to a different response in the aged also require consideration.

Drug absorption

Reductions in gastric acid secretion, splanchnic blood flow and gastric emptying rate accompanying old age might be expected to alter dissolution and absorption rates after oral drug administration, thereby prolonging onset of effect. A similar outcome might be anticipated after extravascular injection owing to lower peripheral blood flow and increased local fat deposition.

However, the few systematic studies of drug absorption in the old that have been done suggest that any changes are not of great clinical significance. For example, studies have found no age-related alterations in the rate or extent of absorption of pethidine (Herman *et al*, 1985), diazepam (Divoll et al., 1983) or lorazepam (Greenblatt et al., 1979) after oral or intramuscular (deltoid) administration. Increases in the oral availability of midazolam (Greenblatt et al., 1984) and chlormethiazole (Nation et al., 1977a) may be attributed to impaired first-pass metabolism rather than greater transfer across the gut mucosa.

After epidural, lumbar and caudal injection there appears to be a small trend to faster systemic absorption of local anaesthetics in the old (Rosenberg et al., 1981; Finucaine & Hammonds, 1984; Freund et al., 1986). This may reflect a greater longitudinal spread of solution owing to the less patent intervertebral foramina.

Drug distribution

The process of drug distribution refers to the reversible transfer of drug between blood and body tissues and is therefore an important determinant of the time-course of drug action. It is convenient to consider it first in terms of extent and then in relation to the more difficult concept of rate.

Extent of distribution

The extent of drug distribution is normally expressed by a volume of distribution, relating the total amount of drug in the body at any time to its concentration in blood or plasma. Thus, the full extent of drug distribution at equilibrium is approximated by the volume of distribution at steady-state (V_{SS}). This can be calculated from blood drug concentration–time data after parenteral administration and may be expressed in physiological terms by:

$$V_{SS} = V_B + \frac{fu}{fu_T} \cdot V_T.$$

Thus, V_{SS} is dependent upon blood volume (V_B), net tissue volume (V_T) and blood and tissue binding, where fu_b = the free (unbound) fraction in blood and fu_T = the free (unbound) fraction in tissue.

The importance of the value of volume of distribution is that if we assume that the distribution of drug throughout all tissues of the body is instantaneous, then the loading dose required to achieve rapidly a particular blood drug concentration associated with optimum effect would be directly proportional to the volume of distribution. The elimination half-life of drug is also directly related to its volume of distribution since a more extensive tissue uptake means that less drug will be delivered by the blood to the liver and kidneys per unit time. Therefore, changes in volume of distribution may also affect (i) the time to reach steady-state on continuous dosing and (ii) the extent of the oscillation between maximum and minimum drug concentrations at steady-state. In turn this may have implications for dosage interval and duration of effect.

All of the determinants of V_{SS} can change with age.

Blood (plasma) binding may decrease or increase depending upon the binding protein involved. In general, acidic drugs are bound predominantly to high capacity sites on albumin, whereas basic drugs (although not benzodiazepines) are primarily associated with low capacity sites on alpha$_1$-acid glycoprotein, one of the 'stress proteins'. Serum albumin tends to decrease with age, explained partly by the relative inactivity of older patients, and augmented by systemic illness. Thus, some studies have shown concomitant decreases in the binding of ligands like thiopentone (Jung *et al.*, 1982) and benzodiazepines (Macklon *et al.*, 1980; Divoll *et al.*, 1981; Divoll & Greenblatt, 1982; Davis *et al.*, 1985). This is not a general finding, however, even for these compounds (Homer & Stanski, 1985; Greenblatt *et al.*, 1984), but discrepancies may in part reflect a confounding effect of sex since changes seem more marked in females. The increased levels of alpha$_1$-acid glycoprotein observed in old age (Verbeeck *et al.*, 1984a; Paxton & Briant, 1984) may be a consequence of underlying pathology and not age *per se*, as it has been shown that the plasma binding of lignocaine and pethidine is correlated significantly with alpha$_1$-acid glycoprotein concentration but not with patient age (Davis *et al.*, 1985; Herman *et al.*, 1985).

In the context of plasma binding it is important that changes in the *fraction* of drug bound in plasma are not necessarily associated with significant changes in free drug *concentration* and, therefore, in effect. The latter will be buffered by extensive extravascular distribution and compensatory increases in clearance. Therefore, in terms of the extent of drug distribution it may be preferable to measure volume of distribution with respect to the concentration of unbound drug in plasma. At steady-state this volume (Vu_{SS}) is given by:

$$Vu_{SS} = \frac{V_B}{fu_b} + \frac{V_T}{fu_T} \simeq \frac{V_T}{fu_T}.$$

Net tissue volume (V_T) tends to decrease with age as body weight declines, and this would be reflected in a decrease in total volume of distribution and hence loading dose requirement. However, significant changes in body composition also occur with age. These will be reflected in the value of fu_T and will either reinforce or oppose the effect of decrease in body weight, depending upon the physicochemical properties of the drug. Thus, as body weight decreases the proportion of water decreases while fat content increases, especially in females. Therefore, lipid-soluble drugs should have greater volumes of distribution (per kilogram of body weight) in the aged while the opposite should be seen with more water-soluble compounds.

Accordingly, increasing age is associated with greater Vu_{SS} values for diazepam (Macklon *et al.*, 1980; Greenblatt *et al.*, 1980; Divoll *et al.*, 1983), chlordiazepoxide (Roberts *et al.*, 1978) and clobazam (Greenblatt *et al.*, 1981), whereas for the closely related but less lipid-soluble derivatives, lorazepam (Greenblatt *et al.*, 1979), oxazepam (Murray *et al.*, 1981) and temazepam (Divoll *et al.*, 1981), the volume of distribution is much the same in young and old subjects. Most data for midazolam, which is relatively lipid-soluble, indicate little or no increase in volume of distribution in the elderly (Avram *et al.*, 1983; Greenblatt *et al.*, 1984; Harper *et al.*, 1985), although in patients over 80 years of age a marked increase was observed (Servin *et al.*, 1987)

Studies of narcotic analgesics in the old indicate an increase or no change in the steady-state volumes of distribution of relatively lipid-soluble agents (pentidine, fentanyl, alfentanil) and a decrease in that of morphine (Holmberg *et al.*, 1982; Herman *et al.*, 1985; Bentley *et al.*, 1982; Helmers *et al.*, 1984; Owen *et al.*, 1983).

There is disagreement as to whether the steady-state volume of distribution of thiopentone (lipid-soluble) increases with age; the positive findings may reflect a preponderance of females in the patients studied (Homer & Stanski, 1985; Jung *et al.*, 1982; Christensen *et al.*, 1982).

Values for the water-soluble neuromuscular blocking agents were found to be either decreased (d-tubocurarine, vecuronium, metocurine) or unchanged (pancuronium) (Matteo *et al.*, 1985; Rupp *et al.*, 1983; Duvaldestin *et al.*, 1982).

Despite some exceptions, therefore, the expected interrelationship between lipid solubility, V_{SS} and age is apparent across a broad range of compounds.

Rate of distribution

Drugs do not distribute instantaneously into a homogeneous volume. Initial rates of distribution and redistribution will therefore be significant determinants of onset and decay of drug effects, particularly after single or loading doses.

Of paramount importance in these processes is blood flow, while the role of plasma protein binding is currently the subject of considerable experimental interest.

Blood flow

Although it has been suggested that cardiac output is maintained in healthy older subjects (Rodeheffer *et al.*, 1984), most old patients would be expected to show some decrease in this function. In an attempt to compensate, there is an increase in sympathetic tone allowing vital organs (heart and brain) to maintain their perfusion at the expense of peripheral and renal blood flow. These haemodynamic adjustments have several implications for drug distribution.

First, a slow circulation time (Hunter, 1947) will tend to delay initial delivery of drug to target organs and tissues after i.v. injection. This probably accounts for delayed muscle fasciculations following the administration of suxamethonium in the aged and, since they precede relaxation, a second (unnecessary) dose of drug might be given if the importance of the prolonged circulation time is not appreciated (Dundee, 1979). Old age has also been associated with a slow onset of pancuronium blockade (Donati & Bevan, 1986). In contrast, induction of anaesthesia with inhalation agents, particularly the more lipid-soluble ones, is faster in the old since, as cardiac output falls, alveolar concentrations approach those of the inspired air more rapidly (Krechel, 1984).

Second, if rate of drug administration is constant, a higher blood drug concentration may be delivered to the systemic circulation in older patients since this concentration should be directly proportional to dose and inversely related both to blood flow in the injected vein and to the duration of injection. Therefore, a lower peripheral blood flow will tend to concentrate an i.v. dose into a sharper bolus. Having left the right atrium the bolus of drug is then attenuated by transit through and uptake in the lungs (Tucker, 1978). However, it is not known whether this buffering effect of the lung on arterial drug concentrations is modified by age.

Third, the fractions of the dose delivered to brain and myocardium will be higher. Thus, dosage to these organs will be in the ratio of their blood flows to cardiac output. Barring gross sclerotic changes, the former tend to be maintained in the aged while the latter may be reduced. Effectively, a lowered perfusion in other organs and in the periphery directs a greater proportion of recirculated drug to the brain and the heart.

Classical pharmacokinetic theory is poorly equipped to describe the events occurring immediately after an i.v. injection of a drug. The parameter which is usually quoted is V_1, the initial volume of distribution, equal to the dose divided by the extrapolated blood drug concentration at zero time. The latter is best defined in terms of measurements in arterial blood since early drug concentrations in the peripheral venous system reflect local distribution and transit within the arm as well as systemic effects. Since the extrapolated drug concentration at zero time is purely hypothetical, the value of V_1, based on arterial blood sampling, represents a rather nebulous descriptor of initial dilution and mixing within the vascular supply on first transit from arm to aorta, modulated by pulmonary distribution with, possibly, a contribution from the disposition of recirculated drug.

Homer & Stanski (1985) concluded that the age-related decrease of thiopentone dose requirement is due to a change in initial distribution of the drug, i.e. V_1 decreases exponentially with age. A similar but weaker inverse correlation between V_1 and age was observed for etomidate using arterial data only (Arden et al., 1986). Relationships reported for other drugs indicate a decrease in V_1 in the old for morphine (Owen et al.,

1983), sufentanil (Matteo *et al.*, 1986), propofol (Nimmo — personal communication), d-tubocurarine and metocurine (Matteo *et al.*, 1985) and neostigmine (Young *et al.*, 1984); no change with fentanyl (Bentley *et al.*, 1982), alfentanil (Helmers *et al.*, 1984), chlordiazepoxide (Roberts *et al.*, 1978), midazolam (Avram *et al.*, 1983; Greenblatt *et al.*, 1984) and lignocaine (Nation *et al.*, 1977b); and an increase for pethidine (Herman *et al.*, 1985) and diazepam (Klotz *et al.*, 1975). These inconsistencies probably reflect the marked sensitivity of the value of V_1 to sampling time and sampling site.

Plasma drug binding

Alterations in plasma protein levels and plasma binding of drugs used in anaesthesia have been associated with changes in the onset of response. Thus, a correlation between the onset time of midazolam and plasma albumin level has been inferred to account for more rapid induction in the old (Halliday *et al.*, 1985), and increased d-tubocurarine requirements have been reported in patients with elevated gamma globulin levels (Dundee, 1979).

Although these correlations are very weak and may not reflect direct causal relationships, it is theoretically feasible that the extent of plasma binding may modulate the initial uptake of drugs by tissues. Recent experiments with a rat model of the brain uptake of drug, involving bolus injection into the carotid artery, demonstrate that extraction on the first-pass may be more or less restricted by plasma binding depending upon the unbound (distributive) clearance into the organ (Pardridge, 1986; Jones *et al.*, 1986). However, the impact of restrictive binding may depend upon the rate of drug injection. Thus, at the high concentrations of drugs circulated to vital organs immediately after a bolus input, considerable saturation of plasma binding sites may occur. Accordingly, the increased free fraction could contribute to greater response seen after fast compared to slow injection of the same dose. Experiments with thiopentone in rats seem to support this view (Kurtz & Fichtl, 1981), although saturable binding could not be demonstrated in patients at arterial plasma concentrations of thiopentone seen after usual induction doses (Burch & Stanski, 1983).

The issue of the role of plasma binding in drug distribution is complicated further by the observation that, depending upon the drug (propranolol, lignocaine, bupivacaine, benzodiazepines) and the binding protein (albumin, alpha$_1$-acid glycoprotein), first-pass brain uptake in rats was much greater than expected based on the unbound fraction (fu) measured *in vitro*, suggesting that binding equilibrium is significantly different and fu is higher within the brain capillaries than in larger blood vessels (Pardridge, 1986; Jones *et al.*, 1986). Therefore, at a given total blood drug concentration entering the brain, this phenomenon would tend to dampen any impact of alterations in plasma binding, as measured *in vitro*, on the initial free concentration of drug within the organ and hence pharmacological response. By the same reasoning, however, it has also been argued that in the case where total drug concentration entering the brain varies, and contrary to current dogma, total rather than free drug concentrations in plasma are better predictors of drug action (Pardridge, 1986). Thus, recent experimental findings on the influence of plasma drug binding on the uptake of drugs are provocative, and further studies are indicated to clarify the role of this phenomenon in pharmacokinetics.

Drug metabolism

Classical pharmacokinetic theory predicts that the maintenance doses of drugs which are predominantly eliminated by metabolism in the liver will depend upon the hepatic clearance of the unbound species (CLu). Any decrease in clearance will also contribute to a prolonged half-life, with implications for less frequent dosage. The physiological determinants of CLu are hepatic blood flow, the intrinsic ability of the enzymes to metabolize the drug and blood drug binding. The relative importance of these three variables changes with the hepatic extraction ratio of the drug and the route of administration (Rowland & Tozer, 1980).

Liver blood flow

Liver weight as a proportion of body weight decreases to half that of a young adult by the age of 80, and this is accompanied by a parallel fall in hepatic blood flow. Therefore, because of reduced perfusion, clearances (based on total blood drug concentration) of drugs with high hepatic extraction ratio (>0.7) would be expected to be lower in the old after parenteral administration. Data for etomidate (Arden *et al.*, 1986) and sufentanil (Matteo *et al.*, 1986) are compatible with this expectation, as are those for morphine (Owen *et al.*, 1983), although in this case extra hepatic metabolism may also contribute to its high systemic clearance. Studies with fentanyl, which is usually considered to be a high extraction drug (although published estimates of its extraction ratio vary considerably), have shown unchanged (Singleton *et al.*, 1985; Scott & Stanski, 1985) or decreased (Bentley *et al.*, 1982) clearance in the aged. Pethidine and lignocaine have intermediate extractions ratios (0.4–0.7) and their systemic clearance will be partially flow dependent. However, again the effect of age is unclear, some studies showing a decrease (lignocaine: Abernethy & Greenblatt, 1983; Cusson *et al.*, 1985; pethidine: Holmberg *et al.*, 1982) and others no change (lignocaine: Nation *et al.*, 1977; Cusack *et al.*, 1985; pethidine: Herman *et al.*, 1985). A study of lignocaine kinetics after lumbar epidural injection indicated a 33% lower clearance and a 10% increase in half-life in patients over 55 compared to those under 40, and suggested that some older patients might show excessive systemic accumulation of the local anaesthetic during continuous block procedures unless dosage is modified (Bowdle *et al.*, 1986). Methohexitone has a moderately high clearance but this was found to be unaffected by age (Ghoneim *et al.*, 1985).

Although hepatic blood flow is the major determinant of the total clearance of high extraction drugs, their unbound clearance should also be directly related to the extent of blood binding. Thus, for example, the effect of reduced liver blood flow in some aged patients might be offset by higher binding owing to raised alpha$_1$-acid glycoprotein levels.

Intrinsic enzyme activity

The decrease in liver weight with age might be expected to be associated with decrease drug metabolism as a result of fewer functioning cells. This may or may not be compounded by a deterioration in actual enzyme activity. In any event, changes in both enzyme capacity or activity should lower the intrinsic clearance of unbound drug (a measure of the $Vmax/K_m$ values of the enzymes involved). In theory, this should be manifest in the systemic (unbound) clearance of drugs with low extraction ratios (<0.4) and in the oral (unbound) clearance of drugs irrespective of their hepatic extraction ratio (Rowland & Tozer, 1980). Any alteration in plasma binding will complicate the interpretation of total clearance values since these are directly proportional to intrinsic clearance and inversely related to the extent of blood binding.

The influence of age on the clearance of low extraction drugs is highly variable. Nevertheless, studies with benzodiazepines have indicated that the clearance of oxidized compounds (e.g. diazepam, chlordiazepoxide, clobazam, midazolam) is impaired in the aged (although this seems to be selective for men, with little change in women), while that of compounds which undergo direct conjugation (e.g. oxazepam, lorazepam, temazepam) or nitro-reduction (nitrazepam) is preserved (Greenblatt *et al.*, 1986). Thiopentone and alfentanil are further examples of low clearance drugs studied in the aged. No clear decrease in the unbound clearance of thiopentone was observed, irrespective of the sex of the subjects (Jung *et al.*, 1982; Homer & Stanski, 1985). The total clearance of alfentanil was found to be lowered in one study (Helmers *et al.*, 1984) but unchanged in another (Scott & Stanski, 1985)

The generally small extent of change in the clearance of low extraction drugs with age should be viewed against the background of normal intersubject variability. Thus, for example, Vestal *et al.* (1975) showed that while there was a 600% variability between subjects in the hepatic clearance of antipyrine, age accounted for only 3% of the variance. On the other hand, benoxaprofen is also a low extraction drug yet it accumulates markedly in aged patients. However, in this case a rather special mechanism may be involved. Thus, in common with other drugs with carboxylic acid groups, including most of the anti-inflammatory agents, benoxaprofen undergoes extensive acyl-conjugation. These conjugates are relatively unstable and if their renal or biliary elimination is impaired, as it might be in the aged, they may undergo significant systemic deconjugation, thereby sustaining levels of the parent drugs (Verbeek *et al.*, 1984b).

A decrease in the intrinsic clearance of high extraction drugs may have a marked effect on the extent of their first-pass metabolism after oral administration, resulting in significantly elevated plasma drug concentrations. Such increases have been observed in aged patients with several compounds including propranolol (Castleden & George, 1979) and chlormethiazole (Nation *et al.*, 1977a). However, these findings were not confirmed by others (Schneider *et al.*, 1980; Hockings *et al.*, 1983). It is possible that raised $alpha_1$-acid glycoprotein levels in sick aged patients included in the original studies were responsible for the raised total plasma drug concentrations and that unbound concentrations, which reflect enzyme activity, were unchanged.

The literature on the relationship between induction and inhibition of drug metabolism as a function of age is confused. However, there is some evidence to suggest that an apparent decline in drug oxidation merely reflects either the decreased use of common enzyme inducers (cigarettes, alcohol, certain foods) in the aged or a lowered capacity for induction (Sellers *et al.*, 1983). Enzyme inhibition has been studied less extensively in the old but it would appear that the effect of cimetidine, as indicated by a decrease in antipyrine clearance, is similar in young and old subjects (Feely *et al.*, 1984).

Smithard & Langman (1977) believe that in the aged poor nutrition is at least partly responsible for decreased microsomal enzyme function. They noted that both vitamin C and folate are often below adequate concentrations in patients admitted to geriatric wards. A deficiency in humans of either of these vitamins has been associated with the impaired metabolism of some drugs.

The activity of extrahepatic enzymes involved in the metabolism of some drugs may change with age. For example, *in vitro* studies indicate a decline in the hydrolysis of suxamethonium by plasma cholinesterase in men but not women (Shanor *et al.*, 1961). This may offset the effect of a slow circulation time on the action of this drug. Thus, although more time would be available for hydrolysis on the way to the neuromuscular end-plate, the intrinsic clearance by the enzyme would be lower.

Blood drug binding

The influence of any changes in blood drug binding on the total and unbound systemic and oral clearances of high and low extraction drugs has been discussed with reference to established pharmacokinetic theory.

Implications for steady-state pharmacokinetics of the new evidence of enhanced free fractions within some vascular beds require clarification since it is suggested that CLu values determined using *in vitro* binding data do not necessarily predict free drug concentrations established in the brain and other organs (Pardridge, 1986).

Drug excretion

Renal function deteriorates by about 1% per year beyond the age of 20. This comprises changes in glomerular filtration rate (GFR), renal blood flow, tubular secretion and the ability to acidify the urine. Corresponding changes in renal drug clearance are anticipated and may be predicted approximately from a knowledge of creatinine clearance. Serum creatinine level is a poor index of renal function in the old since it represents the balance between synthesis and removal of creatinine, both of which may be reduced with age.

In the absence of renal disease, the renal clearance of a drug is likely to decrease by up to half in old age, and such a change may be significant only if a high fraction of the dose is normally excreted unchanged by the kidney and the compound has a low therapeutic ratio.

Most of the drugs used by the anaesthetist are relatively lipid-soluble and are therefore eliminated largely by metabolism rather than excretion. Exceptions include most of the non-depolarizing neuromuscular blocking agents. Thus, it has been shown that the total clearances of d-tubocurarine (Matteo *et al.*, 1985), pancuronium (Duvaldestin *et al.*, 1982), metocurine (Matteo *et al.*, 1985) and vecuronium (Rupp *et al.*, 1983) are lower in the aged, suggesting a smaller maintenance dose requirement. Apart from the case of vecuronium, where the concomitant decrease in volume of distribution compensates fully, these lower clearances are accompanied by increases in elimination half-life and duration of effect. The fractional contribution of renal clearance to the total clearance of the agents varies from 0.2 for vecuronium to 0.4–0.5 for d-tubocurarine, pancuronium and metocurine. Therefore, it is possible that impaired clearance by routes other than renal, notably through the bile, contributes to altered kinetics in aged patients. However, the effect of age on biliary drug clearance is relatively unexplored.

About 70% of a dose of edrophonium is excreted unchanged in the urine and the clearance of this compound was found to be halved in a group of old patients compared to young controls. Its elimination half-life was also prolonged, yet the kinetic changes were not reflected in any alteration in duration of action with respect to reversal of neuromuscular blockade (Silverberg *et al.*, 1986).

Other drugs which require special consideration in the aged owing to impaired renal function include digoxin, aminoglycosides, chlorpropamide, cimetidine and frusemide.

Cimetidine is excreted almost entirely unchanged by the kidney and it ranks high among drugs causing confusion in debilitated aged patients and those with decreased renal function.

Old people have a vulnerable circulatory homeostasis and the administration of high-ceiling diuretics with a prompt onset of action like frusemide can place them at risk of acute hypovolaemia as well as many other side-effects. However, to some extent, the aged patient is protected from the circulatory effects of frusemide in a standard adult dose. This is because it acts from within the lumen of the renal tubule. Thus, any decrease in glomerular filtration of water and electrolytes and reduced renal secretion of the drug itself will attenuate, or at least delay, the diuretic response (Kerremans et al., 1983; Chaudry et al., 1984).

Drug metabolites are generally more water-soluble than their parent compounds and consequently are more likely to have higher renal clearances. Therefore, if they retain pharmacological activity or contribute to toxicity, any impairment of their renal excretion may have to be considered. Possible candidates for greater accumulation under these conditions include the active 6-glucuronide of morphine and norpethidine, the N-desethyl product of pethidine, which has convulsant activity.

Pharmacodynamics

If the response to a drug were shown to be different in old and young subjects at the same steady-state concentration of unbound drug, and any differences in ionization are allowed for, this would suggest the involvement of an age-related pharmacodynamic change. In turn, there would be a need to establish whether the observations resulted from changes in the number of receptors, their affinity for the drug or whether postreceptor events were involved. Also, homeostatic adjustments, or the lack of them, due to age-related changes in receptors or control systems not directly affected by the drug could complicate the issue and might need to be considered.

Several experimental approaches have been used in attempts to quantify pharmacodynamic changes in the old: similar plasma drug concentrations have been established in groups of young and old subjects; non steady-state studies have involved the application of combined pharmacokinetic-pharmacodynamic modelling to calculate indices of the Hill equation relating drug concentration to response (EC50 — the steady-state plasma drug concentration associated with half maximal response, and γ — a power function describing the steepness of the concentration–response curve); isolated human tissues (e.g. pieces of artery) and blood components (e.g. lymphocytes, platelets) have been used as models of tissue receptors.

The limited success achieved with these approaches is illustrated below with data for selected drugs.

Thiopentone

Using a combined pharmacokinetic-pharmacodynamic model and a power spectral analysis of the electroencephalogram (EEG) to measure response, Homer & Stanski (1985) found no difference in EC50 values, based on either unbound or total plasma drug concentrations, or γ values in groups of young and old subjects. They concluded that 'brain sensitivity' to thiopentone is not increased in the old, and that the age-related decrease in dose requirement may be explained by the change in the initial distribution of the drug.

Whether 'anaesthesia' may be equated with EEG changes is debatable. Further studies are required to clarify this point and to see if the findings are common to other anaesthetic agents. Certainly ageing is associated with significant decreases in the quantity and quality of neuronal elements and a depletion of central neurotransmitters, which might be expected to contribute to altered response to drugs acting in the CNS.

Benzodiazepines

Although many studies have established that the benzodiazepines show pharmacokinetic differences in the old, there is some evidence also for age-related pharmacodynamic changes.

One of the better studies providing this evidence is that of Swift *et al.* (1985) who showed that the administration of a single 10 mg oral dose of diazepam to fit, aged subjects resulted in similar plasma drug concentrations to those observed in young controls, but that postural sway was markedly accentuated. Smaller differences were noted in speed-dependent performance tasks. These results are indicative of a selective change in 'receptor sensitivity'. Nevertheless, a kinetic explanation cannot be entirely ruled out since steady-state was not achieved and plasma drug concentrations after a single dose may be insensitive indicators of the rate of drug uptake into the CNS. Also, there may be age-related differences in the distribution of the drug within the brain.

Alterations in benzodiazepine receptors may explain increased 'sensitivity' in the old but no differences in the number or affinity of such receptors have been detected in the brains of senescent mice and rats (Tsang *et al.*, 1982). Alternatively, there might be changes in the CNS levels of the postulated endogenous ligand or in other homeostatic mechanisms within the nervous system.

There is some evidence of adaptation to oversedation in the old during chronic administration of benzodiazepines, despite accumulation of the parent drugs and their active metabolites (Swift *et al.*, 1983).

Opioid analgesics

In a preliminary report, Scott & Stanski (1985) indicate that the decrease in dose requirements of fentanyl and alfentanil in the aged is not explained by a pharmacokinetic mechanism but by a decrease in the EC50 values of the analgesics with age. A combined pharmacokinetic-pharmacodynamic model was used and the effect end-point was based upon EEG power spectrum analysis.

Further work is needed to see how the EEG changes relate to clinical analgesia, sensitivity to ventilatory depression, opioid receptor binding and the turnover of endorphins as a function of age.

Muscle relaxants

There appear to be no significant differences in log plasma concentration–twitch response relationships between 20–80% paralysis in young patients and old patients receiving non-depolarizing neuromuscular blockers (Duvaldestin *et al.*, 1982; Matteo *et al.*, 1985; Rupp *et al.*, 1983). More prolonged blockade in the old can be explained by pharmacokinetic changes.

However, this does not necessarily mean that there are no effects of ageing on events at the neuromuscular junction. Thus, it is possible that peripheral denervation and loss of skeletal muscle mass is compensated for by the proliferation of muscle end-plates and acetylcholine receptors.

Adrenergic agents

Ageing is accompanied by a decrease in the maximum responsiveness of the heart to catecholamines and an increase in vascular loading during exercise. This is associated with a decline in beta adrenoceptor-mediated function, reflected in a reduced response to both agonists (e.g. isoprenaline, terbutaline) and antagonists (e.g. propranolol). Although the issue is complicated by the presence of physiological reflexes which may themselves be altered by age, it is likely that there are direct changes at the receptor or postreceptor level. This is confirmed by studies showing that beta adrenoceptor responsiveness, as measured by isoprenaline stimulation of lymphocytic cyclic AMP production, is decreased in cells from old people. Since there is probably no change in lymphocyte beta adrenoceptor density with ageing but the affinity of the receptors is altered, it appears that a functional uncoupling of the beta receptor-adenylate cyclase system occurs in old age (O'Malley & Kelly, 1983; Feldman *et al.*, 1984).

The effects of ageing on alpha adrenoceptor-mediated events is not so well documented, but there is emerging evidence that some effects mediated by alpha$_2$ receptors postsynaptically are diminished in both animal models and in human veins. These changes may have significance in relation to postural hypotension in the aged.

Atropine

Prolonged sedation after the administration of atropine to aged patients is consistent with observations of a reduced clearance and prolonged half-life. On the other hand, a greater dose is required to accelerate the heart rate in the aged. This may reflect either an age-related change at the cholinergic receptor or the effect of altered cardiovascular reflexes (Virtanen *et al.*, 1982).

Warfarin

Several studies have shown that the dose requirements of warfarin are decreased substantially in the old, although the contribution of other patient variables to this decline is unclear. Since the pharmacokinetics of the anticoagulant are not considered to be different in old age, it appears that pharmacodynamic changes may be involved (O'Malley & Kelly, 1983). As yet, these have not been identified but they could relate to alterations in the kinetics or dynamics of vitamin K.

Local anaesthetics

It is not known whether the old have altered thresholds to the CNS and cardiovascular toxicity of local anaesthetics, independent of pharmaco-kinetic considerations. There are data to suggest that the levels of latent anxiety and sensitivity to pain predict CNS sensitivity to these drugs (Korbon *et al.*, 1984), and pain thresholds may differ in old and young patients.

Lowered local anaesthetic dosage requirements in the aged do not appear to be related to any impairment of the rate of systemic drug uptake. Changes in local distribution and interaction at axoplasmic receptor sites are likely to be more important (Bromage, 1978). Thus, advancing age is accompanied by a steady decline in the neural population, together with a decrease in conduction velocity and deterioration of myelin sheaths and connective tissue barriers. All of these changes are accelerated by arteriosclerosis.

Concluding remarks

For some drugs, lowered dosage requirements and an increased risk of toxicity have been documented in the aged. Also, progress continues to be made towards unravelling the causes of age-related changes in drug response. However, translating this information into precise dosage recommendations for the *individual* patient remains vague. Ageing is only one of the many sources of variability in drug response and indeed in many cases its importance may pall in relation to the contributions from genetic and environmental factors and from the effects of disease, surgery, anaesthesia and drug interactions. At the practical level, prevention is better than cure and the anaesthetist who knows the literature and who can integrate the likely impact of each of these factors may be better at anticipating the 'right' dose. It remains to be seen whether automated approaches to this, based upon the application of 'population pharmacokinetics', rate-controlled drug delivery and the development of flexible control systems, which allow rapid adjustment of plasma drug concentrations and pharmacological response, will improve patient care.

References

Abernethy, D.R. & Greenblatt, D.J. (1983) Impairment of lidocaine clearance in elderly male subjects. *J. Cardiovasc. Pharmacol.* **5**, 1093–1096.

Arden, J.R., Holley, F.O. & Stanski, D.R. (1986) Increased sensitivity to etomidate in the elderly: Initial distribution versus altered brain response. *Anesthesiology* **65**, 19–27.

Arunsalam, K., Davenport, H.T., Painter, S. & Jones, J.G. (1983) Ventilatory response to morphine in young and old subjects. *Anaesthesia* **38**, 529–533.

Avram, M.J., Fragen, R.J. & Caldwell, N.J. (1983) Midazolam kinetics in women of two age groups. *Clin. Pharmacol. Ther.* **34**, 505–508.

Bellville, J.W., Forest, W.H., Miller, E. & Brown, B.W. (1971) Influence of age on pain relief from analgesics. *J. Am. Med. Ass.* **217**, 1835–1841.

Bentley, J.B., Borel, J.D., Nenad, R. & Gillespie, T.J. (1982) Age and fentanyl pharmacokinetics. *Anesth. Analg.* **61**, 968–971.

Boston Collaborative Drug Surveillance Program (1973) Clinical depression of the central nervous system due to diazepam and chlordiazepoxide in relation to cigarette smoking and age. *New Engl. J. Med.* **288**, 277–280.

Bowdle, T.A., Freund, P.R. & Slattery, J.T. (1986) Age-dependent lidocaine pharmacokinetics during lumbar peridural anesthesia with lidocaine hydrocarbonate or lidocaine hydrochloride. *Reg. Anaesth.* **11**, 123–127.

Bromage, P.R. (1978) *Epidural Analgesia.* Saunders, Philadelphia, pp. 40–42; 137–139.

Burch, P.G. & Stanski, D.R. (1983) The role of metabolism and protein binding in thiopental anesthesia. *Anesthesiology* **58**, 146–152.

Castleden, C.M. & George, C.F. (1979) The effect of ageing on the hepatic clearance of propranolol. *Br. J. Clin. Pharmacol.* **7**, 49–54.

Chaudry, A.Y., Bing, R.F., Castleden, C.M. Swales, J.D. & Napier, C.J. (1984) The effect of ageing on the response to frusemide in normal subjects. *Eur. J. Clin. Pharmacol.* **27**, 303–306.

Christensen, J.H. & Andreasen, F. (1978) Individual variation in response to thiopental. *Acta Anaesth. Scand.* **22**, 303–313.

Christensen, J.H., Andreasen, F. & Jansen, J.A. (1982) Pharmacokinetics of thiopentone. A comparison between young and elderly patients. *Anaesthesia* **37**, 398–404.

Cusack, B., O'Malley, K., Lavan, J., Noel, J. & Kelly, J.G. (1985) Protein binding and disposition of lignocaine in the elderly. *Eur. J. Clin. Pharmacol.* **29**, 323–329.

Cusson, J., Nattel, S., Matthews, C., Talajic, M. & Lawand, S. (1985) Age-dependent lidocaine disposition in patients with acute myocardial infarction. *Clin. Pharmacol. Ther.* **37**, 381–386.

Davis, D., Grossman, S.H., Kitchell, B.B., Shand, D.G. & Routledge, P.A. (1985) The effects of age and smoking on the plasma protein binding of lignocaine and diazepam. *Br. J. Clin. Pharmacol.* **19**, 261–265.

Daykin, A.P., Bowen, D.J., Saunders, D.A. & Norman, J. (1986) Respiratory depression after morphine in the elderly. *Anaesthesia,* **41**, 910–914.

Divoll, M. & Greenblatt, D.J. (1982) Effect of age and sex on lorazepam protein binding. *J. Pharm. Pharmacol.* **34**, 122–123.

Divoll, M., Greenblatt, D.J., Harmatz, J.S. & Shader, R.I. (1981) Effect of age and gender on disposition of temazepam. *J. Pharm. Sci.* **70**, 1104–1107.

Divoll, M., Greenblatt, D.J., Ochs, H.R. & Shader, R.I. (1983) Absolute bioavailability of oral and intramuscular diazepam: Effects of age and sex. *Anesth. Analg.* **62**, 1–8.

Donati, F. & Bevan, D.R. (1986) The influence of patient's sex, age and weight on pancuronium onset time. *Can. Anaesth. Soc. J.* **33**, S86.

Dundee, J.W. (1954) The influence of body weight, sex and age on the dosage of thiopentone. *Br. J. Anaesth.* **26**, 164–173.

Dundee, J.W. (1979) Response to anaesthetic drugs in the elderly. In *Drugs and the Elderly. Perspectives in Geriatric Clinical Pharmacology* (Eds J. Crooks & I.H. Stevenson). Macmillan, London, pp. 179–188.

Dundee, J. W., Robinson, F.P., McCollum, J.S.C. & Patterson, C.C. (1986) Sensitivity to propofol in the elderly. *Anaesthesia* **41**, 482–485.

Duvaldestin, P., Saada, J., Berger, J.L., D'Hollander, A. & Desmonts, J.M. (1982) Pharmacokinetics, pharmacodynamics, and dose-response relationships of pancuronium in control and elderly subjects. *Anesthesiology* **56**, 36–40.

Feely, J., Pereira, L., Guy, E. & Hockings, N. (1984) Factors affecting the response to inhibition of drug metabolism by cimetidine — dose response and sensitivity of elderly and induced subjects. *Br. J. Clin. Pharmacol.* **17**, 77–81.

Feldman, R.D., Limbird, L.E., Nadeau, J., Robertson, D. & Wood, A.J.J. (1984) Alterations in leukocyte beta-receptor affinity with aging. A potential explanation for altered beta-adrenergic sensitivity in the elderly. *New Engl. J. Med.* **310**, 815–819.

Finucane, B.T. & Hammonds, W.D. (1984) Influence of age on vascular absorption of lidocaine injected epidurally in man. *Reg. Anaesth.* **9**, 36–37.

Freund, P.R., Bowdle, T.A., Slattery, J.T. & Bell, L.E. (1984) Caudal anesthesia with lidocaine or bupivacaine: Plasma local anesthetic concentration and extent of sensory spread in old and young patients. *Anaesth. Analg.* **63**, 1017–1020.

Ghoneim, M.M., Chiang, C.K., Schoenwald, R.D., Lilburn, J.K. & Dhanaraj, J. (1985) The pharmacokinetics of methohexital in young and elderly subjects. *Acta Anaesth. Scand.* **29**, 480–482.

Greenblatt, D.J. & Allen, M.D. (1978) Toxicity of nitrazepam in the elderly: A report from the Boston Collaborative Drug Surveillance Program. *Br. J. Clin. Pharmacol.* **5**, 407–413.

Greenblatt, D.J., Allen, M.D., Locniskar, A., Harmatz, J.S. & Shader, R.I. (1979) Lorazepam kinetics in the elderly. *Clin. Pharmacol. Ther.* **26**, 103–113.

Greenblatt, D.J., Allen, M.D., Harmatz, J.S. & Shader, R.I. (1980) Diazepam disposition determinants. *Clin. Pharmacol. Ther.* **27**, 301–312.

Greenblatt, D.J., Divoll, M., Puri, S.K., Ho, I., Zinny, M.A. & Shader, R.I. (1981) Clobazam kinetics in the elderly. *Br. J. Clin. Pharmacol.* **12**, 631–636.

Greenblatt, D.J., Abernethy, D.R., Locniskar, A., Harmatz, J.S., Limjuco, R.A. & Shader, R.I. (1984) Effect of age, gender, and obesity on midazolam kinetics. *Anaesthesiology* **61**, 27–35.

Greenblatt, D.J., Abernethy, D.R. & Shader, R.I. (1986) Pharmacokinetic aspects of drug therapy in the elderly. *Ther. Drug Monit.* **8**, 249–255.

Gustaffson, L.L., Schildt, B. & Jacobsen, K. (1982) Adverse effects of extradural and intrathecal opiates: Report of a nationwide survey in Sweden. *Br. J. Anaesth.* **54**, 479–486.

Halliday, N.J., Dundee, J.W., Collier, P.S., Loughran, P.G. & Harper, K.W. (1985) Influence of plasma proteins on the onset of hypnotic action of intravenous midazolam. *Anaesthesia* **40**, 763–766.

Harper, K.W., Collier, P.S., Dundee, J.W., Elliot, P., Halliday, N.J. & Lowry, K.G. (1985) Age and nature of operation influence the pharmacokinetics of midazolam. *Br. J. Anaesth.* **57**, 866–871.

Helmers, H., Van Peer, A., Woestenborghs, R., Noorduin, H. & Heykants, J. (1984) Alfentanil kinetics in the elderly. *Clin. Pharmacol. Ther.* **36**, 239–243.

Herman, R.J., McAllister, C.B., Branch, R.A. & Wilkinson, G.R. (1985) Effects of age on meperidine dispositon. *Clin. Pharmacol. Ther.* **37**, 19–24.

Hilton, P, Dev, V.J. & Major, E. (1986) Intravenous anaesthesia with propofol and alfentanil. The influence of age and weight. *Anaesthesia* **41**, 640–643.

Hockings, N., Stevenson, I.H. & Swift, C.G. (1983) Age-related pharmacokinetics of single doses of chlormethiazole and dichlorphenazone. *Br. J. Clin. Pharmacol.* **15**, 616P.

Holmberg, L., Odar-Cederlof, I., Boreus, L.O., Heyner, L. & Ehrnebo, M. (1982) Comparative disposition of pethidine and norpethidine in old and young patients. *Eur. J. Clin. Pharmacol.* **22**, 175–179.

Homer, T.D. & Stanski, D.R. (1985) The effect of increasing age on thiopental disposition and anesthetic requirement. *Anesthesiology* **62**, 714–724.

Hunter, A.R. (1947) Intravenous anaesthesia and circulation time. *Br. Med. J.* **1**, 16.

Jones, D.R., Hall, S.D., Branch, R.A., Jackson, E.K. & Wilkinson, G.R. (1986) Plasma binding and brain uptake of benzodiazepines. In *Protein Binding and Drug Transport* (Symposia Medica Hoechst 20) (Eds J-P. Tillement & E. Lindenlaub). Schattauer, Stuttgart & New York, pp. 311–324.

142 | *Chapter 8*

Jung, D., Mayersohn, M., Perrier, D., Calkins, J. & Saunders, R. (1982) Thiopental disposition as a function of age in female patients undergoing surgery. *Anesthesiology* **56**, 263–268.

Kerremans, A.L.M., Tan, Y., van Baars, H., van Ginneken, A.M. & Gribnau, F.W.J. (1983) Furosemide kinetics and dynamics in aged patients. *Clin. Pharmacol. Ther.* **34**, 181–189.

Krechel, S.W. (1984) Inhalation agents in the aged. In *Anesthesia and the Geriatric Patient* (Ed. S.W. Krechel). Grune & Stratton, Orlando, pp. 115–126.

Korbon, G.A., Rowlingson, J.C. & DiFazio, C.A. (1984) Sensitivity to pain predicts CNS sensitivity to lidocaine. *Anesthesiology* **61**, 767–769.

Kurtz, H. & Fichtl, B. (1981) Interrelation between plasma protein binding, rate of injection and the anaesthetic effect of thiopental. *Biopharm. Drug Dispos.* **2**, 191–196.

Macklon, A.F., Barton, M., James, O. & Rawlins, M.D. (1980) The effect of age on the pharmacokinetics of diazepam. *Clin. Sci.* **59**, 479–483.

Matteo, R.S., Backus, W.W., McDaniel, D.D., Brotherton, W.P., Abraham, R. & Diaz, J. (1985) Pharmacokinetics and pharmacodynamics of d-tubocurarine and metocurine in the elderly. *Anesth. Analg.* **64**, 23–29.

Matteo, R.S., Ornstein, E., Young, W.L., Schwartz, A.E., Port, M. & Chang, W.J. (1986) Pharmacokinetics of sufentanil in the elderly. *Anesth. Analg.* **65**, S94.

Murray, T.G., Chiang, S.T., Koepke, H.H. & Walker, B.R. (1981) Renal disease, age, and oxazepam kinetics. *Clin. Pharmacol. Ther.* **30**, 805–809.

Nation, R.L., Vine, J., Triggs, E.J. & Learoyd, B. (1977a) Plasma level of chlormethiazole and two metabolites after oral administration to young and aged human subjects. *Eur. J. Clin. Pharmacol.* **12**, 137–145.

Nation, R.L., Triggs, E.J. & Selig, M. (1977b) Lignocaine kinetics in cardiac patients and aged subjects. *Br. J. Clin. Pharmacol.* **4**, 439–448.

O'Malley, K. & Kelly, J.G. (1983) Aging and responsiveness to drugs. In *Recent Advances in Clinical Pharmacology* (Eds D.G. Shand & P. Turner), Churchill Livingstone, Edinburgh, pp. 45–56.

Owen, J.A., Sitar, D.S., Berger, L., Brownell, L., Duke, P.C. & Mitenko, P.A. (1983) Age-related morphine kinetics. *Clin. Pharmacol. Ther.* **34**, 364–368.

Pardridge, W.M. (1986) Transport of plasma-bound drugs into tissues in vivo. In *Protein Binding and Drug Transport* (Symposia Medica Hoechst 20) (Eds J-P. Tillement & E. Lindenlaub). Schattauer, Stuttgart & New York, pp. 277–292.

Park, E.Y., Massengale, M., Kim, S.L., Puck, K.C. & Macnamara, T.E. (1980) Age and the spread of local anesthetic solutions in the epidural space. *Anesth. Analg.* **59**, 768–771.

Paxton, J.W. & Briant, R.H. (1984) Alpha$_1$ acid-glycoprotein concentration and propranolol binding in elderly patients with acute illness. *Br. J. Clin. Pharmacol.* **18**, 806–810.

Roberts, R.K., Wilkinson, G.R., Branch, R.A. & Schenker, S. (1978) Effect of age and cirrhosis on the disposition and elimination of chlordiazepoxide. *Gastroenterology* **75**, 479–485.

Rodeheffer, R.J., Gerstenblith, G., Becker, L.C., Fles, L.C., Weisfeldt, M.L. & Lakatta, E.G. (1984) Exercise cardiac output is maintained with advancing age in healthy human subjects: Cardiac dilatation and increased stroke volume compensate for a diminished heart rate. *Circulation* **69**, 203–213.

Rosenberg, P.H., Saramies, L. & Alila, A. (1981) Lumbar epidural anaesthesia with bupivacaine in old patients: Effect of speed and direction of injection. *Acta Anaesth. Scand.* **25**, 270–274.

Rowland, M. & Tozer, T.N. (1980) *Clinical Pharmacokinetics. Concepts and Applications.* Lea & Febiger, Philadephia.

Rupp, S.M., Fisher, D.M., Miller, R.D. & Castagonli, K. (1983) Pharmacokinetics and the pharmacodynamics of vecuronium in the elderly. *Anesthesiology* **59**, A270.

Schneider, R.E., Bishop, H., Yates, R.A., Quarterman, C.P. & Kendall, M.J. (1980) Effect of age on plasma propanolol levels. *Br. J. Clin. Pharmacol.* **10**, 169–171.

Scott, J.C. & Stanski, D. (1985) Decreased fentanyl/alfentanil requirements with increasing age: A pharmacodynamic basis. *Anesthesiology* **63**, A374.

Sellers, E.M., Frecker, R.C. & Romach, M.K. (1983) Drug metabolism in the elderly: Confounding of age, smoking and ethanol effects. *Drug Metab. Rev.* **14**, 225–250.

Servin, F., Enriquez, I., Fournet, M., Failler, J.M., Farinotti, R. & Desmonts, J-M. (1987)

| *Altered drug effects in the aged*

Pharmacokinetics of midazolam used as an intravenous induction agent for patients over 80 years of age. *Eur. J. Anaesth.* **4**, 1–7.

Shanor, S.P., Van Hees, G.R., Baart, N., Erdos, E.G. & Foldes, F.F. (1961) The influence of age and sex on human plasma and red cell cholinesterase. *Am. J. Med. Sci.* **242**, 357–361.

Silverberg, P.A., Matteo, R.S., Ornstein, E, Young, W.L. & Diaz, J. (1986) Pharmacokinetics and pharmacodynamics of edrophonium in the elderly. *Anesth. Analg.* **65**, S142.

Singleton, M.A., Rosen, J.I. & Fisher, D.M. (1985) Pharmacokinetics of fentanyl in the elderly. *Anesthesiology* **63**, A372.

Smith, D.S., Orkin, F.K., Gardiner, S.M. & Zakeosian, G. (1979) Prolonged sedation in the elderly after intraoperative atropine administration. *Anesthesiology* **51**, 348–349.

Smithard, D.J. & Langman, M.J.S. (1977) Drug metabolism in the elderly. *Br. Med. J.* **2**, 520–521.

Swift, C.G., Ewen, J.M., Clark, P. & Stevenson, I.H. (1985) Responsiveness to oral diazepam in the elderly: relationship to total and free plasma concentrations. *Br. J. Clin. Pharmacol.* **20**, 111–118.

Swift, C.G., Swift, M.R., Hamley, J., Stevenson, I.H. & Crooks, J. (1983) CNS effects of chronic benzodiazepine hypnotic ingestion in the elderly. *Br. J. Clin. Pharmacol.* **16**, 217P–218P.

Tsang, C.C., Speeg, K.V. & Wilkinson, G.R. (1982) Aging and benzodiazepine binding in the rat cerebral cortex. *Life Sci.* **30**, 343–346.

Tucker, G.T. (1978) Pharmacokinetic aspects of the intravenous bolus. In *Adverse Response to Intravenous Drugs* (Eds J. Watkins & A. Milford-Ward) Academic Press, London, pp. 1–15.

Verbeek, R.K., Cardinal, E-J. & Wallace, S.M. (1984a) Effect of age and sex on the plasma binding of acidic and basic drugs. *Eur. J. Clin. Pharmacol.* **27**, 91–97.

Verbeek, R.K., Wallace, S.M. & Loewen, G.R. (1984b) Reduced elimination of ketoprofen in the elderly is not necessarily due to impaired glucuronidation. *Br. J. Clin. Pharmacol.* **17**, 783–784.

Vestal, R.E., Norris, P.K., Tobin, J.D., Cohen, B.H., Shock, N.W. & Andres, R. (1975) Antipyrine metabolism in man: Influence of age, alcohol, caffeine and smoking. *Clin. Pharmacol. Ther.* **18**, 425–432.

Virtanen, R., Kanto, J., Iisalo, E., Iisalo, M., Salo, M. & Sjovall, S. (1982) Pharmacokinetic studies on atropine with special reference to age. *Acta Anaesth. Scand.* **26**, 297–300.

Young, W.L., Backus, W., Matteo, R.S., Ornstein, E. & Diaz, J. (1984) Pharmacokinetics and pharmacodynamics of neostigmine in the elderly. *Anesthesiology* **61**, A300.

Further reading

Caird, F.I. & Scott, P.J.E. (1986) *Drug-Induced Diseases in the Elderly. A Critical Survey of the Literature.* Elsevier, Amsterdam. (Written by geriatricians. Each point is set out in numbered paragraphs. Easy to read for those who want quick and up-to-date information.)

Massoud, N. (1984) Pharmacokinetic considerations in geriatric patients. In *Pharmacokinetic Basis for Drug Treatment* (Eds L.Z. Benet, N. Massoull & J.G. Gambertoglio Raven Press, New York. (Contains extensive tables documenting quantitative changes in the pharmacokinetics of all kinds of drugs in the aged. The rest of the book describes the influence of disease on pharmacokinetics.)

O'Malley, K.(Ed.) (1984). *Clinical Pharmacology and Drug Treatment in the Elderly.* Churchill Livingstone, Edinburgh. (A description of the types and sources of altered responsiveness to drugs and the best way to use drugs in the elderly.)

Brocklehurst, J.C. (Eds.) (1984). *Geriatric Pharmacology and Therapeutics.* Blackwell Scientific Publications, Oxford. (Teachers of geriatric medicine present the principles and practice of drug use.)

Swift, G.G. 1987 *Clinical Pharmacology in the Elderly.* Marcel Dekker Inc., New York. (A multinational survey.)

9 | The milieu interieur in the aged*

M.D.W. LYE

Introduction

One of the hallmarks of the ageing process is a loss of homeostatic regulation so that, with increasing age, the ability to maintain the milieu interieur under stress is impaired. Central to the milieu interieur is the water and electrolyte composition of fluids both without and within metabolically active cells. All healthy aged subjects, even nonagenarians have a 'normal' distribution of water and electrolytes in the unstressed state. It is only when the system is perturbed that disequilibrium is likely to develop. The effects of stress are exaggerated in the old and they take much longer to restore equilibrium following stress than do their younger counterparts. This may be made worse by pre-existing age-related acute or chronic disease(s). The contribution of long-term drug therapy is also important in this regard.

One of the most stressful events in an old person's life is the assault of a surgical operation requiring general anaesthesia. Unfortunately, those surgical conditions which so often afflict the elderly cannot always be anticipated, resulting in a less than ideal situation. It is a triumph of modern anaesthetic practice that mortality of acute surgery has diminished so dramatically in the old. It is almost true to say that now, with good anaesthesia, no aged person is too unfit for a life-saving operation. Whilst much attention has been rightly focused on mortality, morbidity is also important. Here, the anaesthetist has a crucial role, particularly in regard to perioperative management and maintenance of water and electrolyte homeostasis. Serious deviations from the milieu interieur lead to prolongation of recovery and to the development of dependency in aged patients. The consequence of such a state increases overall length of hospital stay, favours the development of secondary complications and prolongs expensive hospital rehabilitation before the patient is able to return to the community.

The objective of this chapter is to acquaint anaesthetists managing aged patients with the effects of 'normal ageing' on homeostatic mechanisms and to alert them to possible pre-existing disease(s) which may hamper efforts to restore homeostatic equilibrium. Decisions taken in the three perioperative stages can lead to a lower immediate mortality and morbidity and shorter length of hospital stay, and thus better utilization of scarce and expensive hospital recourses.

*Claude Bernard used the term 'milieu interieur' for the physiochemical composition and physiological constancy of body fluids.

Ageing and renal function

Increasing age in healthy individuals leads to a significant reduction in renal blood flow (Hollenberg et al., 1974). This may be exacerbated by the presence of arteriosclerosis affecting the renal arteries or, more commonly, by long standing cardiac failure (Dunnill & Halley, 1973). Loss of nutrient supply leads to a progressive loss of functioning nephrons (Fig. 9.1). This decline in nephron numbers is almost linear with age after 40 years and occurs at an approximate rate of 1% per annum (Epstein, 1979). The functional capacity of healthy kidneys is so great that even in advanced old age renal function is able to maintain normal homeostasis at rest. Stress, whether pathological, traumatic or iatrogenic is likely, however, to 'overload' the system, producing variably transient 'renal failure'.

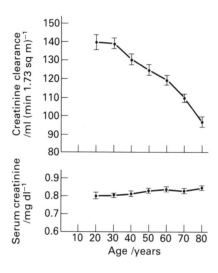

Fig. 9.1 The relationship of creatinine clearance with age. The minimal increase of serum creatinine with age is due to the reduction of active cell mass (from Rowe et al., 1976). (Reproduced with permission of the *Journal of Gerontology.*)

Water balance

The assessment of the hydration of aged patients is extremely difficult. The loose, lax skin due to age changes in the collagen matrix makes skin 'pinching' an unreliable physical sign. Sunken eyes in the aged are commonly due to entropion. Valuable clues can be obtained from the circumstances preceding the patient's admission to hospital. Unfortunately, the patient may be unable or unwilling to give this information, failing to see its relevance in the face of an acute breakdown. A history taken from relatives, neighbours and even ambulancemen can be crucial. Any aged patient living alone who has been immobilized in bed or on the floor for more than eight hours should be assumed to be significantly dehydrated until proved otherwise. They may also be hypothermic and this should be checked in all cases by recording the rectal temperature with a low reading thermometer.

The intracellular fluid (ICF) volume decreases with increasing age in all mammals. In the main, this is due to the loss of metabolically active cells from the lean body mass (Lye, 1981, 1984a) (Fig. 9.2). To a lesser extent, cells also lose fluid (dry-out). This is particularly seen with post-mitotic cells (neurones and muscle cells). The loss of lean body mass and the disproportionate increase in body fat (Durnin & Womersley, 1974) have important consequences, particularly on the pharmacokinetics of various drugs often used in anaesthesia (Saraiva *et al.*, 1977).

Other body fluid compartments change less with age than the ICF. Thus, the extracellular fluid (ECF) and plasma volumes change little with age (Chien *et al.*, 1966; Bruce *et al.*, 1980). Transcellular volumes do not change, with the exception of the cerebrospinal fluid volume which, because of a small loss of postmitotic cells and a greater loss of glial supporting cells, actually increases significantly with increasing age. The total blood volume decreases, primarily due to a decrease in the red cell mass. The overall haemoglobin concentration therefore changes little. The intravascular oncotic pressure is further reduced by a decreased rate of synthesis of albumin by the liver (Hodkinson, 1977). The reduction in the concentration of plasma albumin further affects drug pharmacokinetics, particularly of the protein-bound drugs.

The control of water balance becomes significantly impaired with increasing age. Hypothalamic 'osmoreceptors' are less able to 'drive the aged subject to drink' as they would in a younger individual. The sensation of thirst is markedly blunted and old patients with or without disability may inhabit a water desert. This is particularly seen in patients with hemiplegic strokes who often develop significant and clinically relevant hypernatraemia (Himmelstein *et al.*, 1983).

Renal tubules are less able to conserve water in the presence of dehydration. Somewhat surprisingly, this is not due to any impairment

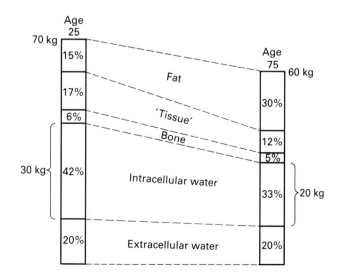

Fig. 9.2. Diagrammatic representation of changes of some major body components in aged females (from Davenport, 1986, fig. 1.10). (Reproduced with permission of Heinemann Medical Books.)

147 | *The milieu interieur in the aged*

of antidiuretic hormone secretion; in fact, rather the opposite. Dehydrated aged patients have an exaggerated anti-diuretic hormone response to various stimuli including dehydration (Kirkland *et al.*, 1984). It seems that the renal tubular response to arginine vasopressin (AVP) — human anti-diuretic hormone — in both animals and man is markedly attenuated. The accumulated effects of reduced water intake and inefficient conservation mechanisms leave the aged patient at great risk of dehydration. These risks are further enhanced by increased water losses from diarrhoea, often associated with chronic laxative abuse, tachypnoea, excessive diuretic therapy, burns and decubitus ulcers and increased sweating, especially seen in patients confined to bed. Deprivation of fluids during prolonged surgical operations and recovery periods may leave a patient with a lot of 'catching up' to restore water balance.

Sodium

The principal cation of the ECF is sodium. Fortunately, the electrolyte composition of the ECF and the intravascular fluid are almost identical, so plasma samples provide an easy method of measuring ECF composition. Total body sodium and its distribution within and between various body compartments do not change dramatically with increasing age. Overall, total body sodium increases slightly with no significant change in its distribution (Luft *et al.*, 1987). Interestingly, there is a significant correlation in aged patients with essential hypertension, but not in younger patients, between exchangeable sodium and blood pressure (Lever *et al.*, 1981). The volume of the ECF is entirely dependent upon sodium balance and there are numerous mechanisms by which the body regulates renal conservation or excretion of sodium (Table 9.1).

The serum or plasma sodium in healthy humans is maintained within very narrow limits. Apart from a small rise in the plasma level at around the menopause in women, the plasma levels do not change with increasing age. Deviations from the normal range in the old are thus the result of pathological, traumatic or iatrogenic insults, many of which may be very subtle.

The ability of the kidneys to control sodium balance decreases with increasing age in healthy humans. Virtually all the dietary and iatrogenic (i.v. infusions) sodium is excreted by kidneys, in temperate climes at least (Luft & Weinberger, 1982). Changes in renal excretion leave the old at risk of becoming overloaded or depleted in sodium during gross changes of intake. Over-zealous infusions of normal or hypertonic saline can usually be accommodated by young kidneys, but the old take much longer to excrete the excess (Luft *et al.*, 1980). Similarly, conservation mechanisms become increasingly less efficient with increasing age (Epstein & Hollenberg, 1976).

Table 9.1. Factors controlling
sodium homeostasis

Water balance*
Dietary sodium
'Trauma'
Intrinsic renal disease
Gastrointestinal balance
Drugs
   Parenteral water
   Diuretics*
   Drugs affecting AVP*
Volume/pressure receptors
   Atrial
   Carotid sinus*
   Intrarenal/intrahepatic
   Intracranial
Hormones
   AVP*
   Aldosterone*
   Angiotensin II
   Prostaglandins
   Noradrenaline (sympathetic)*

*Affected by ageing.

Hyponatraemia

A low plasma sodium may be due to the sodium depletion of a normal
ECF, a normal sodium in the face of an expanded ECF or any
combination of two. The plasma level is but a reflection of the *ratio* of
sodium: ECF volume — the latter being mainly determined by the level
of hydration (Lye, 1984a). Thus, the majority of syndromes of low or
high sodium have nothing to do with sodium *per se* — water balance is
the initiating mechanism of abnormalities.

Modern analytical techniques are now so reliable that laboratory
errors are unlikely, especially if two samples give similar results.
However, it is not unknown for busy doctors to take blood samples
downstream from i.v. infusions, giving rise to the most alarming
electrolyte results (Flear *et al.*, 1981). This is particularly likely to occur
in emergency situations in the operating theatre with an infusion in the
back of the hand of a draped patient. Pseudohyponatraemia occurs
where large molecules in the plasma reduce fractional water content. In
the aged the commonest cause is paraproteinaemia, usually secondary to
multiple myeloma which may be sub-clinical in its early stages (Frick
et al.,1966). A very high erythrocyte sedimentation rate (ESR) is often
present in this condition. The true sodium can be measured by an ion-
specific electrode (Swaminathan & Morgan, 1981). Severe hypoproteinaemia leads to a widening of the anion gap and electroneutrality is only
maintained by losing sodium. Hyponatraemia in these circumstances
does not require direct treatment — protein supplementation orally or
parentally restores normality (Flear *et al.*, 1981).

The prevalence of hyponatraemia is hard to determine because of the
large number of cases in whom it is transitory. There is, however, no

doubt that its frequency increases with increasing age. Whether this increased incidence is due to normal ageing or to the fact that the old are subject to multiple pathology and exposed to more drugs than the young is not known. Up to 11% of unselected admissions to an acute geriatric unit will have sodium levels of less than 130 mmol l^{-1} and 5% of the admissions will have levels of less than 125 mmol l^{-1} (Sunderam & Mankikar, 1983). In this survey, there was a strong association between hyponatraemia and diuretic usage, particularly with amiloride/hydro-chlorothiazide. A number of studies have demonstrated that hypo-natraemia is common in hospital practice, where up to 50% of cases are iatrogenically associated with diuretic therapy or during the course of post-operative fluid therapy (Arieff et al., 1976; Flear et al., 1981; Bouzarth & Shenkin, 1982).

The symptoms and clinical signs of hyponatraemia are difficult to distinguish from those produced by the underlying pathology or therapy. There is no doubt that symptoms are related to the speed of develop-ment of hyponatraemia, with chronic cases tolerating very low levels with seemingly little in the way of clinical manifestations (Morgan, 1984). In the young, where hyponatraemia is secondary to water overload ('dilutional hyponatraemia'), gastrointestinal symptoms pre-dominate, whereas with true sodium depletion, neurological features occur (Demanet et al., 1971; Arieff et al., 1976). In severe cases (values <120 mmol l^{-1}) both types of hyponatraemia are associated with neurological features — confusion, convulsions and coma. In the aged, mental impairment and confusion appear early and dominate the clinical picture (Lye, 1984a).

It now seems clear that the morbidity and mortality associated with hyponatraemia have been unduly exaggerated (Thomas et al., 1978; Flear et al., 1981; Daggett et al., 1982), although in the aged there is no doubt that hyponatraemia is associated with an increase in both morbidity and mortality (Sunderam & Mankikar, 1983). However, it is not known whether this is a direct cause and effect relationship or, as is more likely, a reflection of multiple pathology and polypharmacy seen in aged patients (Lye, 1984a).

Detailed biochemical investigation of patients with hyponatraemia is, in the majority of cases, worthless in terms of aetiological diagnosis and in management (Kennedy et al., 1978; Flear et al., 1981, Thomas et al., 1978). If the hyponatraemia is accompanied by mild uraemia, hyperchloraemia, hyperkalaemia and low blood pressure, the anaesthe-tist should be alerted to the possibility of hypoadrenalism. If there is doubt and this diagnosis is a possibility in an emergency situation, steroids should be given and investigations performed later. Aged patients and/or their relatives may forget to tell staff that the patient has been on long-term steroid therapy. Clinical examination sometimes reveals the 'Cushingoid' features of exogenous steroid use.

The assessment of the likely aetiology of hyponatraemia is best made by consideration of the history and clinical features (Lye, 1985). It may be a struggle to obtain an antecedent history, but it is worth all the trouble — relatives, neighbours, home helps, etc. should be contacted — a telephone may be of more use than the most sophisticated auto-analyser! Hyponatraemia is never primary — it always has a cause which indicates the choice of management. In the main, hyponatraemic patients fall into three main groups, though there may be some over-lapping (Lye, 1984a).

(i) *'Iatrogenic'*: in this condition the plasma sodium is typically between 120 and 130 mmol l^{-1}, accompanied by an overall body depletion of the cation. Urine sodium is markedly reduced, whilst the ECF volume is normal or slightly increased. This is the condition most likely to be seen by anaesthetists or surgical house staff. Basically the patient loses isotonic saline from the gastrointestinal tract — skin, kidneys, pancreas, etc. — and the fluid is replaced by hypotonic saline or dextrose solutions. Unfortunately, many hospital staff are so conscious of the fear of precipitating cardiac failure in aged postoperative patients that normal saline is rarely given intravenously. The solution is simple: during parenteral fluid replacement, the central venous pressure should be frequently monitored. If this procedure cannot be undertaken in a ward, admission to the intensive care unit is necessary. In fact, age may often be an indication *for* admission to either an intensive care or a high dependence unit. Thankfully, ageism is receding from many such units. If it is deemed necessary use major acute or planned expensive surgery and hospitalization in the old then it is wasteful to deny them any intensive postoperative care they require.

Unfortunately, diuretic agents may be inappropriately prescribed to aged patients. Dependent oedema in old people is not a reliable sign of fluid overload due to their relative immobility — indeed, postural oedema is the commonest cause of their swollen ankles. The most appropriate treatment is to mobilize the patient, but often doctors and their patients seem to have more faith in a pill, and diuretics are therefore prescribed. The reduction in effective plasma volume produced by diuretics stimulates AVP secretion, with the consequent development of a dilutional hyponatraemia (Kennedy *et al.*, 1978).

(ii) *'Circulatory'*: the prime 'lesion' in this variety of hyponatraemia is a reduced effective plasma volume. This occurs in the old most often with chronic cardiac failure and more rarely with hepatic cirrhosis or the nephrotic syndrome. Excessive diuresis, especially with thiazide diuretics, may exacerbate the condition. The plasma sodium, on occasions, may be below 120 mmol l^{-1}, but more characteristically is between 120 and 125 mmol l^{-1}. The total body sodium is actually raised, but the ECF volume is disproportionately increased — indeed, there is often peripheral oedema. Urine sodium output may be normal or slightly increased (Stein *et al.*, 1954). The decrease in effective plasma volume further reduces the existing age-related reduction in glomerular filtration rate, reducing fluid delivery to the distal diluting segment of the tubules and hence urine output. The urine is rendered more hypertonic because of the baroreceptor stimulation to AVP release which overrides the normal osmolality control (Riegger et al., 1982).

The treatment of this condition is not easy. If diuretic excess is suspected, judicious withdrawal and monitoring of the ECF volume by daily weighing can be tried. Body weight will rise over the course of the first three to five days, but if it levels off at not more than plus 2 kg, then diuretic excess is likely and a subsequent fall in weight (diuresis) can be expected. If the weight goes higher or symptoms of fluid retention increase, then the diuretics need to be restarted. Changing from a thiazide to a loop diuretic may help (Szatalowicz et al., 1982). Water restriction is poorly tolerated by the aged and is surprisingly unhelpful. Very careful addition of an angiotensin converting enzyme (ACE) inhibitor seems to be the preferred option, but may precipitate severe hypotension in the aged (Montgomery et al., 1982). Reduction of diuretics at the introduction of an ACE inhibitor may lessen hypotension (Reid, 1987).

(iii) 'Inappropriate AVP': the syndrome of inappropriate secretion of antidiuretic hormone (SIADH) was first described by Bartter and Schwartz in 1967. Since then, argument has flourished as to whether the secretion of AVP is appropriate or not. Physiologically the syndrome is characterized by increased levels of AVP, a slightly increased ECF volume, a reduced urinary concentration of sodium and often marked reduction in plasma sodium levels. Total body sodium is usually normal (Lye, 1985).

The aetiology of this condition is protean. Almost any type of stress, especially in an old individual, can lead to an increase in AVP secretion and hence to water retention. The stress can be psychological (Dubovsky et al., 1973), neurological (Mather et al., 1981), traumatic, surgical or accidental (Cochrane et al., 1981). Even the simple expedient of moving old patients from their own homes to residential accommodation may precipitate symptomatic hyponatraemia (Clinch, 1982). We should not therefore be surprised that the AVP levels of aged patients admitted acutely as surgical emergencies are going to be high. Some causes to be considered are shown in Table 9.2.

The commonest cause of preoperative hyponatraemia that the anaesthetist is likely to be confronted with is secondary to an acute respiratory infection which may be quite minor (Thomas et al., 1978). Many aged surgical patients develop respiratory infections because of inhalation and/or recumbency during the prodromal period of their surgical condition. This can be exceedingly difficult to diagnose without the help of a chest X-ray (Lye, 1984b). The treatment of this complication is not water restriction, nor salt loading: antibiotics and physiotherapy resolve the hyponatraemia rapidly (Thomas et al., 1978).

Table 9.2. Aetiology of 'SIADH'

Malignant disease
Small cell carcinoma
Pancreatic
Bladder
Duodenum
Hodgkin's
Prostate*
Pulmonary
Pneumonia
Tubercle*
Abscess
Empyema*
Chronic bronchitis (rarely)
Neurological
Trauma (subdural)*
Subarachnoid haemorrhage
Cerebrovascular accident*
Pituitary adenoma
Encephalitis
Meningitis
Guillain-Barré
Miscellaneous
Psychosis*
Social stress*
Surgical stress*
Drugs*
See text

*Especially in the aged.

Another common cause of preoperative hyponatraemia is drug therapy (Lye, 1984a) (Table 9.3). Diuretic agents, particularly thiazides, used in the treatment of chronic cardiac failure have already been referred to, but a special note should be made of the association between amiloride and chronic hyponatraemia (Sunderam & Mankikar, 1983). Other drugs operate by stimulating AVP secretion or by augmenting activity of AVP on the distal renal tubule. Correction of the hyponatraemia is not urgent — removal of any offending drug is all that is required.

Hyponatraemia is said to be particularly associated with neurological trauma. In the old, acute cerebral vascular accidents (Joynt et al., 1981) often cause hyponatraemia which may be inadvertently 'treated' by poor nursing leading to dehydration (Himmelstein et al., 1983). Water deprivation is not required as the hyponatraemia corrects itself. In the period of postoperative neurosurgical recovery, hyponatraemia is said to be a particular problem (Fox et al., 1971; Lester & Nelson 1981). However, the problem is invariably iatrogenic in origin. As Bouzarth & Shenkin (1982) demonstrated, restricting intraoperative and postoperative fluid infusion to 2.5% glucose in 0.45% saline and limiting daily intake to one litre less oral fluid intake virtually abolishes hyponatraemia.

Chronic hyponatraemia in the old may be due to the elaboration of an AVP-like substance by a tumour (Beardwell et al., 1975) (Table 9.2). Bronchial and prostatic carcinomas may be very small and not easily

153 | *The milieu interieur in the aged*

Chlorpropramide Tolbutamide (rarely) Glipizide Clofibrate Halophenate Carbamazepine Tricyclic antidepressants Vincristine Vinblastine Narcotic analgesics (variable) Nicotine (smoking) Clonidine (variable) Dopamine (variable)	**Table 9.3.** Drugs enhancing AVP release or action

identifiable by the time they are expressing non-metastatic hormone. The treatment here is, where possible, that of the tumour (surgery, radiotherapy and/or chemotherapy). Where it is not practical or possible and the hyponatraemia is giving rise to symptoms with plasma sodium <120 mmol l^{-1}, then treatment with demeclocycline is warranted (De Troyer & Demanet, 1975). Unfortunately, demeclocycline further enchances the age-induced decline in renal function which may limit its usefulness in the aged (Singer & Rotenberg, 1973).

Hypernatraemia

A rise in the serum sodium to above 145 mmol l^{-1} or an increase in serum osmolality to more than 290 mosmol l^{-1} may be due to excess sodium, or decreased body water or a combination of the two (Bay & Ferris, 1976). Most cases are due to the latter and, in the case of the aged in hospital, it is almost invariably due to dehydration (Lye, 1984a). There are other conditions that need to be considered on occasions (Table 9.4).

Signs and symptoms of hypernatraemia are often masked by other

Dehydration
    Immobility (cerebrovascular accident, etc.)
    Mental impairment (dementia)
    Impaired consciousness
    Climatic
    Gastrointestinal loss
    Respiratory loss
Renal
    Diabetes insipidus
    Chronic renal failure
Endocrine
    Hyperosmolar non-ketotic diabetes
    Conn's syndrome
    Cushing's syndrome
Iatrogenic
    Excess saline
    Lactic acidosis
	Table 9.4. Aetiology of hypernatraemia

conditions causing the hypernatraemia. Acute hypernatraemia induced by infusions of sodium as bicarbonate after a cardiac arrest induces extreme lethargy, stupor or coma and convulsions (Katzman & Pappius, 1973). Chronic hypernatraemia, which is much more common and occurs over a time course of 24–48 h, gives rise to much less dramatic signs and symtoms. Thirst is apparent except in markedly confused or semi-conscious individuals. Weakness and confusion are the prime features but are often ascribed to the underlying conditions (Lye, 1984a). As in children, hypernatraemia is a serious condition in itself, being associated with a mortality of around 50%. Treatment of hypernatraemia is easy — give water — with care! If the patient is able to take fluids orally, then water should be prescribed and intake and output monitored (Himmelstein et al., 1983). If, however, the patient is shocked, plasma substitute (polygeline or succinylated gelatin) should be used to stabilize the cardiovascular system. The crystalloids should not be used in the aged because of the risk of volume overload in a compromised circulation (Metildi et al., 1984). In other circumstances, hypotonic solutions should be given with the aim of lowering the serum osmolality by no more than $2 \text{ mosmol l}^{-1} \text{ h}^{-1}$. It may thus take more than 24 h to correct the serum sodium. More rapid correction can lead to cerebral oedema and permanent brain damage (Morris-Jones et al., 1967). A common problem in the aged is the dehydration and hypernatraemia associated with respiratory infections. Here tachypnoea leads to large loss of water from the lungs as well as from the skin due to sweating and this is not replaced because the patient is so ill. The situation is invariably made worse by the injudicious use of diuretics which seemingly few doctors can resist giving to any breathless old patient on the basis that they must 'have a touch of heart failure'.

Potassium

Potassium is the major intracellular cation and is intimately involved in mitochondrial and other metabolic functions of the cell. The cation is also important in membrane activity, particularly of nerve cells where the ratio of intracellular:extracellular potassium concentration determines electrical activity and conductivity. More than 97% of the total body potassium is located within cells, maintained there by continuing function of the Na : K ATPase pump (MacKnight, 1977). Thus, the intracellular pool acts as a vast reservoir of potassium to maintain the ratio. A large drop in extracellular potassium can be compensated for by a very small transfer from the intracellular pool. Unfortunately, many conditions and drugs used in the aged can interfere with this mechanism and lead to problems.

Body potassium and ageing

Total body potassium, however it is measured, falls with increasing age in all healthy mammals (Novak, 1972; Pierson et al., 1974). This has led to the assumption that increasing age is associated with body *depletion* of the cation. However, the content of potassium has to be related to the size of the container. In this case the container is the fat-free mass which has a high concentration of potassium. With normal ageing, the fat-free (lean) body mass decreases largely as a result of muscle atrophy, whilst the proportion of body fat (low potassium concentration) increases. Thus, there is an inevitable decrease in total body potassium with increasing age in healthy humans (Fig. 9.3a), but the decrease is in proportion to the body potassium capacity and does not represent body depletion of the cation (Womersley *et al.*, 1976; Lye, 1981).

Many aged patients suffer from various degrees of chronic cardiac failure; indeed, cardiac failure is a disease of old age (Webb & Impallomeni, 1987). The frequently used isotopic measurement of total exchangeable potassium in aged cardiac failure patients suggests significant depletion (see Novak & Harrison, 1973), but it has only recently been shown that the exchangeable measurement is unreliable in oedematous diseases (Boddy *et al.*, 1978; Lye & Winston, 1979). Whole body counting of ^{40}K is more reliable and has shown smaller, but significant depletion of potassium in cardiac failure (Davidson *et al.*, 1976). In assessing the degree of depletion, reference is made to a predicted normal value but, as we have shown, predicted norms in the aged are valueless (Lye & Faragher, 1982). Again, the recorded value has to be compared with potassium capacity, i.e. total body protein (Davidson *et al.*, 1976) or fat-free mass (Lye, 1982). With these precautions it is evident that cardiac failure and/or its treatment does not lead to body potassium depletion.

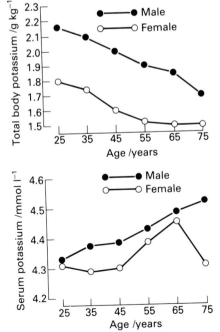

Fig. 9.3. (a) The relationship of total body postassium with age in male and female subjects (from Novak, 1972). (Reproduced with permission of the *Journal of Gerontology*.) (b) The relation of average serum potassium with age in male and female subjects (from Bold & Wilding, 1975).

Plasma potassium

The plasma concentration of potassium is an accurate measure of the cation's concentration in the ECF providing various precautions are observed when taking the blood sample and during analysis. Forearm exercise, often used with old patients to cause venous congestion, leads to an elevated potassium which may even mask hypokalaemia (Skinner, 1961). Haemolysis, particularly with prolonged storage, can be a problem. Marked elevations of white cell or platelet counts associated with clotting problems can lead to falsely elevated plasma levels (Bellavue *et al.*, 1975).

The plasma levels of potassium in healthy subjects show systematic, though small increases with increasing age (Lye, 1985) (Fig. 9.3b) This rise starts at puberty and in men extends well into old age. In women, the rise seems to reverse beyond the age of 65 years (Bold & Wilding, 1975). The latter effect may be due to latent diseases which may be more common in old women, as surveys have shown that with many conditions affecting the old the plasma potassium level falls (Hodkinson, 1977). There is a diurnal variation of plasma potassium, with lower values occurring in the early hours of the morning at a time when many aged patients are undergoing emergency surgery (Bergstrom, 1981). The anaesthetist needs to be aware of this phenomenon, though the level is unlikely to be less than 3.2 mmol l^{-1} unless there are other factors.

Hypokalaemia

The lower limit of 'normal' plasma potassium varies between laboratories, with quoted values between 3.2 and 3.5 mmol l^{-1}. In practical terms, however, the lower limit which prompts investigation and treatment of old people should be 3.0 mmol l^{-1} (Levy & Lye, 1987). It is only below this level that symptoms, signs or electrical problems arise. In the aged, the symptoms and signs are of vague weakness, lethargy, fatiguability and probably confusion. This 'syndrome', however, may be more related to the condition causing the hypokalaemia rather than the level of potassium itself (Judge, 1968). In the aged, constipation is common with chronic hypokalaemia (Pick, 1966). The serious signs of cardiac conduction defects may be a problem with aged patients, especially during surgery (Allison *et al.*, 1972; Steiness & Olsen, 1976). Electrocardiogram (ECG) monitoring is mandatory for hypokalaemic patients undergoing surgery and anaesthesia.

The aetiology of hypokalaemia in the old is the same as for younger patients (see review by Smith *et al.*, 1985), though some points are worth emphasizing. Loss of the cation from the gastrointestinal tract, compounded by accompanying acid-based disturbance, is often associated with hypokalaemia in the old (Crane, 1965). An occult cause of chronic hypokalaemia is laxative abuse (Fleischer *et al.*, 1969). Diuretics used in the treatment of chronic cardiac failure have been implicated in the causation of significant hypokalaemia (British Medical Journal, 1978; Ibrahim *et al.*, 1978). The danger, however, has been much exaggerated. Loop diuretics have less effect on plasma potassium than thiazide agents (Morgan & Davidson, 1980). It is assumed that many older patients have a precarious dietary intake of potassium and are therefore vulnerable to the kaliuretic action of diuretics (Judge, 1968; Williamson & Chopin, 1980). However, controlled studies have suggested that the old are at *less* risk of developing hypokalaemia than young patients (for full discussion see Levy & Lye, 1987).

The management of hypokalaemia demands a full assessment of the likely aetiology and correction where possible (Smith *et al.*, 1985). If the plasma level is less than 2.5 mmol l^{-1} or the patient shows signs of cardiac toxicity, then hypokalaemia should be corrected vigorously. Parental therapy is indicated, but because of the previously described ageing renal changes, caution should be observed. An infusion of 0.75 mmol kg^{-1} body weight per hour should be regarded as a maximum. The plasma potassium and ECG should be monitored throughout the infusion and for several hours after. The potassium is best given in normal or half-normal saline, as dextrose stimulates insulin secretion which enhances transfer of the cation into cells, further lowering ECF and plasma levels (Bia & De Fronzo, 1981). If the hypokalaemia is accompanied by a metabolic acidosis, the potassium chloride normally used should be replaced by potassium bicarbonate — under no circumstances should the acid-base disturbance be corrected before the hypokalaemia (Smith *et al.*, 1985).

Less urgent treatment of hypokalaemia is best accomplished by the oral route — this is always to be preferred and is usually mandatory in patients with oliguric renal failure (Schon *et al.*, 1974). The chloride salt is required in most cases to correct the associated metabolic alkalosis and volume depletion (Schwartz *et al.*, 1968). If the hypokalaemia is due to gastrointestinal loss, there is likely to be an accompanying acidosis, in which case potassium gluconate is to be preferred. The dose of potassium should be titrated against the response, as often the doses given are far too small (Schwartz & Swartz, 1974).

Hyperkalaemia

A plasma potassium of 5.5 mmol l^{-1} or more is abnormally high. Depending upon the rate of increase in the plasma level, signs and symptoms of hyperkalaemia may develop at this level or higher (Kliger & Hayslett, 1978). Neuromuscular and cardiac manifestations predominate. Initially, sensory abnormalities (parasthesiae and diminished sensory perception) are apparent, but these become overshadowed by an ascending flaccid paresis with diminished tendon reflexes (Pollen & Williams, 1960). The paresis can progress to impair respiration (hypoxia and CO_2 retention) and ultimately will produce a flaccid quadriplegia

(Bull *et al.*, 1953). Old patients with hyperkalaemic paresis may be diagnosed as having sustained a brainstem stroke.

Cardiac toxicity is rightly feared in the aged — the first manifestation of hyperkalaemia may be ventricular tachycardia of fibrillation (Smith *et al.*, 1985). Initial changes in the ECG of 'tall tented Ts', lengthening of the P–R interval and/or widening of the QRS complex all herald imminent arrhythmias. Thus, all old patients with a plasma potassium above 5.5 mmol l^{-1} should have the ECG continuously monitored (Ettinger *et al.*, 1974). Treatment should be started immediately (see below).

Hyperkalaemia may be due to a shift of potassium to the ECF from within cells, or to an accumulation of the cation related to a reduction in excretion, or to a combination of the two (Lye, 1984a). The aetiology is the same for old and young patients, though in the old multifactorial aetiology is particularly common (Lye, 1985). Drugs commonly taken by the old, of which the anaesthetist may not always be aware, often underlie an obscure hyperkalaemia (Table 9.5). For example, the aged patient with hypertensive heart failure may be on many such drugs.

It is estimated that 10% or more of aged patients taking potassium-sparing diuretic agents or spironolactone will develop significant hyperkalaemia (Bender *et al.*, 1967; Greenblatt & Koch-Weser, 1973). Indeed, promotion by the pharmaceutical industry has led to a situation where, because of these agents, hypokalaemia is not a problem with aged patients taking diuretics — but hyperkalaemia is (Levy & Lye, 1987). Because potassium-sparing agents lower glomerular filtration rate (Wan & Lye, 1980), they should not be used in patients with a creatinine clearance of less than 30 mmol min^{-1} (Bennett *et al.*, 1980; Lye, 1984a). Most aged patients with chronic cardiac failure are in this category. A sudden stress (surgery, crush injury, revascularization, infection), combined with a degree of dehydration may precipitate development of dangerous hyperkalaemia (Jaffey & Martin, 1981). It is necessary to both anticipate and respond quickly to this serious situation.

The treatment of acute hyperkalaemia should be considered in four-stages (Smith *et al.*, 1985): (i) restabilize cell membranes; (ii) shift potassium into the intracellular compartment; (iii) remove potassium; (iv) identify and treat the cause of the hyperkalaemia. The first two manoeuvres are the most important.

Table 9.5. Drugs leading to hyperkalaemia

Potassium-sparing diuretics
Potassium salts
Prostaglandin synthetase inhibitors
Beta-adrenergic blocking agents
Angiotensin-converting enzyme inhibitors
Digoxin
Heparin
Succinylcholine
Low-salt health food additives

Calcium gluconate (10%) should be given in a 10 ml i.v. bolus (De Fronzo & Thier, 1983). This acts almost immediately and lasts for up to one hour. If it is not effective the dose can be increased to 20 ml and repeated on one occasion only. Aged patients taking digoxin should be given the calcium as a dextrose infusion over 30 min because any hypercalcaemia will potentiate digoxin cardiotoxicity.

A bolus of 50 mmol sodium bicarbonate given over 10 min will cause a shift of potassium from the ECF into cells even in the absence of acidosis (Giebisch & Thier, 1977). Insulin (10 u Actrapid) is an alternative to sodium bicarbonate and is especially useful where the sodium bicarbonate may cause fluid overload (De Fronzo & Thier, 1983). Glucose (500 ml of a 10% solution) should be given to prevent hypoglycaemia. The infusion should be given over one hour and lasts up to four hours. This is particularly useful in the operating theatre as the infusion can be repeated at four hourly intervals.

Encouragement of removal of potassium via the kidney can be attempted using i.v. frusemide (40 mg), though dehydration and renal impairment in the aged may limit an adequate response. Cation exchange resins should be preferred. Sodium polystyrene sulphonate (Resonium A) is effective but may lead to volume overload, in which case the calcium equivalent (calcium resonium) should be used. The latter is contraindicated, however, in hypercalcaemia, e.g. with multiple myeloma or carcinoma metastases. Both agents should be administered rectally. Finally, if there are other electrolyte abnormalities, with or without renal failure, then peritoneal or haemodialysis, when available, should be used (Boen, 1961). However, it must be appreciated that dialysis, especially peritoneal, whilst effective, only removes potassium slowly.

Longer-term therapy includes removing the cause — often drugs, particularly non-steroidal anti-inflammatory analgesics or potassium salts. A low potassium diet combined with high fluid intake is often sufficient. Oral cation-exchange resins will not be tolerated by the aged. For prolonged treatment oral calcium carbonate may be useful as the more popular oral sodium bicarbonate may precipitate cardiac failure in the compromised aged patient (Smith et al., 1985).

Magnesium

Magnesium is, after potassium, the second most abundant cation in the body. As with potassium, it is primarily intracellular, particularly in bone, with only 1% in the ECF (Edelman & Leibman, 1959). Like potassium, it is intimately involved with neuromuscular electrical activity. Unfortunately, unlike potassium, it is not easy to measure body content *in vivo*. Total exchangeable magnesium has been measured by isotopic dilution in man, but the results are conflicting (Aikawa *et al.*,

1960; Jones *et al.*, 1969). The plasma level bears little relation to total body stores (Wacker & Parisi, 1968).

The aged are at greater risk of developing body magnesium depletion by virtue of multiple pathology, polypharmacy and/or dietary insufficiency (Landahl *et al.*, 1980). Surveys have shown that the old, both healthy and patients, consume diets low in magnesium (MacLeod *et al.*, 1975; Peterson *et al.*, 1977). Animal studies have also shown that the cation is less easily mobilized from bone with increasing age (Breibart *et al.*, 1960). Fine regulation of body magnesium rests principally with the kidneys which have an obligatory excretion of the cation even in the face of depletion (Barnes *et al.*, 1958). It is likely that renal ageing impairs this conservation mechanism.

Hypomagnesaemia

The generally accepted normal range of plasma magnesium is 0.70 – 1.00 mmol l^{-1} and levels below 0.65 mmol l^{-1} represent hypomagnesaemia (Sherwood *et al.*, 1986). The prevalence of hypomagnesaemia in a general population is approximately 10% (Whang *et al.*, 1980), but rises to 25% in hospitalized aged patients (McConway *et al.*, 1981). It is likely that these results underestimate the prevalence of body magnesium depletion.

Classically, hypomagnesaemia causes disorientation, memory loss and confabulation, leading on to apathy, lassitude and depression (Hall & Joffe, 1973). Muscle weakness and tremulousness are common, and seizures occur occasionally (Fishman, 1965). Stupor is uncommon and depression of conscious level does not occur. Peripheral vasoconstriction and raised blood pressure are common (Altura, 1982). ECG abnormalities and arrhythmias are unusual except in the presence of digoxin where hypomagnesaemia potentiates any digoxin toxicity (Birch & Giles, 1977).

The aetiology of hypomagnesaemia includes excessive loss from the renal or gastrointestinal tract. Perioperatively plasma magnesium may fall significantly for up to 48 h, though the exact mechanism is not understood (Sawyer, 1970). This will exacerbate any pre-existing chronic hypomagnesaemia in old patients. Diarrhoea, laxative abuse, gastrointestinal aspiration or suction, and small bowel resection or bypass all lead to magnesium depletion. Following parathyroidectomy, the 'hungry bone' leads to a marked deposition of magnesium (and calcium) in healing bone, causing a reduction in plasma levels (Heaton & Pyrah, 1965).

Therapy consists of a search for the causes which differ little between young and old patients. If the deficit is severe or symptomatic, i.v. replacement with magnesium sulphate 3 g in 5% dextrose should be given and repeated as necessary. Oral supplementation with magnesium hydroxide can be continued thereafter for up to five days.

Hypermagnesaemia

This is much less common than hypomagnesaemia and is always either secondary to severe renal impairment or iatrogenic. Excessive administration of antacids, purgatives or enemas are likely causes. Severe burns and tissue trauma may underlie the aetiology in some individuals, but invariably there is an accompanying renal lesion (Lau, 1985).

The early sign of hypermagnesaemia is of generalized muscle weakness which, if the plasma level is particularly high, will progress to marked paresis with absent tendon reflexes (Mordes & Wacker, 1978). Consciousness is not usually impaired, though in the aged confusion is common. In severe intoxication the patient can be in a state of 'suspended animation'. Indeed, in the past, magnesium was used as a sedative and it is of interest that mammals, during hibernation, have very high plasma magnesium levels. Beware of bears with a falling plasma magnesium — they are about to wake up!

Most patients without renal failure require no treatment apart from identifying and rectifying the cause (Lau, 1985). Those with renal impairment or severe hypermagnesaemia will respond to peritoneal or haemodialysis (Mordes & Wacker, 1978).

Acid-base balance

The hydrogen ion content of blood is kept by homeostatic (respiratory and renal) mechanisms within a tight normal range of between 36 and 43 mmol 1^{-1} (pH 3.35–3.45) (Bold & Wilding, 1975). There is no evidence that this normal range changes with increasing age in humans (Shock & Yiengst, 1950). In any evaluation of acid-base abnormalities, the antecedent history of events provides more diagnostic information than any sophisticated biochemical test or its interpretation. This is particularly so in old patients who, because of multiple pathology, often have interacting metabolic and respiratory components in any disturbance (Lye, 1985).

The old take longer to excrete an acidic load whether physiological (severe exercise) or pathological (metabolic/respiratory acidosis) (Dill et al., 1966; Bouhuys et al., 1966). The age-related decline in elimination rate of acid affects both the pulmonary (Altose et al., 1977) and renal mechanisms (Adler et al., 1968). The latter workers found that healthy aged subjects took three times as long to eliminate an ammonium chloride acid load as young healthy individuals. Old patients with further renal impairment (intrinsic or secondary to reduced perfusion) are likely to be even less efficient.

The management of acid-base disturbance in the old follows general principles. It is important, however, to monitor closely the acid-base status and not to be over-zealous in applying corrective measures. This particularly applies to metabolic acidosis where over-correction can do more harm than the original disturbance. If correction is required, the formula of Hazard & Griffin (1982) may be used, namely:

Bicarbonate required $= (0.5\, P_{CO_2} - HCO_3) \times 0.5$ (body weight in kg)

Conclusion

The management of electrolyte and acid-base disorders of old patients by anaesthetists should follow those general principles he/she would follow with younger patients. It is important to have a high index of suspicion and to be moderate in response. A full appreciation of the patient (medical, social, drug histories, etc.) is mandatory before any active treatment — 'first do no harm' is apposite. Finally, with firm knowledge of the patient's condition and the application of good clinical practice there will be few old patients that the anaesthetist cannot prepare for, and steer through, the benefits of modern surgery.

References

Adler, S., Lindeman, R.D., Yiengst, M.J., Beard, E. & Shock, N.W. (1986) Effect of acute loading on urinary acid excretion by the ageing human kidney. *J. Lab. Clin. Med.* **72**, 278–289.

Aikawa, J.K., Gordon, G.S, & Rhoades, E.L. (1960) Magnesium metabolism in human beings: Studies with 28 Mg. *J. Appl. Physiol.* **15**, 503–507.

Allison, S.P., Morley, G.J. & Burns-Cox, C.J. (1972) Insulin, glucose and potassium in the treatment of congestive heart failure. *Br. Med. J.* **3**, 675–678.

Altose, M.D., McCauley, W.C., Kelsen, S.G. & Cherniack, N.S. (1977) Effects of hypercapnia and inspiratory flow resistive loading on respiratory activity in chronic airways obstruction. *J. Clin. Invest.* **59**, 500–507.

Altura, B.M. (1982) Magnesium and regulation of contractility of vascular smooth muscle. *Adv. Microcirc.* **2**, 77–81.

Arieff, A.I., Fllach, F. & Massory, S.G. (1976) Neurological manifestations and morbidity of hyponatraemia. Correlation with brain water and electrolytes. *Medicine (Baltimore)* **55**, 121–129.

Barnes, B.A., Cope, O, & Harrison, Y. (1958) Magnesium conservation in human beings on low magnesium diet. *J. Clin. Invest.* **37**, 430–440.

Bartter, F.C. & Schwartz, W.B. (1967) The syndrome of inappropriate secretion of antidiuretic hormone. *Am. J. Med.* **42**, 790–806.

Bay, W.H. & Ferris, T.F (1976) Hypernatraemia and hyponatraemia disorders of tonicity. *Geriatrics*, **31**, 53–64.

Beardwell, C.G., Geelen, G. & Palmer, H.M. (1975) Radioimmunoassay of plasma vasopressin in physiological and pathological states in man. *J. Endocrinol.* **67**, 189–202.

Bellavue, R., Dosik, H. & Speigel, G. (1975) Pseudohyperkalaemia and extreme leukocytosis. *J. Lab. Clin. Med.* **85**, 660–664.

Bender, A.D., Carter, C.L. & Hansen, K.B. (1967) Use of a diuretic combination of triamterene and hydrochlorothiazide in elderly patients. *J. Am. Geriatr. Soc.* **15**, 166–173.

Bennett, W.M., Muther, R.S., Parker, R.A., Freig, P., Morrison, G., Golper, T.A. & Singer, I. (1980) Drug therapy in renal failure: Dosing guidelines for adults Part II. *Ann. Intern. Med.* **93**, 286–325.

Bergstrom, J. (1981) Determination of electrolytes — methodological problems. *Acta Med. Scand.* **647**, 39–46.

Bia, M.J. & De Fronzo, R.A. (1981) Extrarenal potassium homeostasis. *Am. J. Physiol.* **240**, 257–261.

Birch, G.E. & Giles, T.D. (1977) The importance of magnesium deficiency in cardiovascular disease. *Am. Heart J.* **94**, 649-651.

Boddy, K., Davies, D.L., Howie, A.D., Madkour, M., Mahaffey, M.E. & Pack, A.I. (1978) Total body potassium in chronic airways obstruction: A controversial area? *Thorax*, **33**, 62-66.

Boen, S.T. (1961) Kinetics of peritoneal dialysis. A comparison with the artificial kidney. *Medicine (Baltimore)* **40**, 243-261.

Bold, A.M. & Wilding, P. (1975) *Clinical Chemistry*. Blackwell Scientific Publications, Oxford.

Bouhuys, A., Pool, J. & Binkhorst, R.A. (1966) Metabolic acidosis of exercise in healthy males. *J. Appl. Physiol.* **21**, 1040-1046.

Bouzarth, W.F. & Shenkin, H.A. (1982) Is 'cerebral hyponatraemia' iatrogenic? *Lancet* **1**, 1061-1062.

Breibart, S., Lee, J.S., McCoord, A. & Forbes, G.B. (1960) Relation of age to radiomagnesium exchange in bone. *Proc. Soc. Exp. Biol. Med.* **105**, 361-363.

British Medical Journal (1978) Diuretics in the elderly. *Br. Med. J.* **1**, 1092-1093.

Bruce, A., Andersson, M., Arvidsson, B. & Isaksson, B. (1980) Body composition. Prediction of normal body potassium, body water and body fat in adults on the basis of body height, body weight and age. *Scand. J. Clin. Lab. Invest.* **40**, 461-473.

Bull, A.M., Carter, A.B. & Lowe, K.G. (1953) Hyperpotassaemic paralysis. *Lancet* **2**, 60-63.

Chien, S., Usami, S. & Simmons, R.L. (1966) Blood volume and age: repeated measurements on normal man. *J. Appl. Physiol.* **21**, 583-588.

Clinch, D. (1982) Syndrome of inappropriate antidiuretic hormone secretion associated with stress. *Lancet* **1**, 1131-1132.

Cochrane, J.P.S., Forsling, M.L., Gow, N.M. & Le Quesne, L.P. (1981) Arginine vasopressin release following operations. *Br. J. Surg.* **68**, 209-213.

Crane, C.W. (1965) Observations on the sodium and potassium content of mucus from the large intestine. *Gut* **6**, 439-443.

Daggett, P., Deanfield, J. & Moss, P. (1982) Neurological aspects of hyponatraemia. *Postgrad. Med. J.* **58**, 737-740.

Davenport, H.T. (1986) *Anaesthesia in the Elderly*. Heinemann Medical Books, London, p. 22.

Davidson, C., Burkinshaw, L., MacLachlan, M.S.F. & Morgan, D.B. (1976) Effect of long-term diuretic treatment on body potassium in heart disease. *Lancet* **2**, 1044-1047.

De Fronzo, R.A. & Thier, S.O. (1983) Fluid and electrolyte disturbances: Hypo- and hyperkalaemia. In *Handbook of Renal Therapeutics* (Ed. M. Martinez-Maldonado). Plenum, New York.

De Troyer, A. & Demanet, J.C. (1975) Correction of antidiuresis by demclocycline. *New Engl. J. Med.* **293**, 915-918.

Demanet, J.C., Bonnyns, M. & Stevens-Rocman, C. (1971) Coma due to water intoxication in beer drinkers. *Lancet* **2**, 1115-1117.

Dill, D.B., Phillips, E.E. & MacGregor, D. (1966) Training: Youth and age. *Ann. NY Acad. Sci.* **134**, 760-775.

Dubovsky, S.G., Groban, S., Berl, T. & Schrier, R.W. (1973) Syndrome of inappropriate secretion of antidiuretic hormone with exacerbated psychosis. *Ann. Intern. Med.* **79**, 551-554.

Dunnill, M.S. & Halley, W. (1973) Some observations on the quantitative anatomy of the kidney. *J. Path.* **110**, 113-121.

Durnin, J.V.G.A. & Womersley, J. (1974) Body fat assessed from total body density and its estimation from skin fold thickness: Measurements on 481 men and women aged from 16 to 72 years. *Br. J. Nutr.* **32**, 77-79.

Edelman, I.S. & Leibman, J. (1959) Anatomy of body water and electrolytes. *Am. J. Med.* **27**, 256-277.

Epstein, M. (1979) Effects of ageing on the kidney. *Fed. Proc.* **38**, 168-172.

Epstein, M. & Hollenberg, N.K. (1976) Age as a determinant of renal sodium conservation in normal man. *J. Lab. Clin. Med.* **87**, 411-417.

Ettinger, P.O., Regan, T.J. & Oldewurtel, H.A. (1974) Hyperkalaemia, cardiac conduction and the EKG: A review. *Am. Heart J.* **88**, 360-371.

Fishman, R.A. (1965) Neurological aspects of magnesium metabolism. *Arch. Neurol.* **12**, 562–564.

Flear, C.T.G., Gill, G.V. & Burn, J. (1981) Hyponatraemia: Mechanisms and management. *Lancet* **2**, 26–31.

Fleischer, N., Brown, M., Graham, D.Y. & DeLenna, S. (1969) Chronic laxative-induced hyperaldosteronism and hypokalaemia simulating Bartter's syndrome. *Ann. Intern. Med.* **70**, 791–798.

Fox, J.L., Falk, J.L. & Shalhoub, R.J. (1971) Neurosurgical hyponatraemia: The role of inappropriate antidiuresis. *J. Neurosurg.* **34**, 506–514.

Frick, P.G., Schmid, J.R., Kestler, J.H. & Hitzig, W. (1966) Hyponatraemia associated with hypoproteinaemia in multiple myeloma. *Helv. Med. Acta* **33**, 317–329.

Giebisch, G.H., & Thier, S.O. (1977) Physiological and clinical importance. In *Directions in Cardiovascular Medicine* (Ed. L. Siegel). Hoechst-Roussel Pharmaceuticals Inc., Sommerville, New Jersey, p. 22.

Greenblatt, D.J. & Koch-Weser, J. (1973) Adverse reactions to spironolactone. A report from the Boston collaborative drug surveillance program. *J. Am. Med. Ass.* **255**, 40–43.

Hall, R.C. & Joffe, J.R. (1973) Hypomagnesemia and psychiatric symptoms. *J. Am. Med. Ass.* **224**, 1749–1751.

Hazard, P.B. & Griffin, J.P. (1982) Calculations of sodium bicarbonate requirement in metabolic acidosis. *Am. J. Med. Sci.* **283**, 18–22.

Heaton, F.W. & Pyrah, L.N. (1965) Magnesium metabolism in patients with parathyroid disorders. *Clin. Sci.* **25**, 475–480.

Himmelstein, D.U., Jones, A. & Woolhandler, S. (1983) Hypernatraemic dehydration in nursing home patients: An indicator of neglect. *J. Am. Geriatr. Soc.* **31**, 466–471.

Hodkinson, H.M. (1977) *Biochemical Diagnosis of the Elderly*. Chapman & Hall, London.

Hollenberg, N.K., Adams, D.F., Solomon, H.S., Rashid, A., Abrams, M. & Merrill, J.P. (1974) Senescence and the renal vasculature in normal man. *Circ. Res.* **34**, 309–316.

Ibrahim, I.K. Ritch, A.E.S., MacLennan, W.J. & May, T. (1978) Are potassium supplements for the elderly necessary? *Age Ageing* **7**, 165–170.

Jaffey, L. & Martin, A. (1981) Malignant hyperkalaemia after amiloride/hydrochlorothiazide treatment. *Lancet* **1**, 1272–

Jones, J.E., Shane, S.R., Jacobs, W.H. & Flink, E.B. (1969) Magnesium balance studies in chronic alcoholism. *Ann. NY Acad. Sci.* **162**, 934–946.

Joynt, R.J., Feibal, J.H. & Sladek, C.M. (1981) Antidiuretic hormone levels in stroke patients. *Ann. Neurol.* **9**, 182–184.

Judge, T.G. (1968) Hypokalaemia in the elderly. *Gerontol. Clin.* **10**, 102–107.

Katzman, R. & Pappius, H.M. (1973) Hypernatraemia and hyperosmolarity. In *Brain Electrolytes and Fluid Metabolism* (Eds R. Katzman & H.M. Pappius). Williams & Wilkins, Baltimore, pp. 278–306.

Kennedy, P.G.E., Mitchell, D.M. & Hoffbrand, B. (1978) Severe hyponatraemia in hospital inpatients. *Br. Med. J.* **2**, 1251–1253.

Kirkland, J.L., Lye, M., Goddard, C., Vargas, E. & Davies, I. (1984) Plasma arginine vasopressin in dehydrated elderly patients. *Clin. Endocrinol.* **20**, 451–456.

Kliger, A.S. & Hayslett, J.P. (1978) Disorders of potassium balance. In *Acid-base and Potassium Homeostasis* (Eds B.M. Brenner & J.H. Stein). Churchill Livingstone, Edinburgh, pp. 168–204.

Landahl, S., Graffner, C., Jagenburg, R., Lundborg, P. & Steen, B. (1980) Prevalence and treatment of hypermagnesaemia in the elderly: Studies in a representative 70 year old population and in geriatric patients. *Acta Gerontol.* **10**, 397–402.

Lau, K. (1985) Magnesium metabolism: Normal and abnormal. In *Fluid Electrolyte and Acid-base Disorders* (Eds A.I. Arieff & R.A. De Fronzo). Churchill Livingstone, New York, pp. 575–623.

Lester, M.C. & Nelson, P.B. (1981) Neurological aspects of vasopressin release and the syndrome of inappropriate secretion of antidiuretic hormone. *Neurosurgery* **8**, 735–440.

Lever, A.F., Beretta-Piccolli, C., Brown, J.J., Davies, D.L., Fraser, R. & Robertson, J.I.S. (1981) Sodium and potassium in essential hypertension. *Br. Med. J.* **283**, 1–15.

Levy, D.W. & Lye, M. (1987) Diuretics and potassium in the elderly. *J. Roy. Coll.*

165 | *The milieu interieur in the aged*

Physicians (Lond.) **21**, 148–152.

Luft, F.C., Fineberg, N.S., Miller, J.Z., Rankin, L.I., Grim, C.E. & Weinberger, M.H. (1980) The effects of age, race and heredity on glomerular filtration rate following volume expansion and contraction in normal man. *Am. J. Med. Sci.* **279**, 15–24.

Luft, F.C. & Weinberger, M.H. (1982) Sodium intake and essential hypertension. *Hypertension*, **4**, (Suppl. III), 14–19.

Luft, F.T., Weinberger, M.H., Fineberg, N.S., Miller, J.Z. & Grim, C.E. (1987) Effects of age on renal sodium homeostasis and its relevance to sodium sensitivity. *Am. J. Med.* **82**(Suppl. lB), 9–15.

Lye, M. (1981) Distribution of body potassium in healthy elderly subjects. *Gerontology* **27**, 286–292.

Lye, M. (1982) Body potassium content and capacity of elderly individuals with and without cardiac failure. *Cardiovasc. Res.* **16**, 22–25.

Lye, M. (1984a) Electrolyte disorders in the elderly. *Clin. Endocrinol. Metab.* **13**, 377–398.

Lye, M. (1984b) The deadly or disabling chest infection. *Geriatrics for GPs* **13**, 29–41.

Lye, M. (1985) The milieu interieur and ageing. In *Textbook of Geriatric Medicine and Gerontology* (Ed. J.C. Brocklehurst). Churchill Livingstone, Edinburgh, pp. 201–229.

Lye, M. & Faragher, E.B. (1982) Can body potassium of old people be predicted from anthropometric data? *Clin. Physiol.* **2**, 345–350.

Lye, M. & Winston, B. (1979) Whole body potassium and total exchangeable potassium in elderly patients with cardiac failure. *Br. Heart J.* **42**, 568–572.

MacKnight, A.D.C. (1977) Epithelial transport of potassium. *Kidney Int.* **2**, 391–396.

MacLeod, C.C., Judge, T.G. & Caird, F.I. (1975) Nutrition of the elderly at home III. Intakes of minerals. *Age Ageing* **4**, 49–57.

Mather, H.M., Ang, V. & Jenkins, J.S. (1981) Vasopressin in plasma and CSF of patients with subarachnoid haemorrhage. *J. Neurol. Neurosurg. Psychiatry* **44**, 216–219.

McConway, M.G., Martin, B.J., Nugent, M., Lennox, I.M. & Glen, A.C. (1981) Magnesium status in the elderly on hospital admission. *J. Clin. Exp. Gerontol.* **3**, 367–379.

Metildi, L.A., Shockford, S.R., Virgilio, R.W. & Peters, R.M. (1984) Crystalloid versus colloid in fluid resuscitation of patients with severe pulmonary insufficiency. *Surg. Gynecol. Obstet.* **158**, 207–211.

Montgomery, A.J., Shepherd, A.N. & Emslie-smith, D. (1982) Severe hyponatraemia and cardiac failure treated with captopril. *Br. Med. J.* **284**, 1085–1086.

Mordes, J.P. & Wacker, W.E. (1978) Excess magnesium. *Pharmacol. Rev.* **29**, 273–282.

Morgan, D.B. (1984) Plasma urea and electrolytes: The clinical need. In *Clinics in Endocrinology and Metabolism 13* (Ed. D.B. Morgan). Saunders, London, pp. 399–412.

Morgan, D.B. & Davidson, C. (1980) Hypokalaemia and diuretics: An analysis of publications. *Br. Med. J.* **1**, 905–908.

Morris-Jones, P.H., Houston, I.B. & Evans, R.C. (1967) Prognosis of the neurological complications of acute hypernatraemia. *Lancet* **2**, 1385–1386.

Novak, L.P. (1972) Ageing, total body potassium, fat-free mass and cell mass in males and females between ages 18 and 85 years. *J. Gerontol.* **27**, 438–443.

Novak, L.P. & Harrison, C.E. (1973) Abnormalities of cellular potassium concentration in uncompensated and compensated congestive heart failure. *Mayo Clin. Proc.* **48**, 107–113.

Peterson, B., Schroll, M., Christiansen, C. & Transbol, I. (1977) Serum and erythrocyte magnesium in normal elderly Danish people. *Acta Med. Scand* . **201**, 31–34.

Pick, A. (1966) Arrhythmias and potassium in man. *Am. Heart J.* **72**,295–306.

Pierson, R.N., Lin, D.H.Y. & Phillips, R.A. (1974) Total body potassium in health: Effects of age, sex, height and fat. *Am. J. Physiol.* **226**, 206–212.

Pollen, R.H. & Williams, R.H. (1960) Hyperkalaemic neuromyopathy in Addison's disease. *New Engl. J. Med.* **263**,273–276.

Reid, J.L. (1987) Angiotensin converting enzyme inhibitors in the elderly. *Br. Med. J.* **295**, 943–944.

Riegger, G.A.J., Lieban, G. & Kochsick, K. (1982) Antidiuretic hormone in congestive heart failure. *Am. J. Med.* **72**, 49–52.

Rowe, T.W. *et al.* (1976) The effects of age on creatinine clearance in man: a cross-sectional and longitudinal study. *J. Gerontol.* **31**,155–163.

Saraiva, R.A., Lunn, J.N., Mapleson, W.W., Willis, B.A. & France, J.M. (1977) Adiposity and the pharmacokinetics of halothane. *Anaesthesia* **32**, 240–246.

Sawyer, R.B. (1970) Postoperative magnesium metabolism. *Arch. Surg.* **100**, 343–345.

Schon, D.A., Silva, P. & Hayslett, J.P. (1974) Mechanism of potassium excretion in renal insufficiency. *Am. J. Physiol.* **227**, 1323–1330.

Schwartz, A.B. & Swartz, C.D. (1974) Dosage of potassium choride elixir to correct thiazide-induced hypokalaemia. *J. Am. Med. Ass.* **230**, 702–704.

Schwartz, W.B., Van yperele de Strihou, C. & Kassirer, J.P. (1968) Role of anions in metabolic alkalosis and potassium deficiency. *New Engl. J. Med.* **279**, 630–633.

Sherwood, R.A., Aryamayagam, P., Rocks, B.F. & Mankikar, G.D. (1986) Hypomagnesium in the elderly. *Gerontology* **32**, 105–109.

Shock, N.W. & Yiengst, M. (1950) Age changes in the acid-base equilibrium of the blood of males. *J. Gerontol.* **5**, 1–4.

Singer, I. & Rotenberg, D. (1973) Demeclocycline-induced nephrogenic diabetes insipidus. In vivo and in vitro studies. *Ann. Intern. Med.* **79**, 679–683.

Skinner, S.L. (1961) A course of erroneous potassium levels. *Lancet* **1**, 478.

Smith, J.D., Bia, M.J. & De Fronzo, R.A. (1985) Clinical disorders of potassium metabolism. In *Fluids Electrolytes and Acid-base Disorders* (Eds A.L. Arieff & R.A. De Fronzo). Churchill Livingstone, New York, pp. 413–509.

Stein, M., Schwartz, R. & Mersky, I.A. (1954) The antidiuretic activity of plasma of patients with hepatic cirrhosis, congestive heart failure, hypertension and other clinical disorders. *J. Clin. Invest.* **33**, 77–81.

Steiness, E. & Olsen, K.H. (1976) Cardiac arrhythmias induced by hypokalaemia and potassium loss during maintenance digoxin therapy. *Br. Heart J.* **38**, 167–172.

Sunderam, S.G. & Mankikar, S.D. (1983) Hyponatraemia in the elderly. *Age Ageing* **12**, 77–80.

Swaminathan, R. & Morgan, D.B. (1981) Pseudohyponatraemia. *Lancet* **1**, 96.

Szatalowicz, V.L., Miller, P. D. & Lacher, J.W. (1982) Comparative effectiveness of diuretics on renal water excretion in hyponatraemic oedematous disorders. *Clin. Sci.* **62**, 235–238.

Thomas, T.H., Morgan, D.B., Swaminathan, R., Ball, S.G. & Lee, M.R. (1978) Severe hyponatraemia. A study of 17 patients. *Lancet* **1**, 621–624.

Wacker, W.E.C. & Parisi, A.F. (1968) Magnesium metabolism. *New Engl. J. Med.* **278**, 658–663.

Wan, H.H. & Lye, M. (1980) Moduretic induced metabolic acidosis and hyperkalaemia. *Postgrad. Med. J.* **56**, 348–350.

Webb, S.C. & Impallomeni, M.G. (1987) Cardiac failure in the elderly. *Quart. J. Med.* **64**, 641–650.

Whang, R., Aikawa, J.K., Oei, T.O. & Hamiter, T. (1980) Routine serum magnesium determination — an unrecognised need. In *Magnesium in Health and Disease* (Eds M. Cantin & M.S. Seelig). SP Medical Books, New York, pp. 1–5.

Williamson, J. & Chopin, J.M. (1980) Adverse reactions to prescribed drugs in the elderly: A multicentre investigation. *Age Ageing* **9**, 73–80.

Womersley, J., Durnin, J.V.G.A., Boddy, K. & Mahaffey, M. (1976) Influence of muscular development, obesity and age on the fat-free mass of adults. *J. Appl. Physiol.* **41**, 223–229.

10 | Surgical decisions in the aged

K.D.J. VOWLES

Introduction

Most surgeons, whether general, orthopaedic or other specialty, find they are spending an increasing proportion of their professional time in the out-patient clinic, ward and operating theatre, looking after old people. In general surgery, older patients stay on average two to three days longer as in-patients, though this has been shown to be usually due to a surgical, rather than medical or social cause, and some 80% of them return to their original place of residence. They occupy half the beds available. Twice as many patients over 65 years of age in the UK are admitted to surgical beds as to geriatric wards, and over 75 years of age the same number are admitted to surgical beds as to geriatric and general medical beds combined. They also account for over half of all acute surgical admissions, yet this problem of the 'aged surgical emergency' has received little attention. Anaesthetists, particularly, must be only too aware that it is rare for an operating list not to include at least one octogenarian. Compared with the UK, in the USA almost twice as many common operations, such as hernia repair, cholecystectomy and hysterectomy, are done for the over-65 age group. It is not plain whether this is unnecessary surgery or there is an unmet need in this country. This increased surgical involvement has not yet been matched by an increased acceptance, interest and willingness to study the particular problems of this group.

The care of the old demands a team approach, even more so than some other special groups, yet this often receives only lip-service. The team involves besides nursing staff and all the range of hospital disciplines, the family doctor, the patient's family, friends or those who care for him, and often the social worker. Geriatricians make home visits to assess an elderly patient's quality of life and capabilities, but surgeons rarely take advantage of this approach, though when used it is of great help in subsequent decision-making. The loose concepts of 'biological age', 'quality of life' and 'will to live', though difficult to measure, are very important factors. It is perhaps difficult for anaesthetists to become involved in this way and at this early stage, but certainly, as a vital member of the team with such an important life-or-death part to play, the *results* of such wider social assessment should be available when physical assessment is made by the anaesthetist.

Population predictions show that in the UK the proportion of aged people will continue to increase until the year 2000 and then may begin to decline (Chapter 2). It is important, therefore, to assess how we are using our resources, whether human resources of time, enthusiasm, experience, skill and care, or practical resources of beds, staff and finance. What are we achieving in operating on all these old people? Are we sure that we are not trying to achieve 'the survival of the unfittest'?

The idea of 'aged', 'elderly', 'old', varies with geography, culture and our own viewpoint, and it has been said that 'ageing begins at birth'. The age of retirement, tending to be lowered, hardly seems the right starting point. In 1963, the WHO suggested that we should differentiate between the 'elderly' (60–74 years of age) and 'aged' (75 years and over), mainly because the former still make a valuable contribution to society in knowledge, skill and experience. A study of those over 70 years emphasizes that at 3 score years and 10 the average expectation of life in the UK is over 10 years (females 13.8 years, males 10.4 years) (see Table 10.1). This is important for comparison with the natural history and prognosis of the problem or disease demanding surgical management.

Our aim is to help the patient to achieve a quality of life as good or better, not worse, when he has recovered from surgery. The patient's question 'Is it worth having an operation at my age?' is not always spoken, but looms large in the motivation or 'will to live' which is so vital during recovery from surgery and its complications. Indeed, patients are much more concerned with being well enough to enjoy independent life than whether they will live a long time. This may at times govern surgical decisions and modify surgical management, particularly when dealing with malignant conditions.

A frank discussion concerning the alternatives to surgery is necessary to help a patient decide whether to accept a surgeon's advice. If a well-orientated elderly person decides against surgery, he or she should not be persuaded. The decision should be respected and the patient should be assured of our help in every possible way short of operation. Time spent in discussion is also helpful to the surgeon in deciding how to frame his advice once a full physical, mental and social assessment has been made.

Table 10.1. Average expectation of life in the UK (in years) 1982–84

Males	Age	Female
13.3	65	17.4
10.4	70	13.8
8.0	75	10.6
6.0	80	8.0
4.7	85	5.9

(From Government Actuary's Department Office of Population Censuses and Surveys.)

Surgical decision-making

Anaesthetists must wonder how a decision to operate is achieved, especially when confronted with a very unfit, aged person about whose background and possible future they know little. Ideally, the team — consisting perhaps of family doctor, geriatrician, anaesthetist, and ward sister — should sit down and hold a case-conference. But while it is unusual to achieve this ideal in elective surgery it is clearly impossible in the emergency cases where the aged comprise half the total.

It is not always realized that for a surgeon to operate on someone, carry out the actual assault, and supervise postoperative complications and eventual recovery, requires a decision with emotional as well as intellectual content. Anaesthetists must feel this too. While our assessment leading to decision should be as detached as is feasible, a 'gut-feeling' — especially when shared by surgeon and anaesthetist — should be respected and as far as possible analysed. In the end, the surgeon has to decide, and advise the patient accordingly.

Decisions about, and as a result of, investigations

Much modern high technology investigation is unpleasant, sometimes painful and sometimes disturbing, particularly so for the older patient. The diagnostic specialists and technicians involved, and the anaesthetists when their help is needed, can do a great deal to make these strange and disturbing happenings more bearable. The number of out-patient visits which an older person has to make to the hospital for 'tests', the number of in-patient stays, however brief, for more complicated procedures possibly needing a general anaesthetic, and the worrying days spent as an in-patient before the operation is carried out all contribute to a sometimes unnecessary burden.

A careful plan for investigation and assessment should therefore be made and certain 'routine' screening tests such as blood count, biochemistry, chest X-ray and electrocardiography can be done with the minimum of fuss as an out-patient. It is of little value to repeat them all when the patient is admitted a few weeks later.

A full blood count is usually regarded as essential, and unsuspected anaemia is not uncommon. It should not be forgotten that there are many causes besides the blood loss of gastrointestinal disease. A minimum acceptable level of haemoglobin has varied over the years. Usually 10 g dl^{-1} is regarded as satisfactory, provided the patient is normovolaemic and has reasonable cardiorespiratory function. If the patient has sustained acute blood loss, a haematocrit of 30–35% is adequate. When an elderly patient is discovered to be anaemic the day before surgery, a decision about urgent blood transfusion is required. This depends on whether the anaemia is acute or chronic, the blood volume normal, and whether severe blood loss at operation is likely (Watson-Williams, 1979). Transfusion at this late stage in an older patient may cause circulatory overload. It may be wiser to postpone surgery and treat the anaemia conventionally or give small transfusions of packed cells over several days. Anaemia has not been shown to affect wound healing.

The place of a routine X-ray of the chest is discussed by Seymour *et al.* (1982). Its benefits might be to provide a base-line for postoperative comparison, to discover unsuspected pathology or to predict postoperative problems. Seymour *et al.* found an abnormality in up to 60% of patients over 70 years of age; thus, the preoperative film for comparison is very useful when a postoperative problem develops. Unsuspected neoplastic lesions were found in 2.5% of elderly patients, changing the planned surgery. However, the preoperative film was of no help in forecasting postoperative cardiorespiratory problems.

In 1983, Seymour *et al.* studied whether or not a routine preoperative electrocardiogram (ECG) was useful in elderly patients before surgery. This might provide a useful base-line, discover abnormalities needing a decision to postpone surgery, or help to forecast those who were likely to develop cardiac complications. Some 50–80% of older patients do have an ECG abnormality so that clearly this is useful for postoperative comparison. So many elderly patients have evidence of a silent, painless myocardial infarct postoperatively that the ECG should probably be repeated three days after surgery. The surgical plan will need modification if a silent recent infarct is discovered on the routine preoperative ECG. However, this is probably of no value in predicting which patients will develop a postoperative cardiac problem.

Apart from direct surgical complications, such as anastomotic breakdown and sepsis, most of the serious postoperative complications in the old are indeed cardiovascular. Attempts to forecast complications by careful clinical examination may anticipate problems correctly. Goldman's classic paper from Boston (Goldman *et al.*, 1977) studied patients over 40 years old when he was able to identify nine independent significant correlates of life-threatening and fatal cardiac complications, mainly on clinical examination (Table 10.2).

Del Guercio & Cohn (1980), in New York, used a 'physiologic profile' designed to reveal unsuspected morbidity factors pre-operatively in patients over 65 years old. This involved use of a Swan-Ganz catheter in an intensive care unit. Of the patients cleared for operation by standard assessment, no less than 64% required preoperative adjustment of cardiopulmonary function, requiring 24 h for safe management. Using this approach for patients with hip fractures reduced the mortality from 29% to 2.9%. Just how far is such 'assessment' to go? The financial cost is said to be more than recouped by avoidance of complications and shorter hospital stay.

It has been shown that a proportion of elderly patients coming to surgery are malnourished. This may be dietary or associated with gastrointestinal problems, including lack of teeth, but there may also be more specific causes such as Crohn's disease and carcinoma of the pancreas. There have been many attempts to measure this state of malnutrition preoperatively and to correlate this with postoperative failure to thrive. These include weight loss, triceps skinfold thickness, forearm circumference, grip strength and numerous biochemical measurements, of which assessment of the plasma proteins, particularly serum albumin, is the most useful. Harken (1977) and others have applied the paediatric description of two types of malnutrition — marasmus and kwashiorkor — to elderly surgical patients. The cachexic marasmic patient with inadequate intake of protein and calories has decreased stores of protein and fat but visceral protein and immune functions are unchanged. The serum albumin is normal. The patient with kwashiorkor has protein deficiency but adequate calorie intake. The serum albumin is low, there is oedema, and immunocompetence is compromised. The risks of surgery and sepsis are high.

When malnutrition has been identified preoperatively, and postoperative problems with healing, sepsis and recovery inferred, it is not so certain that a decision to attempt correction of this state will help. Heatley

Table 10.2. Cardiac risk index

	Points
1 History	
Age >70 years	5
Myocardial infarct in previous six months	10
2 Physical examination	
S_3 gallop or jugular venous distension	11
Important valvular aortic stenosis	3
3 Electrocardiogram	
Rhythm other than sinus or premature atrial contractions on last ECG	7
>5 PVCs min^{-1} documented at any time before operation	7
4 General status	
Po_2 <60 or Pco_2 > 50 mmHg	
K <3.0 or HCO_3 <20 meq l^{-1}	
BUN >50 or Creat >3.0 mg dl^{-1}	
Abnormal SGOT, signs of chronic liver disease or patient bedridden from non-cardiac causes	3
5 Operation	
Intraperitoneal, intrathoracic or aortic	3
Emergency operation	4
Possible total	53

Score 13–25 warrants 'medical consultation' and consideration of delay
Score 26 or more — only truly life-saving procedures to be performed

PVCs — premature ventricular contractions; Po_2 — partial pressure of oxygen; Pco_2 — partial pressure of carbon dioxide; K — potassium; HCO_3 — hydrogen bicarbonate; BUN — blood urea nitrogen; Creat — creatinine; SGOT — serum glutamic oxaloacetic transaminase. (Reproduced from Goldman *et al.* (1977), with kind permission.)

et al. (1979) showed in a group of patients with gastric and oesophageal carcinoma treated with i.v. nutrition for 7–10 days preoperatively that there was a significant reduction in wound sepsis compared with the controls, but several patients had the complications of septicaemia and subclavian vein thrombosis. Other workers have not been able to demonstrate significant benefits. The time spent in correction by i.v. hyperalimentation must be balanced against the incidence of side-effects. Whenever feasible it seems better in the aged to use the enteral route, though this too has its side-effects, including nausea, vomiting, aspiration, nasopharyngeal ulceration and skin rashes. Perhaps the most practical approach is to set up an enteral route at the time of surgery, whether small-bore nasogastric tube, gastrostomy or jejunostomy. Postoperatively the help of the dietician, with sip-feeding and superb nursing, are of most value.

Seymour & Pringle (1983) have shown that when the serum albumin is 35 g l^{-1} or less this is associated with a twofold increase in postoperative sepsis and a 10-fold increase in postoperative mortality. This level of hypoalbuminaemia showed a closed statistical association with inoperable malignancy. In patients with resectable malignancy it did not apply. Such a finding should promote a careful search for other evidence of metastases and may lead to a decision, perhaps welcomed by the patient, to advise against surgery.

The acid test to be applied in deciding on any investigation which can be said to be unpleasant, e.g. barium enema, angiography, endoscopy, surely comprises the following questions:

(i) Will this test achieve or alter the diagnosis?

(ii) Will it affect the decision to operate or avoid operation?

(iii) Is there any simpler or less unpleasant test which can be substituted?

Decisions about such investigation must somehow be separated in our minds from the use of techniques which we are developing or in which we have a special interest, so that the patient's interests remain paramount. A total plan can then be made so that all tests are carried out at one visit or with one brief admission, preferably not just before operation. This means that the results can be studied, decisions made, and the patient advised. Every patient should know exactly what he or she is coming into hospital for, when the operation will be done, and the likely date of discharge home. Discussion of plans for any convalescence needed, with family or others involved at this early stage, avoids an unduly prolonged postoperative stay in the ward.

If this 'plan for total care' is to be followed it is clearly unsatisfactory, both for the patient and the anaesthetist, if they meet for the first time the day before the planned surgery. Problems discovered at such a 'last-chance assessment' can often be better elucidated at an earlier meeting, however arranged, and team-agreed assessment tests made available by intelligent anticipation of their likely need.

Decisions about prognosis

A proper appreciation of the natural history of the disease process (or processes) involved is needed. For example, an 85 year old woman with a mild iron deficiency anaemia known to be due to hiatus hernia, with some osteoarthritis of the hips, is referred on account of a breast swelling. This is small, characteristically dimpled and the obvious scirrhous breast carcinoma is confirmed (perhaps unnecessarily) in the out-patient department by needle biopsy.

She is otherwise well, independent, socially active and lively. Apart from her breast cancer, her life expectancy is probably five years and of 'high quality'. Her breast cancer is most unlikely to alter that, being compatible with 10–20 years of symptomless survival. The use of tamoxifen will almost certainly ensure this, and she can be reassured that surgery is not needed and followed up by her family doctor, not by the hospital.

Alternatively, in another patient the iron deficiency anaemia may be new, severe, and accompanied by dyspnoea and ankle swelling without evidence of a cardiac cause. Recent indigestion and marked loss of appetite, energy and 'interest in life' make the diagnosis, by barium meal, of non-obstructing carcinoma of the body of the stomach no surprise. It is known that if operation is undertaken, less than half such patients will have a lesion which is resectable, much less curable, and that very few indeed will survive five years. Though for a very different reason, this patient too should be advised that surgery will not be helpful. With her family and family doctor's help, care can be planned on the basis that the 'dying process' has started. A surgical attempt to alter this is inappropriate. The decision would of course be different if symptoms of obstruction at the cardia or pylorus present.

Such decisions are more difficult in an 'emergency situation' where perhaps a haematemesis has necessitated transfusion and endoscopy. It then becomes important that thoughtful full assessment of the situation is carried out and decisions are made by a clinician of sufficient experience to be aware of the likely outcome with and without an operation.

Prognosis has usually been thought of by surgeons in terms of survival, though early attempts to measure quality of life are now gaining acceptance. A study of patients over 70 years of age admitted to a general surgical ward was carried out with assessment by the family doctor concerned (many in rural practice) (Table 10.3). Of 210 such patients, 163 had an operation and the rest underwent investigations and observation. After surgery the mortality rate was 13.4% in emergencies and 4% in elective cases (Table 10.4). The 150 survivors were assessed after a year and it was found that a quarter of them had died, roughly half of those from their known malignant disease, most of the remainder from cardiovascular disease; a few had just 'faded away'.

Table 10.3. One year follow-up of 163 patients over 70 years of age following surgical operation at The Royal Devon and Exeter Hospital

163 Elective and emergency operations
150 Survivors
  66 Better ⎫
  43 Unchanged ⎬ 73%
   8 Worse (mostly amputees)
 36 Deaths during year (24%)
    13 Cardiovascular
    16 Malignancy
    7 Various
  3 Untraced

Table 10.4. Fate of 210 patients over 70 years of age admitted to a general surgical ward at The Royal Devon and Exeter Hospital

47 — No operation
  35 Emergencies (mortality 10%)
  12 Investigation

163 — Operation
  67 Emergencies (mortality 13.4%)
  97 Elective (mortality 4.0%)

Thus, emergencies formed 49% of the total admissions

Mortality of emergencies without operation — 10%
Mortality of emergencies with operation — 13.4%
Mortality for elective cases — 4%

There were a very few whose quality of life had degenerated, mainly amputees, but nearly three-quarters of the survivors were assessed as enjoying a quality of life better or equally as good as before surgery. Their family doctors were in no doubt that the decision to operate was correct. Even in those who died from their carcinoma in less than a year, e.g. in obstructive jaundice, the comment was often made that surgery had conferred real benefit for the remaining months of life.

Decision about the aim of surgery

Surgical obsession with five year survival figures as opposed to quality of remaining lifespan has led to an attitude that palliative, as opposed to curative, procedures are in some way inferior. However, each has its place, especially in an older patient, where our aim is 'to add life to years'.

Obstructive jaundice in a patient over 70 years is often assumed to be malignant in origin, yet it has been shown that in half such patients the cause is calculous. Courvoisier's 'law' is not infallible, but investigation, preferably by (comfortable) ultrasound and rarely by (uncomfortable) percutaneous cholangiography, will show the probable level of obstruction. If carcinoma of the pancreas is confirmed at laparotomy (with due attention to diuresis, control of sepsis and nephrotoxic antibiotics), it is known that the radical, hopefully curative operation of pancreatico-duodenectomy, while possible in about one-third of patients, carries a mortality rate of some 30% in older patients and a mean survival of 12 months, though palliation is good.

Alternatively, a double bypass procedure (since without gastro-enterostomy half the patients will develop symptoms of duodenal obstruction) carries a much lower mortality and, combined with intra-operative or later postoperative splanchnic nerve block, gives good palliation for an almost equal length of time. However, this worthwhile palliative approach is a major procedure also requiring proper attention to the prevention of sepsis and renal failure. The possibility of a calculous non-malignant cause which can be cured by surgery is always a pleasant surprise. If preoperative investigation has shown a hilar block, percutaneous placement of an endoprosthesis may give weeks or months of relief, since the natural history of cholangiocarcinoma is so much longer than that of the pancreas.

Oesophageal obstruction, whether benign stricture or, more usually, malignant, is a formidable problem for palliation in an aged patient. Classical excision by thoracotomy carries a high mortality, a low cure rate as regards longevity, with a good chance of restoration of normal swallowing. Once we accept that any procedure, however 'radical', is most unlikely to be curative, we must seek a less major approach. Many enthusiasts use intubation but the quality of life is not high, and recurrent dysphagia common. On the other hand, abdominocervical oesophagectomy, without thoracotomy, and with its low-complication anastomosis in the neck, may achieve worthwhile palliation, with a reasonably low mortality rate. In accepting this approach the idea of surgical cure by removing mediastinal nodes and spread is rejected in favour of a less major operation with the aim of normal swallowing alone. Endoscopic laser resection of the stricture may well also offer benefit in this group of patients.

Sometimes the search for worthwhile palliation has given unex-pected benefits. An elderly but active man with iliac arterial stenosis may find his claudication is progressing to rest pain which is spoiling his life. Cardiorespiratory assessment suggests that if his claudication is cured he will instead be crippled by angina. After an angiogram done by image intensification without anaesthesia, he is assessed as unfit for major aortic surgery and a subcutaneous femoro-femoral cross-over graft is planned instead, with minimal risk and good clinical result. The original surgical anxiety that this operation would produce a 'steal' claudication in the opposite donor leg has proved unfounded. There is some evidence that the increased flow through the donor iliac artery protects it from progressive obstructive thrombus to give better long-term outlook.

Decisions on timing of operation

There are many factors beyond surgical control which influence the precise time when operation is advised and planned. The patient initiates the process by seeking help from his family doctor, or by showing overt symptoms such that those around him insist on this. People in their 70s or 80s are remarkably tolerant of symptoms. Thus, colic or change in bowel habit are regarded as 'wind' or 'indigestion', claudication or metastatic bone pain as 'rheumatism' or 'lumbago'. Blood loss per rectum or vaginam or haematuria are either not seen because of poor vision, or dismissed due to fear. These delays lead to presentation of surgical illness often at an advanced stage, so that a higher proportion of carcinoma of colon presents as intestinal obstruction and of appendicitis as peritonitis than is the case in younger people. The family doctor may also procrastinate, though this is changing as it is becoming realized that earlier recognition and treatment of surgical illness is possible and beneficial. In the end, it is the family doctor who decides the time of surgical consultation, whether at home, as an outpatient or as an 'emergency'. Other factors leading to delay include outpatient lists, time consuming and sometimes inappropriate investigation, and waiting-lists for operations.

It is of some value to distinguish between 'elective', 'urgent' and 'emergency' surgery. By proper assessment and planning it is hoped to reduce the large number of elderly patients who form half of our present totals of emergency work (Seymour & Pringle, 1983). This is not merely because such work requires an inordinate resource of time, staff and cost, but mainly because in this age group the mortality is about three or four times greater in an emergency than an elective situation. We have found that in patients over 70 years of age admitted as 'emergencies', one-third did not require emergency surgery — yet the mortality in this group was 10%, since it included such misdiagnoses as coronary thrombosis, advanced carcinomatosis, and uraemia. In the group needing an emergency operation the mortality was 13%, contrasting with 4% mortality in those having elective surgery.

When the surgeon/anaesthetist team are assessing an elderly patient requiring surgery, who has arrived as an emergency, the most important question is whether to operate today (or more often tonight) or to delay for a few hours or a few days. Such a delay may give an opportunity for the correction of heart failure, control of an arrhythmia, restoration of fluid and salt depletion, balance of diabetes, initiation of diuresis in uraemia, or possibly blood transfusion to correct anaemia. During this time diagnostic procedures which may lead to more accurate assessment and a better plan for care, decisions about modified or radical procedures may be carried out. These include upper or lower gastrointestinal endoscopy, 'emergency' contrast enema, image-intensified angiography of the lower limb, and ultrasound examination of abdomen or pelvis.

The benefit to the patient of such an approach may be enormous. He or she can then have an 'urgent' operation, in daylight hours, properly planned, often by an experienced surgeon and an anaesthetist who are used to working as a team. Such problems as availability of operating theatres and staff, surgical and anaesthetic 'training' should be overcome. The concept is not new, since it has been practised for many years with fractured femur, prostatic obstruction and, more recently, gastrointestinal bleeding and acute biliary tract disease. But the latter is a good example of the dictum that undue delay in dealing with sepsis requiring surgical correction in spite of the use of the appropriate antibiotics is harmful. At one time it was thought that in view of the high risk of emergency surgery in the aged patient, it was better to make no attempt to deal with the underlying main problem, but carry out instead a minor procedure, proceeding at a later date to the major operation. An example of this is transverse colostomy for carcinoma or diverticulitis of the sigmoid colon. However, the mortality of transverse colostomy in such cases is the same as that of primary resection, and the patient still has to face a major procedure. Walker & MacDessi (1966) showed that this 'staging' approach involving multiple procedures increases the incidence of cardiovascular problems.

Another emergency with its own problems is that of head injury in an aged patient. The incidence, unlike most trauma, is the same in males and females. They may be complicated by alcohol, and associated with a separate medical condition which obscures or is obscured by the head injury itself, making assessment difficult. When brain trauma is added to an already reduced cerebral reserve, not only are diagnosis and treatment difficult but the outcome is worsened. A computerized axial tomography (CAT) scan may be needed to discover those few with an intracranial or intracerebral haematoma who will benefit from surgery.

Similarly, it has been known since 1900 that mortality from burns is related to age, and even 10 years ago survival over the age of 60 from 30% body-surface burns was very rare. Though this has improved with intensive care and parenteral nutrition, pre-existing medical conditions, poor healing of the atrophic thinner dermis, poor response to infection and prolonged recumbency still lead to a high mortality.

Decisions about elective surgery

At an earlier stage the surgeon often has to decide whether or not to advise an aged person who is only slightly troubled by a surgical condition to put up with it, and run the risk of possible progress to an emergency.

Hernia is the commonest cause of general surgical admission where a true emergency procedure is necessary, because of strangulation which does not permit delay. We found that in 120 patients over 70 years of age needing surgery for strangulated hernia there were 12 deaths. Though 18 patients had required bowel resection, none of these deaths had a surgical cause; they were due to cardiorespiratory or cerebrovascular sequelae. By contrast, the mortality for elective hernia repair in this age group is 1% or less. When assessing an elderly patient with a 'cold' hernia which is a nuisance, the surgeon has to decide whether this particular hernia is likely to strangulate and, if so, advise elective repair. That this can safely be done under regional anaesthetic in almost anyone, with a low recurrence rate, has been amply demonstrated by the records of the Shouldice Clinic (Glassow, 1976). Their approach in turning hernia repair into a minor incident in an elderly person's life could be widely adopted as a useful form of preventive medicine, avoiding emergency surgery.

It is known that gallstones are present at autopsy in a high proportion of elderly people, but studies of patients in whom stones were discovered incidentally during life show that over a period of some years half of them become symptomatic, 15% developing serious complications needing surgery, especially in the older age group, where there is also a higher incidence of stones in the common bile duct. Biliary tract surgery complicated by exploration of the common bile duct, by jaundice, sepsis or pancreatitis, carries under emergency or 'urgent' conditions a mortality of 12%, three times higher than an elective procedure in the aged. We should therefore advise any reasonably fit elderly patient, known to have gallstones which have become symptomatic with pain, cholecystitis, one fleeting attack of jaundice or mild pancreatitis to have properly planned elective biliary tract surgery, rather than just 'hope it will never happen'. In the case of abdominal aortic aneurysm, it has been estimated that once a diameter of 6 cm has been reached (easily monitored by repeated ultrasound examinations) rupture is likely. The mortality of elective repair in an otherwise fit patient over 70 years old is under 10% and the postoperative expectation of life is normal. After rupture, the mortality of those who reach hospital is 50–60%, but many die before doing so.

Decisions about prophylaxis

Sepsis

Compared with younger patients, the elderly are more susceptible to surgical infection which cause greater morbidity and mortality. Cruse & Foord (1973) showed in their study of nearly 25 000 surgical wounds that the sepsis rate for 'clean' wounds was doubled in patients over 65 years of age. (It was also doubled by preoperative shaving, increased sixfold in diabetics and sevenfold in the obese.) This problem in the elderly may be partly due to modified host defence mechanisms, including the mechanical barriers of skin and mucosa, cell-mediated immunity and T-cell dependent humoral immunity. Neutrophil function defects and phagocytosis deficiencies occur in some old people, but poor macrophage activity has not been implicated in altered defence in infections.

Decisions about perioperative antibiotic prophylaxis are therefore even more important in the elderly surgical patient, in spite of the risk of pseudomembranous colitis and other side-effects, than in younger patients. In postoperative sepsis the usual symptoms and signs of fever, tachycardia, leucocytosis and pain may be absent. The patient is just 'not himself'. This may well lead to delay in diagnosis or non-diagnosis of sepsis.

For these reasons, even though many surgeons are not convinced about prophylactic antibiotics for all patients, there is a good case for protecting the elderly in this way. Clean-wound operations need this protection only when the result of infection would be disastrous, especially vascular and orthopaedic procedures where a prosthesis is used. The first dose of antibiotic should be given at the induction of anaesthesia to ensure good blood levels and only one or two postoperative doses need be used. Gastroduodenal procedures (including endoscopy and especially where gastric acidity is reduced), biliary operations where there is known sepsis, where the common bile duct is involved and in jaundice (including percutaneous procedures), appendicectomy, and colorectal procedures all merit the use of perioperative antibiotics. With knowledge of the enteric or other organisms likely to be present, a suitable i.v. drug can be selected, the various cephalosporins being presently favoured. However, the use of prophylactic antibiotics must not, particularly in view of diminished signs and symptoms, give a false sense of security in managing postoperative sepsis. The margin for error is considerably less than in younger patients and the 'biological domino effect' of one complication after another in an older person with diminished 'elasticity' can be devastating. In any older patient who is confused or failing to thrive postoperatively, sepsis is the most likely cause and its detection requires a high index of suspicion, repeated physical examination, wound swabs, urine and repeated blood cultures. Decisions about the timing of judicious aspiration or drainage of abscesses and the use of appropriate antibiotic combinations are matters requiring experience, and often the help of a microbiologist is invaluable. The high incidence of wound sepsis following colorectal surgery, particularly in the elderly and after emergency procedures, makes it important to consider the efficacy of bowel preparation, often exhausting for both staff and patient. There is much variation between surgical units and the ideal has yet to be achieved.

Thromboembolic problems

It is known that about one in twenty general surgical patients over 65 years of age has a history of stroke, though the incidence may be higher. Fortunately, postoperative major stroke is unusual, so that no particular prophylaxis is suggested. If a patient has had a recent stroke, it is usually best to decide on postponing elective surgery.

Postoperative deep vein thrombosis (DVT) and pulmonary embolism (PE) are, however, much commoner in older than younger patients. DVT is detectable in over 50% but few of these become clinically important or embolize, the highest incidence of PE being 3–7% following hip surgery. The event may well be clinically silent and when suspected is difficult to prove except by nuclear ventilation/perfusion scan.

An attempt therefore has to be made to identify a high risk patient and to choose suitable prophylactic measures. The known risk factors include advanced age, previous history of DVT, preoperative and post-operative immobility, obesity, malignancy, long operations, pelvic and hip surgery and oestrogen therapy.

Since several factors apply to so many of our elderly surgical patients, many surgeons decide to use a prophylactic regimen for most, though evidence that this is effective in the older age group is lacking. This being so, the method or combination of methods chosen should be least troublesome to the patient and have a low incidence of side-effects. A combination of compression stockings and low dose s.c. heparin is effective and has fewer problems than oral anticoagulants and i.v. dextran. After PE, a full anticoagulant regimen with i.v. heparin needs to be carefully monitored by activated partial thromboplastin time measurement.

Decisions on the extent of care

Doctors, and perhaps particularly surgeons, are sometimes accused of a lack of both compassion and judgement in knowing how far and for how long to persist in treatment for an ill aged patient. Early decisions to abandon active treatment in favour of 'tender loving care' may lead to accusations of 'playing God'. Similarly, persistence with ventilatory support, parenteral nutrition or chemotherapy is labelled cruel. Paton (1981) has questioned whether intensive care is 'aggressive intervention, therapeutic arrogance, and a mania for measurement'. However, the mortality figures from a number of intensive care units show the same rate, unfortunately high, for all decades from 10 to 90 years. Mortality is related not to age but to organ/system failure, being 98% in triple organ/system failure for more than 24 h. Decisions about the possible need for intensive care in the elderly surgical patient should not be made under stress but should form part of the 'planned total care' for such a patient and usually made preoperatively. Examples might be elective postoperative ventilation for a previously fit man of 75 after a technically successful operation for ruptured aortic aneurysm, or a woman with biliary peritonitis from perforated gallbladder. Similarly, the decision to desist from intensive care is not directly related to age, except in so far as an aged patient after major surgery is more likely to exhibit triple organ/system failure, leading to an irrecoverable state.

Perhaps the most difficult decision of all, one not often directly involving the anaesthetist, is when to advise the patient or his family, that surgery for what appears to be an 'obviously surgical' condition, should not be undertaken. This must be based on a complete and certain diagnosis and assessment of other systems, a knowledge of the natural history of the involved pathological process and an appreciation of the quality of past life and how this is likely to change for the worse and for how long. If some knowledge of the patient's own philosophy and feelings can be added to this, it can sometimes be advised that surgery is not the best treatment, particularly in advanced malignant disease. If such a patient is likely to remain for a while in a surgical ward or is able to attend an out-patient clinic the anaesthetist may have a vital role in the relief of pain.

References

Cruse, P.J.E. & Foord, R. (1973) A five year prospective study of 23649 surgical wounds. *Arch. Surg.* **107**, 206–210.

Del Guercio, L.R.M. & Cohn, J.D. (1980) Monitoring operative risk in the elderly. *J. Am. Med. Ass.* **243**, 1350–1355.

Glasgow, F. (1976) Short stay surgery (Shouldice technique) for repair of inguinal hernia. *Ann. R. Coll. Surg. Engl.* **58**, 133–139.

Goldman, L. *et al.* (1977) Multifactorial index of risk in non-cardiac surgical procedures. *New Engl. J. Med.* **297**, 845–850.

Harken, D.E. (1977) Malnutrition: a poorly understood surgical risk factor in aged cardiac patients. *Geriatrics* **32**(2), 83–85.

Heatley, R.V., Williams, R.H.P. & Lewis, M.H. (1979) Preoperative intravenous feeding — a controlled trial. *Postgrad. Med. J.* **55**, 541–545.

Paton, A. (1981) Aggressive intervention, therapeutic arrogance, and mania for measurement. *World Med.* **16**, 66–68.

Seymour, D.G. & Pringle, R. (1983) Surgical emergencies in the elderly. Can they be prevented? *Health Bull.* **41**, 112–113.

Seymour, D.G., Pringle, R. & Shaw, J.W. (1982) The role of the routine preoperative chest X-ray in the elderly general surgical patient. *Postgrad. Med. J.* **58**, 741–745.

Seymour, D.G., Pringle, R. & MacLennan, W.J. (1983) The role of the routine preoperative electrocardiogram in the elderly surgical patient. *Age Ageing* **12**, 97–104.

Walker, R.L. & MacDessi, B.J. (1966) Myocardial abnormalities following geriatric surgery. *Med. J. Aust.* **1**, 783–786.

Watson-Williams, E.J. (1979) Hematologic and hemostatic considerations before surgery. *Med. Clin. North Am.* **63**, 1165–1189.

Suggestions for further reading

Tindall, G. (1986) High-tech medicine: when to say no. Report of meeting held by Open Section of RSM. *Journal RSM* **79**, 56–57.

Jennett, B. (1985) Benefits and burdens of surgery. *Br. J. Surg.* **72**, 939–941.

Johnson, J.C. (1984) Surgery in the elderly. In *Medical Care of the Surgical Patient* (Ed. L. Goldman *et al.*). Harper & Row, London.

Crosby, D.L. (1987) Management of the elderly surgical patient. *Br. J. Hosp. Med.* **38**, 135–138.

11 | Preparations for anaesthesia for the aged

H.T. DAVENPORT

Introduction

The ageing process has been described as 'a decreasing ability to survive stress' (Kenney, 1982). If aged patients are to maintain homeostasis they need more support to compensate for this decrease. Before any operation it is necessary to determine what risk factors are present that will affect homeostasis. This must be done by clinical examination, with non-invasive and invasive technological measurements, and an analysis of collected data. While it is rare for surgical operations to be aborted due to excessive anaesthesia risk, facilities and expertise are not so widely available that we can deny surgery to no one (Babu *et al.*, 1980). Attempts to undertake elective (protective) surgery rather than emergency operations are laudable (Gerson-Greenberg *et al.*, 1981) but they are of least consequence in treating the very seriously ill (Fig. 11.1).

The timing of common urgent procedures, such as the treatment of fractured hips, is controversial. While it is logical that there should be sufficient time for assessment and preparation, as for patients to recover from some of the stress caused by their injuries, further deterioration due to immobilization must also be avoided. This has been indicated by one follow-up report (Fig. 11.2). Others have maintained that immediate

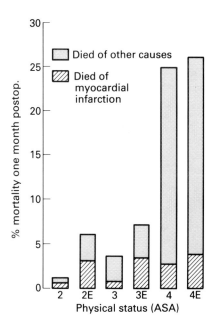

Fig. 11.1. Preoperative American Society of Anesthesiologists score related to 1 month mortality postoperation in patients over 80 years of age. (Reproduced from Djokovic & Hedley-Whyte, 1979, with kind permission.)

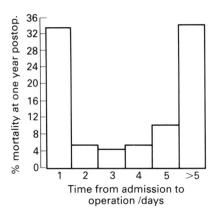

Fig. 11.2. One year mortality related to time of operation after hospital admission for fractured hip. (Reproduced from Kenzora *et al.*, 1984, with kind permission.)

operations are desirable as delays in admission to hospital have led to poorer rehabilitation (Villar *et al.*, 1986). For more urgent procedures, optimal timing of operations, which should be undertaken by senior staff, is desirable, as are structured recoveries and rehabilitation (Sikorski *et al.*, 1985).

In anaesthesia literature generally, preoperative evaluation and assessment of patients are described at great length. However, the amount of preparation which can be undertaken in the light of this knowledge is limited. Anaesthetists only have a little time with patients before their operations, even where arrangements for preoperative clinics or in-patient visiting are good. The recommended amount of time spent on preoperative preparation is likely to be an ideal rarely achieved in practice.

In an emergency situation, even obvious preparatory requirements may not be fulfilled. When it is suggested that an operation should be postponed or cancelled the inconvenience is often unduly stressed by all concerned. In such cases it is salutary to bear in mind that, where a second surgical opinion is obtained, indications for surgery are not always clear cut, particularly when dealing with the old. For example, where prostatectomy and cataract extraction operations were recommended by one surgeon a second surgeon only concurred for 15–30% of the sample of patients (Finkel *et al.*, 1982).

It is quite clear that older patients may have de-compensated physiological systems and a greater incidence of concurrent disease. The American Society of Anesthesiologists system (ASA score) has proved to be of consistent use in classifying the physical state of patients so as to predict likely postoperative complications or death. There is, however, a subjective element in assigning patients to different classes, which this system entails, and old patients are less often assigned to Class 1 or 2 (Djokovic & Hedley-Whyte, 1979). The degree of mobility and independence of such patients (Wallace *et al.*, 1986) or the simple question of whether they do their own shopping or not are also valid indicators of the time required for preparation, and of the monitoring and support that they are likely to need after their operation. Mortality figures indicate the degree of support which patients require when undergoing different operations but risk factor studies rarely agree. The latest for patients of all ages (Duncan & Cohen, 1987) implicates the duration of the operation, the seriousness of the patient's medical condition (ASA score) and the amount of the anaesthetist's experience.

Anaesthetists can become more expert at assessment if, by following up their patients, they learn what problems to anticipate. Anticipation of likely postoperative progress will help in organizing the amount of medical and surgical special care required. Patients and their relatives should always be informed if there is an intention to use high dependence or intensive care facilities. Ideally, rehabilitation programmes should be discussed and pre-arranged in preparatory assessment.

In making any decision as to what preparation is required complete medical histories, thorough examinations and appropriate laboratory tests are necessary. All three must be particularly stringent when dealing with old patients as they are not as straightforward as in the treatment of other age groups. Details concerning acute and chronic diseases and impairments, drug experience and past perioperative history may be more complex and less readily remembered. Natural ageing problems are often unremarkable to the patients. Falls and postural blood pressure changes, nocturnal dyspnoea, angina or sudden excessive tiredness or mental confusion are all important points to be considered in taking medical histories. These vague symptoms may point to serious disease in the aged. It is also important to gauge their degree of physical activity as the sedentary have diminished cardiac and respiratory reserves and prolonged bedrest can have dire consequences.

Physicians are too ready to prescribe bedrest for patients suffering from symptomatic heart failure or ischaemia and refractory oedema, despite the absence of any formal study of its effects upon the aged. Bedrest can cause decreased intravascular and extracellular fluid volume through diuresis, decreased calf blood flow and increased venous compliance, diminished muscle strength, glucose intolerance, negative nitrogen balance, orthostatic hypotension and increased clotting, all of which are detrimental perioperatively (Hogan, 1985).

Over-prescription of drugs for the aged is widespread and their administration and the patients' compliance is particularly irregular in this age-group. For years anaesthetists were concerned about the effects of preoperative medication on the conduct of anaesthesia, and many possibly interacting drugs were withdrawn. Now the tendency is to continue any appropriate medication as withdrawal may be more detrimental. As long as interactions are appreciated (Table 11.1) they are controllable and less hazardous than the effects of withdrawal. The anticholinergic effects of drugs may be more dramatic in the old (Bartus *et al.*, 1982) and drugs with these effects are widely used (Table 11.2). When there are no parenteral products available for essential medica-

Table 11.1. Important interactions of drugs

Preoperative drug	Caution required with:	Because this may cause:
Warfarin	Barbiturates	Bleeding
Cortisone	Barbiturates	Hypotension
Cytotoxics	Succinylcholine	Prolonged relaxation
Ecothiopate (eye-drops)	Succinylcholine	Prolonged relaxation
Narcotics	Barbiturates and sympathomimetics	Exaggerated responses
Glyceryl trinitrate	Pancuronium	Prolonged relaxation
Quinine, aminoglycosides and polymyxins	Relaxants	Extra relaxation
Beta adrenoceptor blockers	Ether or cylopropane	Cardiac depression
Potassium-sparing diuretics	Succinylcholine	Hyperkalaemia (cardiac effect)
Potassium-loosing diuretics	Non-depolarizing blocker	Hypokalaemia (prolonged)
Levodopa, methyldopa	Anaesthetic or sympathomimetic	Depressed blood pressure
Lithium	Relaxants and barbiturates	Depressed central nervous system
Tricyclic antidepressants	Sympathomimetics	Excess pressor response
Amitriptyline	Neostigmine	ST and T abnormality
Tetracycline	Methoxyflurane	Marked renal depression (*avoid*)
Monamine oxulase inhibitors (MAOI)	Narcotics, barbiturates and sympathomimetics	Exaggerated response (*avoid*)
Verapamil	Beta adrenergic blockers	Marked reduction of cardiac output (*avoid*)

tion, e.g. levodopa and oral hypoglycaemic agents, alternatives may be required. In the case of parkinsonism, this may require the use of anticholinergic drugs, keeping in mind their effect on mentation, glaucoma or prostatism. Where oral anticoagulants have been administered for a long time preoperatively, and particularly when patients are undergoing neurosurgical or eye operations, the anaesthetist must decide whether to discontinue them or substitute heparin.

Drug withdrawal or the introduction of new treatment should take days rather than hours in the treatment of older patients. This is also true of electrolyte and fluid balance correction (Chapter 9), as of nutritional adjustments. Over- or under-nutrition, while they are clearly important risk factors, are little affected by preparation, and allowance must be made for their effects. In obese patients, thrombosis and emboli, atelectasis and pneumonia, bleeding and sepsis are all more evident. Undernourished patients become more so in hospital, so protein, vitamins and minerals should be supplemented to assist their recovery. The value of artificial feeding, enterally or parenterally, in the treatment of wasted patients is questionable. Indications of alcoholism, with its

Table 11.2. Anticholinergics effects and commonly used drugs with these effects

Anticholinergic effect	Drugs with these effects
Bladder dysfunction	1. Anticholinergics, e.g. atropine,
Urinary obstruction	hyocine, orphenadrine,
Pupillary disorders	cyclopentolate propantheline,
Refraction changes	glycopyrronium
Mydriasis	2. Anti-depressants, e.g. MAIO and
Dry eyes	tricyclics
Constipation	3. Anti-Parkinsonism, e.g. amantidine,
Ileus — decreased small bowel	selegidine and levodopa
mobility	4. Antipsychotic, e.g. phenothiazines,
Fever — especially with a	butyrophenones, thioxanthenes,
combination of drugs	5. Antihistamines, e.g. hydroxyzine,
Impaired drug absorption due to	cyclizine trimeprazine, promethazine
gastric emptying delay and intestinal	6. Others, e.g. alcohol, disopyramide
motility change	and nitroflurantoin
Delirium (confusion)	

effect upon liver and coagulation activity perioperatively, plus the problems of withdrawal, e.g. delirium tremens, confusion, etc., are often overlooked.

Cardiopulmonary system

The cardiovascular and pulmonary systems are usually considered separately (Chapters 3 and 4). A satisfactory perioperative course is much more likely when patients have a properly functioning combined cardiopulmonary system. With increasing age, lung volumes and flow rates decrease and the protection and clearance of airways are less effective. As a result, serious peri-operative dysfunction is a constant threat to aged patients. Functional tests, X-rays and blood gas checks, which should allow for normal ageing changes, provide useful baselines by which to measure potential changes (Chapter 14). Precise counting of the breathing rate (McFadden *et al.*, 1982; Gravelyn & Weg, 1980) provides a good indication of respiratory disease. Conditions which are unrelated to the lung but which affect ventilation, e.g. stroke, parkinsonism, ascites, etc., are also important considerations in the treatment of old patients.

Bronchitic (blue bloater) and emphysematous (pink puffer) patients are now rarer and decreasing in number as air pollution declines. However, pollution caused by smoking must be proscribed (Jones *et al.*, 1987). If patients can be induced to stop smoking four to six weeks before their operations bronchorrhoea will be decreased, the cilial cleansing process will be revived and there will be a crucial improvement in their cerebral circulation (Roger *et al.*, 1985). Even a more brief cessation of smoking before an operation will reduce the carboxyhaemoglobinaemia and the tendency of alveoli walls to leak with certain stimuli, e.g. endogenous catecholamines. For these reasons, patients should be strongly urged to stop smoking before an operation.

Lack of research has meant that measures needed to identify those patients who require extra respiratory care have not been modified for treatment of the aged. Studies have shown perioperative hypoxaemia in old patients, due to ventilation perfusion mismatch areas in their lungs, and this mismatching is accentuated by anaesthesia and surgery. The relationship of age and postoperative respiratory complications has not been proved but prophylaxis should be liberally used to prevent the dire results of such complications in aged patients. Complications can be anticipated when patients have histories of chest disease, smoking, limited mobility, effort intolerance, obesity or pulmonary oedema and a high ASA score, or if examination reveals acute or chronic lung disease with sputum, especially if it is purulent, or if there is X-ray evidence of chest disease. In such cases, more intense assessment of respiration may be necessary, particularly if the projected operation is thoracic or upper abdominal, and patients should be advised as to the administration of oxygen, when this is feasible, and urged to improve their mobility, reduce their weight and/or give up smoking.

The simpler tests which have been validated in the treatment of the aged are FEV1, FVC, FEV1/FVC, and PEFR (the 'abnormals' of which are respectively <2 l, less than 70% of predicted, less than 60%, and <250 l min^{-1}) (Chapter 14). Arterial gas analysis is required as indicated. For major procedures, doxapram administration, appropriate antibiotic cover, heparinization and planned operative and postoperative regional anaesthesia with artificial ventilation support are called for (preferably in a high dependency or intensive care unit).

It is salutory to note that, after years of search for objective measures, the patient's subjective account of dyspnoea may be the best indication of risk (Nunn, et al., 1988). If a patient has bronchospasm, a bronchodilator, e.g. salbutamol, should be used. If sputum culture indicates pathogens susceptible to a particular antibiotic, then the antibiotic should be given prophylactically. Physiotherapy, improved posture and suction should be attempted in an effort to reduce sputum production. Cor pulmonale, as indicated by right heart enlargement, heavy hilar and pale peripheral markings in chest X-rays, finger clubbing, etc., presents a risk of serious complications.

When chest or abdominal operations are planned, patients must be told to deep-breathe and cough frequently, emphasizing that this will not be detrimental to the operation. Whenever respiratory insufficiency is apparent preoperatively, there should be prolonged monitoring, ventilatory support, oxygen administration and sputum control. The cardiovascular contribution to respiration must not be forgotten. This includes the propulsion, conduction, carriage and exchange of the gases in the periphery. Each of these may be awry in any aged patient and needs investigation.

Heart disease most commonly occurs among the old (Fig. 11.3). A history of smoking, extreme obesity or thinness, gross physical inactivity, previous myocardial infarction or unstable angina, hypertension or serious arrhythmia, or indeed any preoperative cardiovascular problems, are possible risk factors for cardiovascular complications. The routine electrocardiogram (ECG) provides an essential base-line and may indicate clinically unsuspected myocardial infarction. ECG results can also be included in a multivariate risk index (Chapter 10). The chest X-ray will predict functional left ventricular morbidity when gross cardiomegaly or pulmonary oedema are present. The ASA score will also correlate with the cardiovascular outcome.

Extra risk caused by other cardiovascular diseases, e.g. hypertension and diabetes mellitus, is surprisingly unproven. When all old patients are viewed in the light of these factors, with such simple laboratory tests as a blood count, urea and electrolytes, urine analysis, etc., we are faced with the dilemma of how much further to investigate. The simple expedient of monitoring the pulse strength and temperature of the big toe has been shown to indicate the state of the circulation (Ross *et al.*, 1969; Joly & Weil, 1969) and this deserves more study in relation to the aged. Clearly, surgery should be postponed following recent myocardial infarction. If this is not possible, a very high level of attention must be maintained in order to avoid the risk of re-infarction and death (Sheen *et al.*, 1978; Rao *et al.*, 1983).

Uncontrolled right or left heart failure severely limits the patient's ability to cope with the stresses of major surgery. Diuretics, wisely administered so as to avoid low potassium and hypovolaemia, and inotropes are often required to combat heart failure. Digoxin, however, is inherently toxic and as a prophylactic it is of little value in improving myocardial contractility. However, when the patient has atrial fibrillation or other supraventricular arrhythmia it can be beneficial.

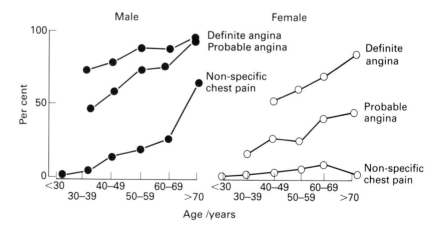

Fig. 11.3. Relation of age, sex and type of chest pain to presence of coronary artery disease. (Reproduced from Maille *et al.*, 1986, with kind permission.)

| *Preparations for anaesthesia for the aged*

Current research also appears to support the continuation of digoxin in those already taking it for a definite cardiac indication. The same applies to antihypertensive drugs and a present view, formed from studies of young patients, is that the untreated hypertensive patient with a diastolic pressure of >110 mmHg may encounter problems and should, if possible, be treated before undergoing an operation. Antibiotics should also be administered in preparing patients with valvular lesions, prosthetic heart valves or congenital heart anomalies, so as to prevent infected endocarditis. A current regimen, which should be regularly updated, is suggested in Table 11.3. Prophylactic anticoagulants being administered to those with prosthetic heart valves are sometimes best discontinued and replaced by heparin, which can itself be discontinued, for 18–30 h perioperatively.

The proportion of cardiac output supplied to the heart muscle is, to a great extent, dependent on the patency of the patient's coronary arteries. This is even more important than intrinsic heart wall changes as a contributory factor in cases of insufficient cardiac output and dysrhythmia. In post-mortem examinations, significant coronary artery narrowing (>60%) has been found in 60% of men at 55 and 60% of women at 80 years old. We must, therefore, diligently seach for, and treat, heart failure and important arrhythmias. A past history of leg oedema, dyspnoea or foaming sputum indicates previous de-compensation. Angina, central cyanosis, neck vein distention and pulsation, pulmonary

Table 11.3. Antibacterial prophylaxis for infective endocarditis in patients with heart valve lesion, septal defect, patent ductus or prosthetic valve

1 With dental procedures under general or local anaesthetic:
  (i) Oral amoxycillin 3 g four hours before induction of anaesthesia and then oral amoxycillin 3 g as soon as possible after the procedure
  (ii) Intramuscular amoxycillin 1 g before the induction of anaesthesia and oral amoxycillin 500 mg six hours later
  (iii) For those with special risk (e.g. those who have had endocarditis, who are gravely ill or diabetic), i.m. amoxycillin 1 g, plus i.m. gentamicin 1.5 mg kg^{-1} immediately before induction of anaesthesia, and oral amoxycillin 500 mg six hours later
  (iv) For patients who are penicillin sensitive or who are already taking penicillin, i.v. vancomycin 1 g over 60 min and then i.v. gentamicin 1.5 mg kg^{-1} before induction of anaesthesia

2 For genitourinary and colonic procedures:
  (i) Intramuscular amoxycillin 1 g plus i.m. gentamicin 1.5 mg kg^{-1} immediately before induction of anaesthesia, and then oral or i.m amoxycillin 500 mg six hours later
  (ii) If penicillin-allergic, i.v. vancomycin 1 g over 60 min before and i.v. gentamicin 1.5 mg kg^{-1} before induction. Metronidazole may also be added 500 mg i.v.

Note: Prophylaxis should be used freely, remembering that the classic signs of infective endocarditis, e.g. fever, murmur, rash or splenomegaly, may not be observed and the presentation may be the signs and symptoms of congestive cardiac failure, stroke or mental upset congestion with basal creps, hepatomegaly, ascites or peripheral oedema should never be considered to be normal ageing stigmata. Unfortunately, diagnosis from symptoms and signs is not straightforward (Table 11.4).

Because myocardial dysfunction may be so covert in the old it is necessary to consider the likely aetiology of failure and the precipitating factors in each instance. Three-quarters of old patients will have hypertension. Valvular dysfunction and heart enlargement (with faint heart sounds or pansystolic murmur) may also be harbingers of heart failure. The heart's pumping capacity can be gauged by giving the patient a small infusion of crystalloids and observing their effect upon their central venous pressure. Steroid administration (causing sodium retention and potassium loss), atrial fibrillation, tachycardia, anaemia, thyrotoxicosis, pulmonary embolism and myocardial infarction or infections may all precipitate heart failure. In such cases further examinations should be undertaken in order to determine whether or not there is heart failure.

The use of sophisticated invasive and non-invasive methods will depend on the availability of such tests and their expert interpretation. It is difficult, in the light of their fallibility and sequelae, to justify routine invasive investigations, e.g. pulmonary artery catheterization or coronary angiography, at any age (Whittmore et al,, 1980; Shoemaker et al., 1983; Kalman et al., 1986; Hertzer et al., 1984; Shultz et al., 1985). The pulmonary artery catheter is of only limited use in treating aged patients as the change in heart wall compliance will influence pressure readings and complications are likely (Robin, 1985; Nadeau & Noble, 1986). Non-invasive impedance cardiography, ballistocardiography and the carbon dioxde rebreathing methods of measuring cardiac output have all been used with limited success and popularity. Other non-invasive diagnostic techniques may also be applied, e.g. 2D-echocardiography or radionuculide ventriculography, but to date they have proved disappointing.

Positron emission tomography, nuclear magnetic resonance imaging and cine-computerized tomography scanning are still in the experimental stages. Whilst an ECG is essential as a base-line for change and an in-

Table 11.4. Diagnostic dilemmas with myocardial ischaemia

1 Symptoms:
    (i) Mental confusion may cause poor history and obscure diagnostic pointers
    (ii) Pain perception changes lead to disregard or acceptance of condition
    (iii) Dyspnoea and fatigue arise from deconditioning, obesity or lung problems as well as heart failure
    (iv) Anorexia and nausea can be due to medication or other illness than ischaemia

2 Signs:
    (i) Rales are present with atelectesis or lung disease
    (ii) Ankle oedemas arise from varicosities and stasis
    (iii) Hepatomegaly may be misdiagnosed with a low diaphragm with chronic obstructive airway disease
    (iv) Jugular distension can be due to unfolding aortic arch entrapment

dicator for further study, e.g. enzyme assay for ischaemic change, it is rarely of diagnostic use in treating old patients. It can, of course, define a heart block which requires pacing. Pacing is now suggested for those with a bifascicular, permanent or intermittent complete heart block (especially with faints or dizzy spells) and a first degree arteriovenous (AV) block. If pulmonary artery catheterization is to be performed on a patient with a left bundle branch block, a pacing device should be used because instrumentation may cause a right bundle branch block. There should be cardiological consultation if a pacemaker is to be used as a prophylactic for sick sinus syndrome or as an 'inotropic technique.' Clinical examination of heart murmurs is very important. Many are innocent, particularly when less distinct or localized, and echocardiography helps to define them. Subacute bacterial endocarditis or carditis is not uncommon in the aged and, if they are suspected, blood cultures should be ordered to ensure prompt treatment.

Other dysrhythmias should be controlled. For example, fast atrial fibrillation should be treated with digoxin. The administration of digoxin should not be rushed (Liu & Collis, 1984) and a loading dose is not recommended for older patients. Therefore, the initiation of treatment may entail a two to three day postponement of operation. Raised blood pressure is, as I have noted, common in older patients and, if this is gross, the effects of the usual associated arteriosclerosis on the brain, kidneys or heart should be determined. If one is proficient with an ophthalmoscope, examination of the fundi may, by defining the amount of retinal hypertensive changes present, help assessment. It is important to exclude secondary, as opposed to idiopathic, causes of hypertension. The commonest cause of this hypertension in the aged is renal artery stenosis, but thyrotoxicosis, aortic insufficiency and complete heart block are other possibilities.

If a patient still has marked fluctuations of raised blood pressure after resting for two or three days before surgery, an appropriate hypotensive agent should be used to stabilize them perioperatively. Beta receptor blocking drugs appear to be particularly effective in limiting a major drop in blood pressure during general, and even more during regional, anaesthesia (Dagnino & Prys-Roberts, 1986). Patients who are shown to have high blood pressure prior to an emergency operation should be particularly closely observed and the anaesthetist should be prepared to treat them by parenteral means if necessary. When diuretics have been taken, the patient's serum potassium level should be checked several times before they undergo an operation as sudden changes have serious repercussions. Chronic mild hypokalaemia (<3.5–3.0 mmol l^{-1}) or hyperkalaemia (>5.5 mmol l^{-1}) may present vague symptoms or signs which require therapy. The usual respective therapy, i.e. potassium or calcium bicarbonate, glucose with insulin (Vitez, 1987), may be given, with caution, parenterally.

When the old patient is seriously ill it is difficult to assess their degree of shock as the usual evaluation factors are all less precise. The older the patient, the more morbidity and mortality will be caused by burns (Howie, 1971). This is also true of serious trauma, the severity of which should be gauged by a scoring system (Baker *et al.*, 1974). Thus, aged patients with major burns and those who have had accidents need meticulous preparation before an operation. Their skin perfusion is already diminished by age and their extremities will also often be cold. As axillary and oral temperatures are fallible, core measurements must be used more frequently. Because postural hypotension, hypertension and less variable pulse rates are normal for older patients, levels of heart rate and blood pressure signs are unreliable. Sunken eyes and less turgor of the skin may be present without hypovolaemia. While apathy and drowsiness or reduced urine output may not be significant they indicate the need for further studies.

It is widely accepted that central venous and arterial canullation is helpful in the management of patients jeopardized by grave disease or major procedures. Other clinical, statistical or haemodynamic techniques which might assist cardiovascular management have yet to be fully explored. Promising developments involve the measurement of patients' exercise tolerance (Gerson *et al.*, 1985) and dipyridamole-thallium scanning (Boucher *et al.*, 1985). However, the generally poor predictive value of exercise ECGs (Petch, 1987) indicates the need for careful assessment of these tests. Some medical centres are trying to prove the value of the prophylactic use of coronary artery bypass surgery, as of carotid endarterectomy by preoperative tests for severe coronary or carotid artery obstruction. However, in such difficult cases, clinical acumen is still invaluable.

Deep vein thrombosis

Old age is always listed as a verified risk factor for postoperative deep vein thrombosis. Multi-centre trials have clearly indicated that heparin administration can reduce the incidence of this complication, and consequent pulmonary embolism, after general surgery. Therefore, in the absence of contraindications, aged patients should receive 5000 u heparin s.c. two hours before any major operation and every 8–12 h postoperatively until they are fully mobile (Kiil *et al.*, 1978). With this regimen, bleeding should not increase appreciably during the operation but there may be more wound haemorrhages afterwards.

This regimen has not proved successful in hip operations. In such instances, dextran 40 should be administered at the rate of 10 mg kg^{-1} on the day of operation and 5 mg kg^{-1} daily until the patient is mobile. Pneumatic compression or pressure graduated elastic stockings (so-called antiembolism stockings) should also be applied to the patient's legs perioperatively. If such regimens are not routine, patients most prone to this condition, i.e. those with heart disease, obesity, varicosities, previous deep vein thrombosis or embolism, blood dyscrasias or immunosuppressive therapy, must undergo regular clinical checks and Doppler flow studies so that they can receive immediate treatment as required. Before their operations, patients should be instructed in deep breathing and leg exercises which will be of great benefit postoperatively.

Renal system

We can compensate for the diminished lung ventilation reserves of old patients but we cannot do the same for the decrease in their kidney function. However, their diminished glomerular filtration rate (GFR) can be protected by ensuring a good blood supply, as by careful maintenance of fluid and electrolyte balances (Chapter 9). Creatinine clearance indicates GFR but it is tedious to measure. Creatinine levels and the application of the Cockcroft/Gault formula are preferable indicators (Cockcroft & Gault, 1976).

$$\text{Male creatinine clearance (ml min}^{-1}) = \frac{(140 - \text{age}) \times \text{body wt. (in kg)} \times 1.2}{\text{serum creatinine } \mu\text{mol l}^{-1}}$$

Female creatinine clearance is 15% less. Electrolytes, acid-base and inappropriate antidiuretic hormone problems, which are discussed in Chapter 9, need to be corrected with caution and this may require some postponement of the operation. Anaesthetists must give thought to kidney and liver action in preparing patients for operations, principally because of their effect on drug metabolism (Chapter 8).

As many aged patients suffer renal impairment, their reduced GFR will cause cumulation of drugs normally excreted through the kidney. For this reason, anesthetists should consider reducing or discontinuing the dose of such drugs. Renal drug toxicity, which is not always obvious in older patients, is likely when there is concurrent salt or water depletion. As I have indicated, postural hypotension, hypertension, a less variable heart rate, limited skin turgor and peripheral vascular disease generally afflict the elderly and can make it difficult to detect volume depletion.

Patients should be consulted as to their use of diuretics, whether they are subject to diarrhoea or vomiting and how much fluid they are accustomed to drink. The inability to concentrate or dilute urine will make deficiencies or excesses of fluids and electrolytes poorly tolerated, and for this reason perioperative balance must be more carefully controlled. Because pH adjustment is less efficient in old patients, changes produced by trauma, sepsis, or respiratory insufficiency will be less promptly dealt with and the results of this poorer control will be more common. Although the incidence of acute renal failure rises perioperatively in older patients, it is not very common. However, renal insufficiency of varying degrees is often apparent.

When renal failure does occur in old patients its consequent mortality is high, although the ultimate cause of death may be sepsis or cardiovascular collapse rather than uraemia *per se*. As acute tubular necrosis is the commonest perioperative cause of acute renal failure, attention must be directed to hypovolaemia. While haemorrhage and vomiting are easily observed as causes there may also be subtle reductions of intake due to the patient's loss of will, immobility or chronic disease or even because of the hospital's excessively prolonged *nil per os* (NPO) rules before investigations or surgery.

Other reasons for extra monitoring and planned intensive care are anaesthesia which may produce serious hypotension, cardiotomy during heart surgery, aneurysm excision, unrelieved obstructive jaundice and the misuse of radiocontrast material or other nephrotoxic drugs. The prophylactic value of mannitol prior to operation is not established, but up to 25 g is unlikely to be harmful. The same applies to the prophylactic use of i.v. dopamine (2 mg kg^{-1} min^{-1}). The guidelines for correcting pre-existent deficits and the replacement of losses preoperatively are similar to those for younger patients, as is the regimen to be followed for the oligaemic. If, after various causes of oligaemia (such as blocked catheter or simple bladder neck obstruction requiring catheterization) have been eliminated, a patient's urine output is still less than 30 mlh^{-1} and decreasing, further attention is required. Because of the seriousness of kidney dysfunction, consultation with a nephrologist must be encouraged so that, by combined efforts, we can learn more about the older patient's kidney action in stress. To avoid renal depression with obstructive jaundice, oral administration of bile salts and/or i.v. mannitol is recommended (Chapter 14).

Central nervous system

The incidence of postoperative strokes appears to rise with ageing but any preventable factor which may be controlled preoperatively is not yet known. To avoid mental upset the best that can be done is to give the patient a full explanation of their circumstances preoperatively, re-peated, if need be, by other staff and relatives. The use of inappropriate drugs should also be discontinued. If there is a history of the patient fall-ing, an underlying medical cause should be sought. The patient's orientation in time, place and person should be checked (Chapter 5) to show the extent of preoperative confusion, which may entail further tests. Success in obtaining consent from older patients is related to their age and level of education (Taub *et al.*, 1986) and has certain problems which are dealt with in Chapter 17.

Full assessment of a patient's mental state and autonomic com-petence, while clinically helpful and of much investigative value, is practically difficult and infrequently used. A very brief 'composite decision rule' has been proposed (Klein *et al.*, 1985) for when there is little time for such a check. This consists of asking the patient what the date is (day, month and year), getting them to subtract 7 from 100 five times (or to spell 'world' backwards) and asking them to repeat three memorized words after five minutes. Two and a half minutes are allowed for the patient to complete 10 questions and a score of less than 7 is thought to require a supportive history from someone who knows the patient well. However, such a test seems too stringent to me, particularly in dealing with vulnerable people who are likely to get stressed and confused if they feel they are 'on trial' and threatened with institutionalization. More 'conversational' questions are less alarming.

As older patients may suffer a physical and intellectual decline which will require prolonged rehabilitation after major surgery, such convalescent care as may be needed should be considered and discussed preoperatively. Older patients should also be forewarned of the mental aberrations that may occur after anaesthesia so that they will be less anxious should they arise. If surgeons, nurses and anaesthetists made more of an effort to orientate old patients they would be less likely to require sedation. Confusion and delirium after operations is quite common in all age groups, particularly the old and especially when intensive care is required. Moreover, visual and auditory functional changes which have not been noticed by patients or their relatives may become apparent for the first time when they are exposed to new stresses. Intermediate care facilities should be more frequently used for the prolonged convalescence which most older patients require.

Biochemistry

The reference range of biochemical test is not markedly different for the aged. Serum albumin changes are among the most marked but only amount to 2–3 g l^{-1} in the fit aged and this is far exceeded by the dramatic fall in albumin levels which occurs when old people become ill (Fig. 11.4). The degree of reduction of the serum albumin level has consist-

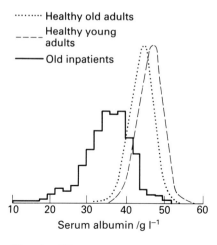

Fig. 11.4. The fit young and old subjects (probability) and old in-patients (distribution) serum albumin levels. (Reproduced from Hodkinson, 1984, with kind permission.)

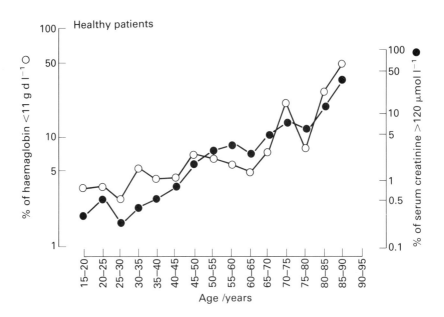

Fig. 11.5. The incidence of low haemoglobin and high serum creatinine levels related to age in healthy surgical patients. (Reproduced from Jacobsen *et al.*, 1987, with kind permission.)

ently been shown to be directly related to increased morbidity and mortality with medical and surgical disease (Seymour, 1986). An exceptional 'normal' reference range is that for serum phosphate in old men (0.65–1.23 mmol l^{-1}). Renal impairment, multiple pathology and drug therapy are associated with illness in the aged and they can all affect biochemical test results. In essence, the discriminatory powers of each test is much reduced when applied to the aged, and over-diagnosis on the evidence of small changes is common. Laboratory investigations of old patients more often produce 'abnormal' results (Fig. 11.5) but these should be interpreted with circumspection.

Endocrine systems

Ten per cent of people over 65 years old have diabetes mellitus. A random measure which shows a blood sugar level higher than 11 mmol l^{-1} (or a fasting blood sugar level higher than 7.2 mmol l^{-1}) is usually diagnostic. Diabetic control involves the use of many oral hypoglycaemic agents and the anaesthetist must decide whether it is permissible to discontinue them for a short time or whether insulin therapy is required. Due to impaired renal function, hyperglycaemia may lead to hyperosmolar non-ketotic coma and the diabetic patient's sensitivity to hypoglycaemia is also heightened. The use of thiazide diuretics or corticosteroids should be stopped if possible as they can cause diabetes.

In preparing a patient who is not insulin dependent for a minor

Preparations for anaesthesia for the aged

operation the usual oral hyperglycaemic agent should be omitted on the day of the operation. For the insulin dependent patient a glucose drip and a blood sugar estimate should be arranged before their operation. When blood sugar is above 12 mmol l^{-1} the rate of insulin should be increased; when it is below 6 mmol l^{-1} it should be decreased accordingly. The usual intraoperative fluids and transfusions, etc. must be administered by a separate infusion. If the patient's renal function is seriously compromised, he or she may need to be given a concentrated glucose solution which can be administered through a central venous catheter. Serum potassium levels should be regulary checked (6–12 hourly) and corrected.

Indications of low or high thyroid activity are very indistinct in older patients, so hormones must be assayed more often than when treating younger patients. There is conflicting advice concerning steroid supplementation. One idea is that any patient who has had steroid administration of a week's duration within one year of an operation should receive supplementation perioperatively. Others maintain that administration of hydrocortisone is only necessary when otherwise unexplained hypotension is observed. Because the older patient is particularly vulnerable, and monitoring can be variable, a regular regimen is advisable for patients who have had steroids within three months of an operation. The usual regimen is 50 mg hydrocortisone hemisuccinate, first administered with premedication and then every six hours for one or two days.

Haematology

Anaemia due to iron deficiency, megaloblastic changes or chronic disease occurs in up to 40% of patients in geriatric wards. Treatment is often prolonged and sometimes tedious. Therefore, the anaesthetist has to reply more heavily on transfusions than when treating younger patients. The detection of anaemia in relationship to dehydration haemoconcentration is important. Haemoglobin level and the freshness of transfused blood (2–3 dpg content) must be maintained to ensure efficient respiration. Alkalosis, hypothermia or hypocarbia, all of which can adversely affect the oxygen dissociation curve, should receive particular attention when treating older patients.

Hypothermia, hypotension and hypoxia, which particularly afflict this age-group , are all potentially crisis-creating conditions for patients with sickle cell anaemia. Coagulation problems, apart from those associated with liver disease, may arise through blood diseases which occur more frequently in older patients, i.e. polycythaemia, multiple myelomytosis and chronic lymphatic leukaemia. A thorough coagulation study should be obtained and a haematologist's advice should be sought in order to correct a patient's increased viscosity, platelet numbers and hypogammaglobulinaemia. Where an autologous blood transfusion service exists, older patients may use it provided there is sufficent time for weekly bleedings which should ensure that their haemoglobin levels will not fall below 11 g dl^{-1} (James & Smith, 1987).

Malnutrition

In paediatrics, malnourished patients have long been identified as either marasmic or kwashiorkor type and these terms are equally valid for old patients. The marasmic exhibits marked reduction of fat stores and skeletal muscle and is easily identified clinically, while the kwashiorkor patient has depleted visceral protein, reduced immunocompetence and may, due to oedema, appear to be obese rather than wasted. In older patients such oedema is often attributed to cardiac or postural causes. For verification, serum albumin levels and cutaneous sensitivity testing may be used.

The extent of malnutrition in preoperative patients is difficult to determine, as is the value of supplementary enteral or parenteral feeding perioperatively. There are indications that, for the most seriously malnourished patients, supplementary nutrition over a prolonged period does produce better wound healing and probably decreases morbidity (Heatley et al., 1979; Muller et al., 1986). In the light of complications, oral/enteral supplementation is preferable for those patients with poor intake of food, burns or sepsis. Elemental diets, rather than i.v. hyper-alimentation, are also acceptable for most other indications apart from oesophageal obstruction or head and neck pathology.

A special team should document the use and control of parenteral feeding regimens (Chapter 15). The relationship of sepsis to nutrition and immunological response is important to anaesthetists but the use of prophylactic antibiotics is usually decided by surgeons. However, when the risk of sepsis is heightened, anaesthetists should be particularly careful about cleanliness, using asepsis techniques in some instances.

Thermoregulation

Balancing the temperature of older patients is not a refinement but a crucial element of their care. Frequently, body temperature will fall due to impaired mechanisms which will be further disrupted by the administration of drugs and the exposure of the patient's body and viscera. At all times the temperature of the body should be maintained. Temperature regulation is paramount in reducing the risks of depressed cardiorespiratory function with hypotension, impaired ventilation and cardiac dysrhythmias. The correction of developed hypothermia can be a major insult involving may complications.

Pressure-sores present another insidious, but no less debilitating, problem. There is evidence that a hard surface, immobility, shearing or rough movement can initiate damage within a brief period and produce a dreadful complication (Vershuysen, 1986). We must ensure that patients rest on a hard surface for a minimum of time and that sliding or lifting of them is undertaken with extreme care.

Aspiration problems must be considered in relation to the gastro-intestinal tract. H-blockers and antacid are useful in dealing with such problems. Hiatus hernias, oesophageal pouches and bowel obstructions are fairly common in aged patients and they should be detected before an operation, as they all pose aspiration risks. Teeth and jaws, which are particularly prone to decay in aged patients, must be carefully examined pre-operatively with a view to airway management. Patients with oral sepsis may develop parotitis when debilitated perioperatively.

Premedication

Most anaesthetists are rightly cautious about using the usual premedi-cants on older patients. Older patients, with experiences of a long life, are often more sanguine than expected and sedatives act excessively upon them, producing prolonged amnesia, anxiety and confusion. A very drowsy patient can still be anxious, and for this reason the value and im-portance of preoperative visits cannot be over-emphasized. On such visits the anaesthetist should attempt to allay the patient's anxiety due to unfamiliar surroundings, uncertainty and concern over the future and worry about anaesthesia and discomfort after the operation.

An appropriate benzodiazepine, such as temazepam (Salomen et al., 1986), triazolam or oxazepam given an hour before the operation or diazepam or lorazepam given the evening before, is the commonest premedication choice. When night sedation with limited after-effects is required, Chlormethiazole or Lormetazapam appear to be most satisfac-tory (Overstall & Oldman, 1987). The place of midazolam as a premedicant is still not defined but its potency for sedation and anxiolysis is two or three times that of diazepam. All benzodiazepines should be given in a decreased dose for older patients as they have enhanced central nervous system depression.

Droperidol is strongly antiemetic and, with its dissociative action, it is used by some anaesthetists, but its strong dopaminergic receptor blocking effect can lead to unwanted extrapyramidal syndrome symp-toms. Hydroxyzine is an antiemetic and a tranquillizer and also has minimal analgesic properties. In small doses, both of these drugs may be helpful options for premedication. Methotrimeprazine, a tranquillizer with an analgesic action, is sometimes useful.

Unfortunately, the euphoric effects of narcotics are not dominant and dysphoria can be upsetting for patients. However, for those in pain, small preoperative doses of narcotics cannot be contraindicated and they will greatly assist induction and maintenance of anaesthesia — 'normal' doses can be safely used only as a part of an anaesthetic directly controlled by the anaethetist. Routine use of narcotics in other than quite small doses is clearly dangerous for old patients (Arunasalam et al.,

1983), particularly when they are suffering from renal insufficiency (McQuay & Moore, 1984).

Anticholinergic drugs are now considered unnecessary and unacceptable because of their side-effects, which range from restlessness, confusion and hallucinations to delirium or coma. It is also possible that they precipitate tachycardia, bowel stasis, urinary retention and unpleasant mouth dryness, together with less obvious relaxation of lower oesophageal sphincter, mydriasis and cycloplegia, increased respiratory dead space and increased body temperature (the latter is sometimes beneficial).

Current use of H blockers, cimetidine and ranitidine to reduce acid gastric secretions is pertinent to the treatment of older patients. Ranitidine is probably preferable to cimetidine, which has been shown to prolong diazepam, propranolol and lignocaine action and to cause arrythmias, hypotension and central nervous system depression on occasions. I recommend 150 mg ranitidine given orally two to four hours before an operation, followed by 5 mg metoclopramide given intramuscularly one hour before the operation, but this needs full investigation. Metoclopramide may also cause unwanted extrapyramidal syndrome symptoms, particularly when repeated postoperatively as an antiemetic. Perphenazine and promazine have both been favoured as premedication antiemetics in some circumstances, e.g. eye surgery.

The use of day care surgery for older patients is problematic. While reduction of hospital admission is theoretically sound, assistance must be ensured for the ageing patient, alone or with an ageing partner, who may experience difficulties immediately after an operation. However, with the correct screening process, day care can be beneficial for older patients and should be encouraged. It is commonly taught that preoperative medication should be avoided in day care procedures. However, there is no clear evidence to support such a practice. Much is gained by sensible premedication which should not affect a patient's street fitness after an operation but should limit their postoperative discomfort (White, 1986).

Envoi

Medical scientists argue about, and have not yet proved, the value of complex techniques in preparing old patients for operations. If present general standards of care were perfected and assiduously applied, the majority of clinicians could achieve a major improvement in this regard. One of the most important and irreplaceable aspects of that care is an understanding and sympathetic approach to the old.

References

Arunasalam, K. *et al.* (1983) Ventilatory response to morphine in young and old subjects. *Anaesthesia* **38**, 29–33.

Babu, S.C. *et al.* (1980) Monitor guided response. *Arch. Surg.* **115**, 1384–6.

Baker, S.P. *et al.* (1974) The injury severity scores — a method of describing patients with multiple injuries and evaluating emergency care. *J. Trauma* **14**, 187–196.

Boucher, C.A. *et al.* (1985) Determination of cardiac risk by dipyridamole-thallium imaging before peripheral vascular surgery. *New Engl. J. Med.* **312**, 389–394.

Bartus, R.T. *et al.* (1982) The cholinergic hypothesis of geriatric memory dysfunction. *Science* **217**, 408–16.

Cockcroft, D.W. & Gault, M.T. (1976) Prediction of creatinine clearance from serum creatinine. *Nephron* **16**, 31–41.

Dagnino, J. & Prys-Roberts, C. (1986) Anesthesia in the hypertensive patient. In *Geriatric Anesthesia, Principles and Practice* (Ed C.R. Stephens & R.A.E. Assaf). Butterworths, Boston, p. 243.

Djokovic, J.L. & Heldley-Whyte, J. (1979) Prediction of outcome of surgery and anaesthesia in patients over 80. *JAMA* **242**, 2301–2306.

Duncan, P.G. & Cohen, M.M. (1987) Post-operative complicators — factors of significance to anaesthesia practice. *Can. J. Anaesth.* **34**, 2–8.

Finkel, M.L. *et al.* (1982) The current status of surgical second opinion programs. *Surg. Clin. North Am.* **62**, 705–19.

Gerson, M.C. *et al.* (1985) Cardiac prognosis in non-cardiac geriatric surgery. *Ann. Intern. Med.* **103**, 832–837.

Gerson-Greenberg, A. *et al.* (1981) Mortality of gastrointestinal surgery in the aged. Elective vs emergency procedures. *Arch. Surg.* *166*, 788–791

Gravelyn, T.R. & Weg, J.G. (1980) Respiration rate as an indicator of acute respiratory dysfunction. *JAMA* **244**, 1123–1125.

Heatley, R.V. *et al.* (1979) Preoperative intravenous feeding — a controlled trial. *Postgrad. Med. J.* **55**, 541–545.

Hertzer, N.R. *et al.* (1984) Coronary artery disease in peripheral vascular patients. A classification of 1000 coronary angiograms and the result of surgical management. *Ann. Surg.* **199**, 223–233.

Hogan, D.B. (1985) Imposed activity restriction for the elderly. *Ann. CRMCC* **18**, 410–412.

Howie, C. (1971) In *Research in Burns* (Ed Matter), Herlag Hans Huber, Berne, pp. 162–165.

James, S.E. & Smith, M.A. (1987) Autologous blood infusion in elective orthopaedic surgery. *J. R. Soc. Med.* **80**, 284–285.

Jones, R.M. *et al.* (1987) Smoking and anaesthesia. *Anaesthesia* **42**, 1–2.

Joly, H.B. & Weil, M.H. (1969) Temperature of the great toe as an indication of the severity of shock. *Circulation* **39**, 131–138.

Kalman, P.G. *et al.* (1986) Cardiac dysfunction during abdominal aortic operation. The limitations of pulmonary wedge pressures. *J. Vasc. Surg.* **3**, 733–781.

Kenney, R.A. (1982) *Physiology of Aging.* Year Book Medical Publications, Chicago, p. 11.

Kiil J. *et al.* (1978) Prophylaxis against post-operative PE and DVT by low dose heparin. *Lancet* **1**, 1115–1116.

Klein, L.F. *et al.* (1985) Diagnosing dementia: Univariate and multivariate analyses of mental status examination. *J. Am. Geriatr. Soc.* **33**, 483–488.

Liu, S. & Collis, G. (1984) Pre-operative evaluation and preparation of the aged patient with cardiovascular disease. *Int. Anesthesiol. Clin.* **3**, 31–37.

McFadden, J.P. *et al.* (1981) Raised respiratory rate in elderly patients: a valuable physical sign. *Br. Med. J.* **284**, 624–627.

McQuay, H. & Moore, H. (1984) Beware of renal function when prescribing morphine. *Lancet* **2**, 284–285.

Muller, J.M. *et al.* (1986) Indications and effects of pre-operative parenteral nutrition. *World J. Surg.* **10**, 53–63.

Nadeau, S. & Noble, W.H. (1986) Misinterpretation of pressure measurements from the pulmonary artery catheter. *Can. Anaesth. Soc. J.* **33**, 353–363.

Nunn, J.F. *et al.* (1988) *Anaesthesia* in press.

Overstall, P.W. & Oldman PM 1987. A comparative study of Lormetazepam and chlormethiazole in elderly in-patients. *Age Ageing* **16**, 45–51.

Petch, M.C. (1987) Misleading exercise electrocardiograms. *Br. Med. J.* **295**, 620.

Polson, R.T. *et al.* (1987) The prevention of renal impairment in patients undergoing orthoptic liver grafting by infusion of low dose dopamine. *Anaesthesia* **42**, 15–19.

Rao, T.L.K. *et al.* (1983) Re-infarction following anesthesia in patients with myocardial infarction. *Anesthesiology* **59**, 499–505.

Robin, E.D. (1985) The cult of the Swan-Ganz catheter. *Ann. Intern. Med.* **103**, 445–449.

Roger, R.K. *et al.* (1985) Abstention from cigarette smoking improves cerebral perfusion among elderly chronic smokers. *JAMA* **253**, 2970–2974.

Ross, B.A. *et al.* (1969) Observation on central and peripheral temperatures in the understanding and management of shock. *Br. J. Surg.* **156**, 877–882.

Salomen, M. *et al.* (1986) Oral temazepam as a premedication in elderly surgical patients. *Acta Anaesth. Scand.* **30**, 703–708.

Seymour, G. (1986) *Medical Assessment of the Elderly Surgical Patient.* Croom Helm, London, p. 53.

Sheen, P.A. *et al.* (1978) Myocardial infarction after anaesthesia and surgery. *JAMA* **239**, 2566–2570.

Shoemaker, W.C. *et al.* (1983) Use of physiologic monitoring to predict outcome and to assist in clinical decisions in critically ill post-operative patients. *Am. J. Surg.* **146**, 43–50.

Shultz, R.J. (1985) The role of physiological monitoring for patients with fracture of the hip. *J. Trauma* **25**, 309 –316.

Sikorski, J.M. *et al.*(1985) The rapid transit system for patients with fracture of proximal femur. *Br. Med. J.* **290**, 439–443.

Taub, H.A. *et al.* (1986) Informed consent for research: effect of readability, patient age and education. *J. Am. Geriatr. Soc.* **34**, 601–606.

Vershuysen, M. (1986) How elderly patients with femoral fracture develop pressure sores in hospital. *Br. Med. J.* **292**, 1311–1313.

Villar, R.N. *et al.* (1986) Hip fracture in healthy patients: operative delay versus prognosis. *Br. Med. J.* **293**, 1203–1204.

Vitez, T. (1987) Potassium and the anaesthetist. *Can. J. Anaesth.* **34**, 530.

Wallace, R.G.H. *et al*, (1986) A simple grading system to guide the prognosis after hip fracture in the elderly. *Br. Med. J.* **293**, 665.

White, P.F. (1986) Pharmacologic and clinical aspects of pre-operative medication. *Anesth. Analg.* **65**, 963–971.

Whittmore, A.D. *et al.* (1980) Aortic aneurysm repair. *Ann. Surg.* **192**, 414–421.

Further reading

Brocklehurst, J.C. (Ed.) (1985) *Geriatric Medicine and Gerontology.* Churchill Livingstone, Edinburgh. (This is the standard British text book for trainee geriatricians and therefore a prime reference book.)

Seymour, G. (1986) *Medical Assessment of the Elderly Surgical Patient.* Croom Helm, London. (This is an excellent review of present knowledge concerning assessment and the related postoperative complications, written by an academic geriatrician.)

Wright, W.B. (1986) *The Elderly Patient.* Springer-Verlag, London.

Kenny, R.A. (1985) *MCQs in Geriatric Medicine.* Churchill Livingstone, Edinburgh. (These presentations of multiple choice questions are enhanced by the answers appearing on the reverse pages. They provide refresher and test questions on basic medical matters.)

Goldman, D.R. *et al.* (Eds) (1982) *Medical Care of the Surgical Patient. A problem orientated approach to management.* Lippincott, London. (This is a systemized American account of pre- and postoperative management.)

12 | Modifications of general anaesthesia for the aged

M.E. DODSON

Introduction

Most surgical procedures in the aged are carried out under general anaesthesia. There is on the whole a preference on the part of patients, certainly in the UK, to be unconscious during an operation. General anaesthesia is also often preferred by the surgeon and anaesthetist because it is the quickest way of presenting the patient to the surgeon ready for the operation, without delays while a nerve block is performed and the local anaesthetic becomes effective.

There has been a tendency in the past to regard a spinal or epidural anaesthetic as more suitable for the less fit patient than a general anaesthetic. However, the advent of new drugs, together with a better understanding of their effects and also of the effects of anaesthetic procedures such as intermittent positive pressure ventilation and endotracheal intubation, has enabled the anaesthetist to use general anaesthetic techniques in any patient. In fact, many anaesthetists will prefer a general anaesthetic to a regional technique in the very ill or very unfit.

As the ability to adapt to any sort of stress decreases with increasing age, especially in the patient with pathological changes in addition to the physiological changes of age, the anaesthetist will need to pay careful attention to detail in the conduct of an anaesthetic in order to minimize the impact of the stress of anaesthesia and surgery.

Drugs

For some drugs, the responses of the elderly are clearly different from those of younger patients, whereas for others, the differences are less obvious. These differences may be related to pharmacokinetic and pharmacodynamic changes, or a mixture of the two. Even if there are no measurable pharmacokinetic changes with age, pharmacodynamic differences can still exist and necessitate a modification in drug dosage. It is of considerable interest to the anaesthetist that, when extensive traumatic surgery is carried out, there can be a loss of age-related pharmacokinetic changes which are seen in older patients undergoing minor surgery. This has been shown for alcuronium (Stephens *et al.*, 1984) and midazolam (Harper *et al.*, 1985).

Increased sensitivity is a feature of most drugs which affect the central nervous system (CNS), especially those with sedative, analgesic or anxiolytic actions. Thus, the drug effect is more profound and often also of longer duration. Although data are only available for some drugs, it can be stated as an important general principle that smaller doses of drugs which depress the CNS will usually be needed with increasing age. It is also possible that, with the heterogeneity of the ageing population, the range of doses required will be larger than for the more homogeneous younger population, and it may thus be less easy to predict the dose which will be required. Increased sensitivity to the side-effects of drugs can also be shown: e.g. the incidence of muscle rigidity after fentanyl is higher in older patients, and central anticholinergic effects of drugs are more common with increasing age.

Decreased sensitivity tends to be shown by drugs which act on the autonomic nervous system (ANS), such as anticholinergics, beta adrenergic blocking drugs, and vagal and sympathetic stimulants. This decrease in effect is related to the decreased activity of the ANS which occurs with age. It may to some extent be counteracted by pharmacokinetic changes, such as a decrease in the initial volume of distribution, which tend to increase the bioavailability of the drug at its receptor site.

Intravenous induction agents

In the following brief account of anaesthetic drugs, some age-related changes in volume of distribution, clearance and the elimination half-life ($t_{1/2}\beta$) are mentioned. The changes should be viewed in the light of information on pharmacokinetics provided in Chapter 6.

For most i.v. induction agents, studies have shown a decreasing requirement with increasing age (Table 12.1). Although the average dose clearly decreases, the values given in this table will not help greatly in predicting the actual dose required by an individual older patient because of the variability of response between individuals. It may be possible to increase predictability by relating dose to lean body weight, but this measurement is not usually available in clinical practice. The best criterion for the dose which a patient needs must still be the dose which will produce the desired effect, in this case anaesthesia. For some patients this dose will be small; for others, the dose will differ little from that required by younger patients.

The physiological and pathological changes in the cardiovascular system (CVS) must be borne in mind when administering i.v. induction agents. The drug must be given more slowly to older patients in order to allow time for the slower circulation to transfer drug to the brain. This slower rate of administration will also tend to reduce the hypotensive effects of some of the i.v. induction agents, which can be profound and worrying in older patients.

The choice of i.v. induction agent now lies between thiopentone, methohexitone, a benzodiazepine (usually midazolam or diazepam), etomidate, or disoprofol. Opioids are occasionally used.

Thiopentone is widely used as anaesthetists are familiar with the reduced requirements of aged patients. The study of Homer & Stanski (1985) suggests that this increased sensitivity is largely due to pharmacokinetic factors, particularly a decrease in the initial volume of distribution (V_1), no evidence being found of increased sensitivity of the brain to the dose used for induction of anaesthesia. There is also a longer recovery period after thiopentone anaesthesia in older patients (Oduah, 1969).

The range of dose requirements of a group of older patients will be wide. A recent study of patients aged 70–86 years found that the dose of thiopentone given over a minimum period of 2 min until the eyelash reflex disappeared ranged from 0.9 to 4.0 mg kg^{-1}.

Methohexitone is a barbiturate and, although it is more rapidly metabolized than thiopentone, redistribution is still the main cause of its short duration of action. It has a $t_{1/2}\beta$ of 240 min, considerably shorter than that of 700 min for thiopentone (Hudson *et al.*, 1982). There is thus a good pharmacokinetic reason for preferring methohexitone to thiopentone in the old, especially if repeat doses are used. A disadvantage of methohexitone is that it can cause pain on injection, and it is preferable to give it into a larger vein. This is contrary to the more usual practice of giving an i.v. injection into an indwelling needle in a vein on the dorsum of the hand.

Diazepam is a benzodiazepine which has minimal depressant effects on the CVS. Cook *et al.* (1984) have produced a regression formula for the dose of diazepam which includes age, body weight and factors related to regular sedation and daily alcohol consumption. A clear correlation between age and dose of diazepam has been shown by Giles *et al.* (1978)

Table 12.1. Doses of i.v. induction agents in younger and older patients

Drug	Younger	Older	Reference
Thiopentone	6.0 mg kg^{-1} (Females 20–40 years)	4.5 mg kg^{-1} (Females 60–85 years)	Christensen *et al.* (1983)
Methohexitone	1.5 mg kg^{-1}	No recommended doses	
Midazolam	May need >0.5 mg kg^{-1} (Age 16–60 years) Wide range of doses	0.2–0.3 mg kg^{-1} (62–76 years) Wide range of doses	Gamble *et al.* (1981)
Diazepam	10.0 mg Age 20 years	3.0 mg Age 80 years	Cook *et al.* (1984)
Etomidate	0.6 mg kg^{-1} Age 20 years	0.2 mg kg^{-1} Age 80 years	Arden *et al.* (1986)
Propofol	2.25–2.5 mg kg^{-1} <60 years	1.5–1.75 mg kg^{-1} >60 years	Dundee *et al.* (1986)

and these authors also observed that previous users of diazepam required a larger dose. The onset of action of diazepam is faster in older patients (Dundee *et al.*, 1985). Pharmacokinetic changes with increasing age have been observed: increases in $t_{1/2}\beta$ and volume of distribution at steady state (V_{SS}), and decrease in clearance (Kanto *et al.*, 1979). A decrease in the concentration of the active metabolite desmethyldiazepam was also observed.

Midazolam is a water-soluble benzodiazepine and, like diazepam, has little depressant effect on the CVS and so is a valuable drug in older patients. Bell *et al.* (1987) have clearly shown the decreasing requirement for this drug with increasing age (Fig. 12.1), and this would appear to be related to an increase of $t_{1/2}\beta$, and V_{SS} with possibly also a decrease in clearance (Harper *et al.*, 1985). The onset of action is faster in older patients. There are theoretical advantages in using midazolam rather than diazepam because no active metabolites are produced by midazolam metabolism. However, comparative studies of recovery after these two benzodiazepines have not been able to detect any differences which could be due to the presence of active diazepam metabolites. In fact, in the study of Kortilla & Tarkkanen (1985), recovery after midazolam 0.1 mg kg^{-1} was slower than after diazepam 0.2 mg kg^{-1}, and this could be a

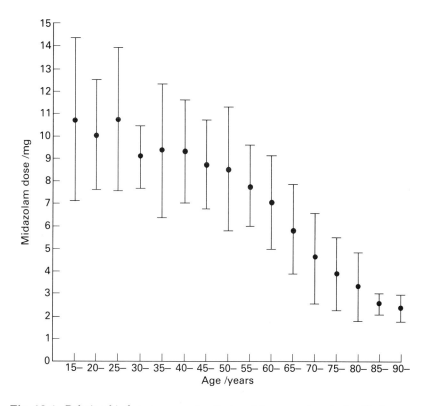

Fig. 12.1. Relationship between age of patient and the mean dose (± 1 s.d.) of i.v. midazolam required to produce adequate sedation prior to upper gastrointestinal endoscopy (Reproduced from Bell *et al.* (1987), with kind permission.)

Modifications of general anaesthesia

disadvantage when midazolam is used for short procedures in the aged. Recovery after midazolam has also been shown to be slower than after both methohexitone and thiopentone when these drugs were used alone for short procedures.

Etomidate is an imidazole. It has a less depressant effect on the CVS and respiratory system (RS) than thiopentone, and a shorter duration of action. These features make it a potentially useful drug in the older patient. There is no evidence that the incidence of minor complications, such as pain on injection or muscle movement, differ with age or that the major problem of depression of corticosteroids will assume a greater or lesser importance in older patients.

Older patients require lower doses of etomidate than younger patients and it is thought that this increased sensitivity is the result of a decrease in V_1 (Arden *et al.*, 1986). There is also a decrease in clearance and increase in $t_{1/2}\beta$.

Propofol is the latest i.v. induction agent with a very short duration of action. It does, however, cause considerable though usually transient depression of both CVS and RS.

As age increases over 40 years, the requirement for this drug begins to decrease, but the change becomes more obvious in those over 60 years of age (Dundee *et al.*, 1986). These authors observed that if the dose of propofol exceeded 1.75 mg kg^{-1}, or a smaller dose was given rapidly, there was a higher incidence of hypotension and apnoea. The use of this drug in older patients remains to be fully evaluated.

Competitive neuromuscular blocking drugs

There is no evidence for any age-related changes in initial dose requirement for these drugs, though some studies have shown that lower rates of infusion for maintenance of muscle relaxation are required with increasing age. The deterioration in renal function which occurs with age will affect the clearance and duration of action of those muscle relaxants which rely to any extent on the kidney for their elimination, such as alcuronium and pancuronium. As with i.v. induction agents, cardiovascular side-effects assume greater importance with increasing age.

Atracurium is normally free from effects on the CVS but it can release sufficient histamine to cause hypotension when larger doses are used (Lowry *et al.*, 1985). No age-related changes in dose requirement for this drug have been observed, nor is there any increase in duration of action (d'Hollander *et al.*, 1983).

Vecuronium is free from cardiovascular side-effects and causes virtually no histamine release. D'Hollander *et al.* (1982) found that the recovery of twitch height was significantly longer in patients over 60 years of age compared with patients below 60 years. They also observed a reduced dose requirement in older patients when using an i.v. infusion to maintain a constant degree of twitch depression.

Pancuronium can cause a tachycardia and increase in blood pressure and this may be advantageous or disadvantageous in older patients (see later). The duration of action of this drug is prolonged in older patients (Duvaldestin *et al.*, 1982; Lowry *et al.*, 1985).

Alcuronium can cause hypotension and tachycardia, and it is the author's experience that a combination of thiopentone and alcuronium in older patients can rapidly be followed by profound hypotension. This combination of drugs should therefore not be used without an i.v. infusion *in situ*. The $t_{1/2}\beta$ in older patients having minor surgery is prolonged (Stephens *et al.*, 1984; Walker *et al.*, 1980). However, when elderly patients are subjected to major surgery with considerable blood loss, alcuronium pharmacokinetics do not differ from those in younger patients.

d-Tubocurarine can readily cause hypotension. In a recent study in young adults, it was shown that this hypotension was sometimes reversed by endotracheal intubation, but that this reversal was only transient (Lavery *et al.*, 1987). It is probable that hypotension caused by this drug will be even less readily reversed in older patients. As would be expected, the clearance of this drug decreases with age, with an increase in $t_{1/2}\beta$ and decreased V_1 and V_{SS}. Recovery of twitch tension is slower in older patients (Matteo *et al.*, 1985).

Drugs used for reversal of neuromuscular blockade

Anticholinesterases   *Neostigmine* is still the most commonly used drug, and dose requirements do not differ with age. All the anticholinesterases are less likely to cause a bradycardia in older patients.

The use of *pyridostigmine* with atropine was followed by a reduced incidence of cardiac arrythmias when compared with neostigmine and atropine (Owens *et al.*, 1978). The difference was most obvious in patients who had been anaesthetized with halothane (Table 12.2).

Edrophonium displays no difference in time of onset or duration of action in older patients, even though the $t_{1/2}\beta$ is increased.

Anticholinergic drugs   Although the $t_{1/2}\beta$ of *atropine* is prolonged in patients over 65 years of age, the chronotropic response of the heart is reduced (Virtanen *et al.*, 1982). An important disadvantage of this drug in the aged is that it crosses the blood–brain barrier and can cause central anticholinergic effects such as drowsiness, hallucinations and memory loss. A dose of 2 mg has been shown to impair memory in younger patients (Wetherell, 1980) and there are clinical reports of coma after the intraoperative use of more than 2 mg i.v. (Erikssen, 1969; Smith *et al.*, 1979). Central anticholinergic effects of drugs will be more likely to occur in patients who already have some degree of central

Table 12.2. Incidence of arrhythmias after reversal of competitive neuromuscular blockade in the elderly (numbers in parentheses refer to total numbers in each group)

Drugs	N + A*	P + A*	N + G[†]	P + G[†]
Overall incidence	15 (43) 35%	7 (50) 14%	3 (21) 14%	5 (29) 17%
Patients with cardiovascular disease	14 (28) 50%	7 (33) 21.2%	2 (5) 40%	2 (10) 20%
Patients with hypertension	8 (20) 40%	4 (17) 23.5%	1 (3) 33%	2 (7) 29%
Patients with no cardiovascular disease			0 (12)	0 (8)
Use of halogenated agent (halothane in 93%)	10 (20) 50%	2 (22) 9.1%	1 (8) 13%	1 (17) 6%

N — neostigmine 0.07 mg kg^{-1} (maximum 5 mg); A — atropine 0.02 or 0.03 mg kg^{-1} (maximum 2 mg); P — pyridostigmine 0.28 mg kg^{-1} (maximum 20 mg); G — glycopyrrolate 0.015 mg kg^{-1} (maximum 1.2 mg).
*Owens et al. (1978).
[†]Muravchick et al. (1979).
(Reproduced from O'Malley (1984) with kind permission of publisher and editor)

cholinergic dysfunction, which may be shown by preoperative episodes of confusion or even dementia.

Hyoscine has undesirable central anticholinergic effects that are more readily recognized than those of atropine, and this drug has long been considered unsuitable for the elderly.

Glycopyrrolate has several advantages over atropine in the older patient: (i) it does not cross the blood–brain barrier (see above), and its use with neostigmine in younger patients was followed by less postoperative memory loss than atropine with neostigmine (Simpson et al., 1985); (ii) there are probably fewer arrhythmias after glycopyrrolate (Table 12.2); (iii) glycopyrrolate with neostigmine was followed by faster recovery of neuromuscular blockade (Sheref, 1985).

Succinylcholine   There is no evidence for any change in the effects or side-effects of this drug with increasing age, except that postoperative muscle pain appears to be less common.

Inhalation agents

Nitrous oxide is the only anaesthetic gas which is widely used. Of the volatile agents, halothane, enflurane and isoflurane have, in the developed countries, almost entirely replaced the older agents, trichloethylene and diethyl ether.

The minimum alveolar concentration (MAC) for halothane, for

enflurane and for isoflurane have been shown to decrease with age, the value at 80 years of age being about 20% lower than at 20 years of age. It can be assumed fairly confidently that the MAC for nitrous oxide and for other volatile agents will decrease in a similar manner.

Nitrous oxide, a weak anaesthetic, is a good analgesic in concentrations which do not produce anaesthesia. Because MAC decreases with age, this drug will be a more effective anaesthetic in older patients.

Its use can be accompanied by signs of sympathomimetic stimulation, such as increases in heart rate and systolic arterial pressure, pupillary dilatation and sweating. Systemic vascular resistance can also increase. There is some evidence that when nitrous oxide is added to volatile agents or administered with opioids there is a depressant effect on the CVS which is greater in patients with cardiac disease. This could have implications for the older patient with less effective cardiovascular function, and with a higher incidence of ischaemic heart disease.

An important side-effect of nitrous oxide is that it causes abnormalities of vitamin B_{12} metabolism, which can occur in ill patients after as little as 2 h of anaesthesia. The exposure needed for toxic effects to appear in fit patients is much longer. No information is available about the incidence of this toxic effect in the aged.

Nitrous oxide can diffuse into closed body cavities. One consequence of this arises if the Eustachian tube is blocked: the changes in pressure in the middle ear as nitrous oxide diffuses in and out can cause a period of postoperative deafness, and this could contribute to postoperative disorientation.

Halothane, enflurane and isoflurane: the debate continues about the place of each of these agents in anaesthesia, and many of the arguments apply equally to any patient irrespective of age. However, all these agents decrease the blood pressure and their cardiovascular effects will assume a greater importance with increasing age.

Halothane: the well known ability of this drug to cause cardiac arrhythmias is a disadvantage in older patients, in whom arrhythmias are more common before surgery, and who seem to be more likely to develop arrhythmias when halothane is given. The systemic vascular resistance (SVR) of older patients was reduced to a greater extent by halothane compared with younger patients, and there was also a decrease in cardiac index (CI). These decreases in SVR and CI interacted together so that there was no evidence of tissue, including myocardial ischaemia (Tokics *et al.*, 1986). Halothane does not appear to dilate the coronary vasculature and coronary flow tends to decrease as arterial pressure decreases.

It is not known whether the metabolism of halothane changes with age, or whether the older liver differs in sensitivity to the hepatic damaging effect of halothane. In younger patients, it is known that halothane is metabolized to bromide which is excreted in the urine for several days after a halothane anaesthetic. The bromide ion can depress the CNS, a potential disadvantage in the old, should such depression persist for some time after the anaesthetic has ended.

Enflurane, a methylethyl ether, is much less likely to cause arrhythmias than halothane. It does cause a fall in blood pressure, and this is reported to be accompanied by a rise in SVR which is greater in older patients than in younger (Haldemann *et al.*, 1975). An increase in SVR would increase the afterload, and this could adversely affect myocardial function in the elderly. However, other studies have shown a decrease in SVR with enflurane. Enflurane causes coronary vasodilatation, so that there is the possibility of 'coronary steal', i.e. the more normal coronary vessels are dilated by this agent, and the increase in blood flow through these vessels diverts blood away from myocardium supplied by diseased and narrowed vessels which cannot dilate (Rydvall *et al.*, 1984).

Isoflurane seems to cause a greater decrease in SVR than halothane, thus causing a decrease in afterload which may or may not be an advantage in the patient with myocardial disease. It does also cause coronary vasodilatation, with no decrease in coronary blood flow. Despite this, evidence of myocardial ischaemia was found in 10 of 21 patients aged 55–80 years with ischaemic heart disease during isoflurane anaesthesia (Reiz *et al.*, 1983). This could be due to coronary steal (see above) and further evidence for this is found in the study of Moffitt *et al.* (1986).

A clear difference between isoflurane and the other two fluroninated agents is that isoflurane does not increase cerebral blood flow (Eintrei *et al.*, 1985).

Trichloroethylene: no specific studies of this drug have been carried out in older patients. The ability of trichloroethylene to cause cardiac arrhythmias will be a disadvantage in the old, and slow recovery may result from its high fat solubility. Its place in anaesthesia for the aged is probably limited.

Diethyl ether can be safely used in older patients and has some advantages compared with other volatile agents. It causes less depression of blood pressure as its direct myocardial depressant effect is at least partially offset by an increase in sympathetic nervous system activity. It does not depress respiration at light levels of anaesthesia, and the Pa,co_2 may decrease. It should not be used with air alone as the Pa,o_2 usually falls, even in the presence of hyperventilation.

Opioid analgesic drugs

The older patient is clearly more sensitive to the effects of these drugs, with a more intense and often more prolonged duration of action. This is at least partly due to pharmacokinetic factors, and Table 12.3 gives a summary of some age-related pharmacokinetic parameters for the most commonly used intraoperative opioids. These pharmacokinetic changes with age are related to factors such as the decrease in lean body mass, decreased hepatic and renal blood flow, and less efficient renal function.

There is now evidence for the involvement of the kidney in the elimination of morphine and possibly other opioids, e.g. dihydrocodeine. This must be borne in mind in older patients in whom renal function will be deteriorating, and whose renal function may deteriorate more as a result of anaesthesia and surgery.

The first dose of all opioid analgesic drugs should be reduced in the aged and a longer duration of action expected. No dose recommendations are given here as the range of requirements is large, and body weight is very unreliable as an indicator of the dose which an individual older patient will require. When it is wished to use morphine i.v. to provide analgesia during surgery, an i.m. dose of morphine can be given first as a premedicant. The i.v. dose which is then given is based on the response of the patient to the initial premedicant dose.

Smaller doses of opioids will also cause more severe respiratory depression in the elderly, and apnoea can result if the usual doses for younger patients are given to the elderly. Other side-effects may be more common, e.g. rigidity after fentanyl (Bailey et al., 1985), and hypotension after pethidine. However, it is the author's clinical impression that opioid-induced emetic effects are less common with increasing age.

There is no clear evidence that any particular opioid has substantial advantages over any other opioid in the older patient, and the same indications and contraindications apply as in younger patients. The more long acting buprenorphine should probably be avoided especially as its respiratory depressant effect cannot be reversed by naloxone. The main consideration for the other opioids is the need for a smaller dose, and in some individuals a very small dose can provide effective pain relief for a considerable period of time. *Naloxone* is always available to reverse any respiratory depressant effects of many opioid drugs. This drug can, however, cause hypertension and arrhythmias, especially if larger doses are used, and the initial dose should not exceed 0.1 mg i.v. when attempting to reverse opioid induced respiratory depression at the end of an anaesthetic.

Table 12.3. Effects of increasing age on volume of distribution, $t_{1/2}\beta$ and clearance of some opioids

Drug and i.v. dose	Volume of distribution	$t_{1/2}\beta$	Clearance	Reference
Morphine 10 mg per 70 kg	↓ V_{SS}	↓	↓	Owen et al. (1983)
Pethidine 25 mg	↑ V_1 and V_{SS}	→	→	Herman et al. (1985)
Fentanyl 10 μg kg^{-1}	→ V_1 and V_D	↑	↓	Bentley et al. (1982)
Alfentanil 50 μg kg^{-1}	→ V_{SS} V_1 and V_{area}	↑	↓	Helmers et al. (1984)
Sufentanil 2 μg kg^{-1}	↓ V_1 and V_{area}	→	↓	Matteo et al. (1986)

V_1 — initial volume of distribution; V_{SS} — steady state volume of distribution; V_D — unspecified volume of distribution; V_{area} — volume of distribution of the area under the curve.

Modifications of general anaesthesia

Induction of anaesthesia

Induction of anaesthesia in older patients will often be easier because of the increased sensitivity to CNS depressant drugs with increasing age. However, induction will be more likely to be accompanied by hypotension, which will be related to the following factors.

(i) *Hypovolaemia:* there may be an obvious pathological or pharmacological cause for hypovolaemia, e.g. vomiting or blood loss, or the use of diuretics. These drugs may have been used as part of the preparation of the patient for surgery, an example being mannitol used to reduce the intraocular pressure, or as part of bowel preparation. However, there can be some degree of hypovolaemia in even the fit because, with increasing age, there is decreasing ability to sense when fluid intake needs to be increased to meet the needs of the body (Phillips, 1983). Thus, older patients may simply not drink enough. If access to fluids is further reduced by immobility for any reason, a considerable fluid deficit can be present. Sometimes an intravascular fluid deficit is present even in patients with oedema, or with an apparently good urine output.

(ii) *Depression of the CVS:* many anaesthetic drugs cause myocardial depression and vasodilatation; the ability of the older CVS to respond to such changes is reduced, and persistent and more profound hypotension will occur in the older patient.

(iii) *Intermittent positive pressure ventilation:* when this is instituted, the rise in intrathoracic pressure reduces venous return and thus cardiac output decreases. The hypotension which results will be more common and more severe in older patients.

Intravenous induction

Some of the advantages and disadvantages of the more commonly used i.v. induction agents have already been discussed, and the necessity for slow administration of a dose of drug tailored to the patient's need and not necessarily to the body weight, has been stressed. Midazolam, with its minimal effects on the CVS, is useful, especially for longer operations. The author gives a dose of 2.0 mg and then waits for at least 2 min to observe the response. Anaesthesia is then deepened in one of several ways — further midazolam can be given or a dose of thiopentone, and usually a small dose of this drug will be needed. Occasionally, the initial small dose of midazolam will send the patient to sleep, and an inhalation anaesthetic only is required.

Inhalation induction

As the MAC for all agents is reduced with age, it follows that it will often be easier to carry out an inhalation induction or to introduce an inhalation agent after only a small dose of an i.v. agent. The inspired concentration should be increased slowly and high concentrations avoided by allowing a longer period of time for anaesthesia to deepen. Although in younger patients halothane seems to give a smoother induction of anaesthesia than either enflurane or isoflurane, it may be that the difficulties with induction using the last two agents may be overcome more easily in the aged.

Endotracheal intubation

As the old have weaker musculature, are often edentulous and have less active laryngeal reflexes, endotracheal intubation is usually easy even when an inhalation agent has been used without a muscle relaxant. Problems in older patients will arise as a result of arthritis of the neck or disease of the larynx or pharynx.

In younger patients, endotracheal intubation is usually followed by some evidence of increased activity of the autonomic nervous system. The stimulation is usually sympathetic, with increases in heart rate and blood pressure. As the activity of the ANS is obtunded with age, a less marked rise in heart rate occurs (Bullingham *et al.*, 1987) but no relationship between increase in blood pressure and age was observed in this study. However, if sympathetic stimulation does occur, the rise in heart rate and arterial pressure will increase the work of the heart. In the presence of coronary vascular disease, the resultant increase in oxygen requirement may not be met by increased oxygen delivery and the myocardium will become ischaemic. It is thus wise to consider whether to try to reduce the extent of any sympathetic response to intubation in older patients. Many methods have been used, e.g. vasodilators, adrenergic blocking drugs, analgesics, local anaesthetic spray. The method chosen for old patients must not itself have adverse effects in these patients, and drugs with potent cardiovascular effects should possibly be avoided. The author advocates the use of a small extra dose of thiopentone (25–50 mg) just before intubating, after a competitive neuromuscular blocking agent has been used. Alternatively, alfentanil 600–800 μg can be given, but as this drug causes a bradycardia, atropine should also be given if the patient is receiving any other drug which can reduce the pulse rate, e.g. succinylcholine or beta adrenergic blockers.

For longer operations, and perhaps for all procedures in the aged, endotracheal tubes with low pressure cuffs should be used. The low cuff pressure will interfere less with blood supply to, and function of, the tracheal mucous membrane, than will a high cuff pressure. As the tracheal mucous membrane membrane plays an important role in the protection of the lungs from infection, it would seem wise to try to maitain its proper function in these patients in whom immune responses may be depressed. The use of a heat and moisture exchanger (HME) will also assist proper mucosal function by maintaining warm moist mucus within which cilia can function effectively.

Choice of muscle relaxant

The indications for the use of succinylcholine in the aged are similar to those in younger patients.

Of the competitive neuromuscular blocking agents, atracurium and vecuronium have clear advantages in older patients because of their lack of effects on the CVS. Recovery from these drugs is also faster, with much less chance of residual muscle weakness. Alloferin and d-tubocurarine can cause hypotension. Pancuronium is useful in the ill hypotensive patient, but the hypertension and tachycardia which can accompany its use may be undesirable in some older patients.

Rapid sequence induction   In most instances, an i.v. infusion should be sited before a rapid sequence induction in the older patient, as it has been shown that the administration of succinylcholine with thiopentone is followed by a higher incidence of hypotension in patients over 66 years of age compared with younger patients (Roizen *et al.*, 1985). Before induction, a decision has to be made about the dose of i.v. induction agent which will be required, and assessment of this dose will be made on the age and general condition of the patient. Occasionally, in the very ill patient it may be considered inadvisable to use an i.v. induction agent. In such a patient, induction with an inhalation agent will be very rapid and it will be possible to apply cricoid pressure and give succinylcholine at an early stage. Rapid sequence induction will be used more often in older patients because of the increasing incidence of hiatus hernia with age.

Other drugs at induction

Antibiotics may be required for prophylaxis against subacute bacterial endocarditis in patients with lesions of the heart valves (Chapter 11). The incidence of aortic stenosis increases with age, and antibiotics should be given to all patients in whom there is a suspicion of such valve disease.

Maintenance of anaesthesia

Awareness will be a very rare event in older patients because of the reduction in MAC which occurs with age, and the increased sensitivity of older patients to injected anaesthetic drugs, including opioids. Inspired concentrations of inhaled drugs and doses of injected drugs can therefore be reduced without fear of this complication, and with the beneficial effect of a decrease in undesirable side-effects. There is no information which clearly points to the preferential use of either volatile agents or opioids during maintenance of anaesthesia in the older patient. When using controlled ventilation, over-ventilation must be avoided, as a decrease in Pa_{CO_2} is a potent cause of a reduction in cerebral blood flow (see later). A decrease in Pa_{CO_2} will also cause an increase in systemic vascular resistance, thus increasing afterload and increasing the work of the heart. A further disadvantage of a low $Pa\text{CO}_2$ is that it increases haemoglobin–oxygen affinity, thus decreasing tissue oxygen delivery. As the lungs of older patients tend to have altered ventilation/perfusion ratios, a slow inspiration and prolonged expiration during controlled ventilation will contribute towards optimum gas exchange of areas of lung in which ventilation is reduced. The peak inspiratory pressure should be as low as possible as this pressure has been shown to correlate positively with the incidence of postoperative deep venous thrombosis (Takunnen & Takunnen, 1982).

Septicaemia and endotoxaemia can have serious consequences in older patients because of their reduced resistance to infection. Antibiotics should, therefore, be given when there is any suspicion of bacteraemia during the surgery.

Reversal of competitive neuromuscular blocking drugs

Glycopyrrolate will often be preferred to atropine (see above). If atropine is used, the dose should not exceed 2.0 mg during the perioperative period. The elderly seem to require smaller doses of an anticholinergic to prevent the bradycardic effects of neostigmine, and the author uses doses of glycopyrrolate 0.4 mg with neostigmine 2.5 mg, and of glycopyrrolate 0.6 mg with neostigmine 5.0 mg.

A longer recovery of twitch height was observed in older patients in whom the effects of pancuronium had been reversed by neostigmine and atropine, recovery taking up to 30 min (Marsh *et al.*, 1980). Thus, a longer period of time must be allowed after giving reversal drugs for recovery of adequate neuromuscular activity, and extubation must not be rushed.

Despite the apparent advantages of pyridostigmine in causing fewer cardiac arrhythmias than neostigmine (Table 12.2), this drug is rarely used to reverse competitive neuromuscular blocking drugs.

The early postoperative period

Oxygen should be given postoperatively to all patients. An inspired concentration of 36% will be suitable for most patients though higher or lower concentrations may be preferred in some circumstances. Additional indications for oxygen administration include hypothermia, especially if the patient is shivering, hypotensive, hypovolaemic, or septicaemic.

If the elderly patient is cold and peripherally vasoconstricted, rewarming will be accompanied by vasodilatation with a fall in blood pressure. Fluid input will then have to be increased. In most patients, adequacy of fluid intake will be shown by a good urine output, but monitoring of central venous pressure or even of left ventricular function using a pulmonary artery catheter may be required (see later).

Postoperative controlled ventilation, used for a few hours after major surgery has several advantages: the patient can be warmed without the problem of shivering; hypoxia due to hypoventilation will be avoided; there will be no residual neuromuscular blockade when the patient is extubated; pain relief can be provided using opioids without fear of respiratory depression. For a smaller number of patients, a more prolonged period of artificial ventilation may be required.

Pain relief   The old are just as likely to experience postoperative pain as are younger patients. If an injection of an opioid analgesic is required, it must *not* be given by the i.m. route if the patient is cold or hypovolaemic. Not only will such a dose be ineffective as it will not be absorbed, but it will provide a reservoir of unabsorbed drug which will enter the circulation later when the muscle becomes warm and perfused. This is potentially dangerous. Thus the most effective way of providing analgesia using a parenteral injection of opioid is to give the drug i.v. until pain is relieved. The dose given can then be used as a guide to prescribing further i.m. doses. The choice of opioid is largely one of personal preference though perhaps the more potent sedative effects of pethidine should be avoided. The long-acting partial agonist opioid buprenorphine has the disadvantage that its effects are not readily reversed by naloxone, and it occasionally causes unconsciousness with twitching and even neck stiffness in older patients. Any respiratory depressant effects of the agonist and of most partial agonist opioids can be reversed by naloxone, but the initial dose of this drug should not exceed 0.1 mg (see above). When opioid drugs are not required, oral aspirin or paracetamol are usually effective and avoid sedative side-effects of other stronger analgesics such as dihydrocodeine and dextropropoxyphene.

Good postoperative analgesia after abdominal, thoracic, perineal and lower limb surgery can be provided by drugs injected into the lumbar epidural space. Local anaesthetics via this route are very effective but have the disadvantages of causing hypotension and weakness of the legs. These drugs must be injected adjacent to the nerves which are to be blocked and the analgesic effect will only last for a few hours and will then wear off with rapid return of unabated pain. Opioids can also be injected into the epidural space and provide prolonged analgesia with no effects on blood pressure or mobility. However, occasional cases of marked depression of respiration and consciousness have occurred several hours after the injection of some opioids, and the incidence of this complication is greater in older patients. Thus, the dose of opioid given by this route must be small in such older patients, and the author uses morphine 0.5–2.0 mg. An i.v. infusion of naloxone can reduce the incidence of late respiratory depression, and a dose of 5 μg kg^{-1} h^{-1} has been recommended. A combination of local anaesthetic and opioid can be used, the latter drug providing less intense but more prolonged analgesia, while the former can provide shorter periods of more intense analgesia when required.

Postoperative confusion can be reduced by sitting patients up and encouraging them to return to a 'normal' life as soon as possible. Restoration to the patient of hearing-aid and spectacles will improve orientation, and of teeth will improve morale. There should be no unnecessary delay in returning the patient from the postoperative recovery area to the more familiar ward surroundings, and in allowing intake of food and fluid. Intravenous infusions and oxygen should be discontinued as soon as it is safe to do so.

Care in positioning and handling the aged patient

The physiological and pathological changes which must be borne in mind when handling aged patients are as follows:

(i) *Joint diseases*, which are very common and result in stiffness, and occasionally joint instability;

(ii) *Skin fragility*, due to loss of collagen in the tissues thus making the skin more vulnerable to both shearing stresses and to pressure, especially over bony prominences; skin fragility will increase in the patient on corticosteroids;

(iii) *Osteoporosis*, resulting in fragile bones, especially if the osteoporosis is pathological rather than physiological.

It is necessary to try to prevent damage associated with these conditions, and this will require vigilance in several respects. It may be necessary to discuss the position of the patient with the surgeon where safe positioning will reduce surgical access.

The head The neck is often permanently flexed, with the head requiring support in this position during the whole of the procedure. Forcible or extreme movement of the head or neck must be avoided, especially if there is any preoperative history of pain or paraesthesia in the arms. If the neck is very stiff, endotracheal intubation may be difficult, and in patients with rheumatoid arthritis, cervical joints can be unstable.

The arms If the arms are abducted, they must rest easily on well padded arm boards. It may not be possible to abduct the arms to a position that does not interfere with the surgical access, and in these cases, the arms may have to be positioned over the patient's chest, or supported from a screen over the patient. If shoulder joints are very stiff, abduction can interfere with arterial flow to the arms. The elbow must be padded if the arm is placed by the patient's side to reduce the chance of injury to the ulnar nerve.

The body Operating tables can exert high pressure on the body, sufficient to cause anoxic necrosis, and further damage can be done by shearing stresses when moving the patient. The treatment of pressure-sores is long and expensive, and these injuries must be avoided whenever possible. Ripple mattresses exert a pressure only a little lower than the operating table mattress, but problems are avoided as the site at which this pressure is exerted is constantly changing. Such mattresses should therefore always be used in surgery in the very thin and frail elderly, and in more robust patients for operations of longer duration.

Shearing stresses are applied to the skin if sheets are pulled out from underneath the patient, or when strapping is pulled off, and both can cause subcutaneous damage.

The legs It may be difficult to place the patient in the lithotomy position if hip joints are stiff. When there is a recent history of leg ulceration, the legs must be padded throughout the procedure, until the patient is fully awake.

The back Backache is not uncommon after surgery. The lithotomy position increases the frequency of this complaint, especially when the hip joints are very fully flexed. Severe lumbar extension by the use of the bridge and breaking the operating table can cause distressing backache. The surgeon must be told if the anaesthetist considers that these extreme positions are unwise because of back problems. The use of a three litre bag inflated with air beneath the back in lithotomy position has been recommended to reduce backache in younger patients, but its use has not been evaluated in older patients.

Maintenance of tissue oxygen supply

The organs with which the anaesthetist is most concerned are heart, brain and kidney. Tissue oxygen supply depends on several factors, including Pao_2, haemoglobin content and saturation, and tissue blood flow. Pao_2 and haemoglobin saturation are in turn governed by the inspired oxygen concentration and the ventilation/perfusion ratio in the lungs. Tissue blood flow will be altered by changes in the perfusion pressure and the size of the blood vessels.

In younger patients, important adjustments can be made to ventilation, cardiac output and vessel diameter in order to maintain tissue oxygen supply, and these adjustments can still be made, though sometimes less effectively, under anaesthesia. The older patient is much less able to make these adjustments. Even when not anaesthetized, perfusion pressure falls more easily as a result of physiological and pathological changes in the heart and blood vessels and obtunded autonomic reflexes, and rigid and diseased vessels cannot dilate in order to maintain blood flow with a reduced perfusion pressure. Thus, changes in haemoglobin, Pao_2 or arterial pressure which would be of no consequence in younger patients can cause tissue hypoxaemia in older patients. The anaesthetist must be aware of this, and be more ready to increase inspired oxygen, administer blood and restore arterial pressure in older patients.

Cerebral oxygen supply   Cerebral blood flow (CBF) is affected by the arterial pressure and the intracranial pressure, and the latter will also affect the diameter of the cerebral vessels. In the normal subject, autoregulatory mechanisms can maintain the cerebral blood flow regardless of falls in the arterial pressure until a certain critical level of arterial pressure has been reached. Below this level, CBF falls as arterial pressure falls. It has been clearly demonstrated that this critical level is increased in hypertensive patients and many old patients have some degree of hypertension. However, oxygen flux may be maintained until the CBF has fallen to even lower levels, and it has been estimated that in younger patients, cerebral hypoxia does not occur until the mean arterial pressure has fallen by 50%. Anaesthetics may affect cerebral autoregulation, but this is not proven.

The effects of changes in blood pressure will interact with anaesthetically induced changes in the diameter of the cerebral blood vessels. These vessels respond readily to changes in Pao_2 and $Paco_2$. The latter is a particularly important factor in anaesthesia, as reducing the $Paco_2$ by hyperventilation will reduce the cerebral blood flow. An increase in CBF results from hypoxia, hypercarbia and the use of halothane and enflurane. The ultimate effect of the interaction of arterial pressure, Pao_2, $Paco_2$ and volatile agent will not always be easy to predict, but it can be said that a combination of hypocarbia and hypotension has the potential for seriously affecting the cerebral oxygen supply.

Myocardial oxygen supply.   Myocardial blood flow is intermittent, being reduced during contraction of the myocardial muscle. The flow to the subendocardial area of the left ventricle occurs only during diastole, though flow to other areas of the myocardium occurs during both systole and diastole, as in these areas it is related to the pressure difference between the systolic arterial pressure and the pressure in the right ventricle and atria.

In the normal myocardium, coronary blood flow is maintained relatively constant irrespective of perfusion pressure, though it is now recognized that neurogenic stimuli can cause constriction of the coronary blood vessels. However, in most circumstances, vasodilatation occurs as perfusion pressure decreases from 120 mmHg to about 50 mmHg, due to the effects of local vasodilators and adrenergic stimulation. The increasing incidence of disease of coronary vessels with age will reduce the effectiveness of these responses in older patients, and a higher arterial pressure may be needed to maintain myocardial oxygen supply. In the presence of diseased coronary vessels, it will also be more difficult to increase myocardial oxygen supply in response to an increasing workload. Workload increases when the SVR is increased by anaesthetic drugs or by a decrease in $Pa,_{CO_2}$ during artificial ventilation. Workload also increases with rises in heart rate or systolic pressure, which can be caused by drugs, such as pancuronium, or by sympathetic stimulation. However, as adrenergic activity is reduced in older patients, large increases in pulse rate and arterial pressure are less likely than in younger patients.

Although increasing afterload has disadvantages, it is not always beneficial to the myocardial oxygen supply to decrease afterload by vasodilatation. Vasodilatation will also decrease preload, and with reduced cardiac filling, cardiac output and arterial pressure will decrease and the coronary flow will be reduced. In the presence of congestive cardiac failure, when coronary blood flow is decreased by the high venous pressure, some decrease in preload may improve myocardial oxygenation. However, cardiac de-compensation can readily occur in such patients, and vasodilators should only be used when it is possible to monitor patients intensively, including pulmonary artery balloon catheterization.

All the three commonly used volatile anaesthetic agents depress myocardial contractility and thus lower the arterial pressure. They do, however, have different effects on systemic vascular resistance and coronary blood flow (see above), but experimental work has produced conflicting results when considering whether any particular inhalation agent can cause an improvement or deterioration in the oxygen consumption/availability ratio in ischaemic myocardium.

Renal oxygen supply   Renal blood flow (RBF) is normally maintained by autoregulatory mechanisms irrespective of falls in systolic arterial pressure down to 90 mmHg. Below this, RBF falls as the systolic arterial pressure falls. RBF can also be reduced by sympathetic nervous stimulation causing renal vasoconstriction. With increasing age, RBF decreases, and it is also likely that autoregulation is less effective, so that RBF starts to decrease at a higher level of systolic arterial pressure. However, as sympathetic nervous system activity may be obtunded with age, renal vasoconstriction will be a less important influence on RBF.

The use of induced hypotension

It will be apparent from the foregoing discussion that, as the arterial blood pressure is reduced, tissue oxygen supply is more likely to be compromised in older patients. In any individual patient, however, we have little idea of the state of the myocardium or the blood vessels, or of the activity of compensatory autonomic or other reflex mechanisms. Thus, the effect of lowering the arterial pressure can rarely be predicted with any degree of accuracy. Monitoring of electrocardiogram (ECG) and of urine output can give warning of adverse effects on heart and kidneys, but evidence of severe tissue hypoxia, especially myocardial, can appear without warning. Monitoring of cerebral function is not easy and rarely carried out routinely. Thus, evidence of intraoperative cerebral hypoxia is usually only seen after surgery, when it is realized that the patient has deteriorated mentally or has had a stroke.

The value of hypotension in reducing bleeding is widely accepted, but the relationship between reduced arterial pressure and reduced bleeding has not in fact been established unequivocally (Donald, 1982). The incidence of deaths attributable to induced hypotension during anaesthesia over all age groups is about 1:160, with a morbidity of 1:39. The main morbidity is cerebral thrombosis, shown by failure to recover consciousness or neurological deficits. Other morbidity includes myocardial infarction and retinal artery thrombosis. In the old, the margin of safety for all these complications is reduced, and thus severe problems are more likely. Hypotensive techniques in the aged should be reserved for those patients in whom surgery will be very difficult or indeed impossible unless arterial pressure is reduced to a level which reduces bleeding.

Maintenance of function of the central nervous system

The simple procedure of placing an old person in unfamiliar surroundings can cause confusion. Thus it is not surprising that illness, together with transfer to hospital and an anaesthetic and operation can be followed by a deterioration in the mental state of old patients. Smith et al. (1985) describe significant deficits in concentration and orientation in time and place in older patients two days after surgery. These were not seen in younger patients, though memory deficits were found in patients of all ages. In addition to transient mental changes, there is always the suspicion that in rare cases, anaesthesia and surgery can result in permanent mental deterioration.

As has already been discussed, early postoperative confusion can be reduced by ensuring restoration of orientation, memory, sight, hearing and normal activity as soon as possible after anaesthesia. In order to provide this, and to avoid long-lasting mental deterioration, the anaesthetist must consider two important factors during general anaesthesia: drugs and cerebral oxygen supply.

Drugs Short-acting CNS depressant drugs should be used, and drugs which are rapidly metabolized to inactive metabolites have theoretical advantages over drugs which are redistributed or which are metabolized to active metabolites. The duration of the amnesic and sedative effects of benzodiazepines can be considerably prolonged in the old and these drugs should be used carefully, especially for short surgical procedures. The undesirable central anticholinergic effects of atropine and hyoscine have already been described. It must be remembered that many other drugs have central anticholinergic effects, including phenothiazines, droperidol and antidepressants.

Cerebral oxygen supply Attention must be paid to maintaining this at all times. The systolic arterial pressure must be controlled, and normal oxygen and carbon dioxide contents of the blood maintained. This will include maintenance of the haemoglobin. It is increasingly considered that it is very important to avoid passive hyperventilation in older patients. A drop of the Pa,co_2 to 26 mmHg will reduce cerebral blood flow by two-thirds, and therefore the end-tidal or arterial Pco_2 should be monitored to prevent such levels occurring during artificial ventilation.

Day case surgery

The patient having surgery and anaesthesia as a day case avoids the disorientating procedure of overnight admission to hospital, and many patients over 70 years of age can be most satisfactorily treated in this way. In such patients, it is even more important that the anaesthetist can ensure rapid restoration of an alert, orientated and active patient as soon after the anaesthetic as possible. For many patients, an inhalation technique, with avoidance of all injected or oral drugs, will prove entirely satisfactory.

Maintenance of body temperature

The mean body temperature of patients of any age falls if the ambient temperature during surgery is less than 24 °C. If the ambient temperature does not fall below 21 °C, the body temperature falls only initially and then stabilizes. Unfortunately, in the UK, surgeons are rarely prepared to tolerate an ambient temperature over 21 °C and so the body temperature of patients operated upon will be expected to fall progressively throughout the procedure. The fall is greater in patients over 65 years of age, who arrive in the recovery room with lower temperatures than younger patients. Recovery of a normal body temperature takes longer in older patients even when they are shivering, and so body temperatures are still lower on leaving the recovery room (Carli *et al.*, 1985). Despite the large fall in body temperature, the oxygen consumption of older patients does not increase to the same extent as that of younger patients with a similar drop in temperature (Roe *et al.*, 1966). Little work has been carried out to establish the importance of body temperature in relation to recovery after surgery. One study in younger patients demonstrated a faster recovery after anaesthesia for day case surgery when body temperature was not allowed to fall during the procedure (Conahan *et al.*, 1985). It would be of considerable interest to know whether hypothermia delays recovery in older patients.

It would thus seem sensible to try to maintain the body temperature of older patients during surgery, and the possibility of raising the ambient temperature should be discussed with the surgeon. Several simple measures can be used by the anaesthetist to try to reduce heat loss, including a warming blanket, covering all areas of the body not involved with the surgery, keeping the patient's arms close to the body and use of a heat and moisture exchanger. The use of a heated humidifier to warm the inspired gases can be effective, and hypothermia has also been prevented by circulating water at 37°C into the oesophagus (Kristensen *et al.*, 1986). There may be advantages in allowing the patient to warm before discontinuing artificial ventilation as this will prevent shivering. However, the absence of muscle activity will tend to slow the rate of rewarming. Flacke & Flacke (1986) have provided a full account of hypothermia in the aged surgical patient.

Immediately after surgery, the cold patient is vasoconstricted. With rewarming there is vasodilatation, and this can cause hypotension unless fluid input is increased. Injections of drugs via the i.m. route are likely to be ineffective in the cold vasoconstricted patient. If shivering occurs, the patient should be given a high inspired oxygen concentration. Such shivering can be distressing to the patient and it is worth considering whether to give a small dose of pethidine — Pauca *et al.* (1984) have shown that a dose of 20 mg can stop shivering, and the author has found that 10–15 mg may be sufficient in older patients.

Hydration and fluid balance

Some causes of hypovolaemia in the older patient have already been discussed. Fluid overload and possibly pulmonary oedema will be easy to induce in the patient who has recently been in cardiac failure or is in chronic cardiac failure. Such patients may require invasive monitoring using pulmonary artery catheterization if major surgery is required.

Intraoperative fluid requirements

It is unwise to apply hard and fast rules in the older patient about the volumes of i.v. fluids which should be given during surgery in order to maintain homeostasis. As much as 15 ml kg^{-1} h^{-1} may be required during major abdominal and other surgery, especially if fluid output has been increased before surgery, e.g. by the use of mannitol for bowel preparation (Tweedie *et al.*, 1986), or if fluid deficits due to other causes are present (see above). Monitoring of urine output provides a useful guide to the adequacy of fluid replacement and it may be judicious to insert a urinary catheter before any major surgery in the aged.

The choice of fluid for infusion remains debatable (Chapter 9). The adminstration of dextrose was accompanied by higher intraoperative urine output than the use of saline 0.9% but, after surgery, urine output was less well maintained using the dextrose solution (Tweedie *et al.*, 1986). The use of saline will also reduce the possibility of postoperative hyponatraemia, a serious complication which is more likely to occur in patients given too little saline during and after surgery (Swales, 1987). The adminstration of colloids, which remain longer in the circulation than crystalloids, may predispose to congestive cardiac failure in the elderly.

Blood transfusion

The younger patient, with a healthy CVS, will be able to maintain good tissue oxygen supply even after the loss of 1000 ml of blood, provided that the intravascular volume is maintained. In contrast, as tissue perfusion is more easily decreased in older subjects with consequent reduction in tissue oxygen supply, a decrease in haemoglobin will be less readily tolerated. The assumption cannot be made that, in the old, decreased viscosity will compensate for the decreased oxygen capacity. Blood transfusion should therefore be started when the blood loss has reached 500 ml and is likely to continue. Perhaps more attention should be paid in older patients to the re-transfusion of blood lost during surgery.

The use of autologous blood transfusion is likely to increase, and it has been used in fit patients up to 65 years of age (Kay, 1987). The criteria for the inclusion of aged patients in an autologous blood transfusion programme will need to be clearly established, and may differ from the criteria for inclusion of younger patients.

Urine output

Maintenance of good urine output during surgery can best be ensured by the administration of adequate volumes of fluid. Low dose dopamine, infused up to the dose of 5 μg kg^{-1} min^{-1} is a useful drug, but is best infused into a catheter in a central vein. Mannitol can be given if such access is not available; a dose of 0.3–0.5 g kg^{-1} is used, but the initial increase in intravascular volume caused by this drug can induce cardiac failure. Frusemide is not recommended during anaesthesia, as a dose of 20mg i.v. can cause such a large diuresis (up to one litre during the first hour after the drug has been given) that hypovolaemia occurs.

The patient with a pacemaker

The following problems have arisen during surgery in patients with pacemakers:

(i) *Demand pacemakers* are inhibited by diathermy. Most will then revert automatically to a fixed rate, but some will not and will cease to pace.

(ii) *Triggered pacemakers* may respond to diathermy with production of a fast atrial or ventricular rate, and ventricular fibrillation has been described. A magnet placed over the pacemaker will change it to a fixed device.

(iii) *Programmed pacemakers* may be reprogrammed by electromagnetic induction from the use of the diathermy, and reprogramming can also occur if a magnet is placed over the pacemaker in an attempt to convert it into a fixed rate device. The resultant reprogramming can cause varying and irregular heart rate or rhythm.

It is recommended that the indifferent electrode of the diathermy is sited distant from the heart or pacemaker, and that the diathermy itself should not be used within 10 cm of the heart or pacemaker. Initially, the diathermy should be used for very short periods only, until any effect on the pacemaker has been evaluated. The type of pacemaker should be determined before the operation, and a magnet used only for those which do not revert automatically to a fixed rate if they are inhibited by the diathermy. It may be necessary to reprogramme a programmed pacemaker to the asynchronous mode before the start of surgery, and then the pacemaker is reprogrammed to the required mode after the operation.

The aged diabetic

The incidence of diabetes increases with increasing age, and it may be that the number of older diabetics who require insulin is increasing. On the whole, the intraoperative management of the old diabetic is similar to that of the younger diabetic, with the same indications for the use of an Alberti regime or of an insulin infusion. However, it must be remembered that the aged are more likely to develop *non-ketotic hyperosmolar coma*. This can occur in non-insulin dependent diabetics, and even in those on dietary control alone. The blood sugar in this condition can rise very rapidly to high levels, and thus it is advisable to measure the blood sugar more frequently in all older diabetics during the perioperative period, and intraoperative blood sugar measurements should be made during long operations.

The use of invasive monitoring

The indications for the use of central venous pressure and arterial catheters are similar in old and young patients.

Invasive monitoring using a pulmonary artery balloon catheter may come to be more widely used in the management of the older patient having major surgery in the presence of heart disease. It has been found possible to reduce the mortality after major surgery in patients with ischaemic heart disease by using intensive monitoring, including pulmonary artery catheters, for 72 h after surgery. In many countries, some selection will have to be made of the patients who will benefit most from such monitoring, which is expensive in equipment, time and staff. The measurement of pulmonary capillary wedge pressures, together with the central venous pressure, will provide information which can be used intraoperatively by the anaesthetist to maintain optimum cardiac function by the use of i.v. fluids, and drugs such as inotropes and vasodilators. Cardiac output and vascular resistance of both systemic and pulmonary circulations can also be measured and these can be useful additional information (Chapter 1).

Afterthought

The effects of a general anaesthetic can outlast the duration of the surgical procedure. Postoperative complications which can be related to aspects of the anaesthetic range from minor transient problems such as deafness or confusion to major complications including pulmonary embolus or cerebrovascular accident. The anaesthetist must consider these more distant effects as well as the immediate intraoperative responses when conducting a general anaesthetic in an aged patient.

References

Arden, J.R., Holley, F.O. & Stanski, D.R. (1986) Increased sensitivity to etomidate in the elderly: Initial distribution versus altered brain response. *Anesthesiology* **65**, 19–27.

Bailey, P.L., Wilbrink, J., Zwanikken, P., Pace, N.L. & Stanley, T.H. (1985) Anesthetic induction with fentanyl. *Anesth. Analg.* **64**, 48–53.

Bell, G.D., Spickett, G.P., Reeve, P.A., Morden, A. & Logan, R.F.A. (1987) Intravenous midazolam for upper gastrointestinal endoscopy: a study of 800 consecutive cases relating dose to age and sex of patient. *Br. J. Clin. Pharmacol.* **23**, 241–243.

Bentley, J.B., Borel, J.D., Nenad, R.E. & Gillespie, T.J. (1982) Age and fentanyl pharmacokinetics. *Anesth. Analg.* **61**, 968–971.

Bullingham, J., Rigby, J., Pinkerton, M., Rogers, D., Lewis, T., Preganz, P., Mouton, S., Wood, A.J.J. & Wood, M. (1987) The effect of age on the adrenergic response to endotracheal intubation. *Anesth. Analg.* **66**, S23.

Carli. F., Gabrielczyk, M., Clarke, M.M. & Aber, V.R. (1985) Postoperative hypothermia: factors affecting rewarming. *Br. J. Anaesth.* **57**, 820P.

Christensen, J.H., Andreasen, F. & Jansen, T.A. (1983) Thiopentone sensitivity in young and elderly women. *Br. J. Anaesth.* **55**, 33–40.

Conahan, T.J., Williams, G.D., Apfelbaum, J.L. & Lecky, J.H. (1985) Airway heating reduces recovery time (cost) in outpatients. *Anesthesiology* **63**, A166.

Cook, P.J., Flanagan, R. & James, I.M.(1984) Diazepam tolerance: effect of age, regular sedation and alcohol. *Br. Med. J.* **289**, 351–353.

D'Hollander, A., Massaux, F., Nevelstein, M. & Agoston, S. (1982) Age-dependent dose-response relationship of Org NC 45 in anaesthetised patients. *Br. J. Anaesth.* **54**, 653–657.

D'Hollander, A.A., Luyckx, C., Barvais, L. & De Ville, A. (1983) Clinical evaluation of atracurium besylate requirement for a stable muscle relaxation during surgery: lack of age-related effects. *Anesthesiology* **59**, 237–240.

Donald, J.R. (1982) Induced hypotension and blood loss during surgery. *J. Roy. Soc. Med.* **75**, 149–151.

Dundee, J.W. Halliday, N.J., Loughran, P.G. & Harper, K.W. (1985) The influence of age on the onset of anaesthesia with midazolam. *Anaesthesia* **40**, 441–443.

Dundee, J.W., Robinson, F.P., Collum, J.S.C. & Patterson, C.C. (1986) Sensitivity to propofol in the elderly. *Anaesthesia* **41**, 482–485.

Duvaldestin, R., Raada, J., Berger, J.L., d'Hollander, A. & Desmonts J.M. (1982) Pharmacokinetics, pharmacodynamics, and dose-response relationships of pancuronium in control and elderly subjects. *Anesthesiology* **56**, 36–40.

Eintrei, C., Leszniewski, W. & Carlsson, G. (1985) Local application of ^{133}Xenon for measurement of regional cerebral blood flow (CBF) during halothane, enflurane and isoflurane anesthesia in humans. *Anesthesiology* **63**, 391–394.

Erikssen, J. (1969) Atropine psychosis. *Lancet* **1**, 53–54.

Flacke, J.W. & Flacke, W.F. (1986) Impaired thermoregulation and perioperative hypothermia in the elderly. *Clin. Anesthesiol.* **4**, 859–880.

Gamble, J.A.S., Kawar, P., Dundee, J.W., Moore, J. & Briggs, L.P. (1981) Evaluation of midazolam as an intravenous induction agent. *Anaesthesia* **36**, 868–873.

Giles, H.G., MacLeod, S.M., Wright, J.R. & Sellers, E.M. (1978) Influence of age and previous use on diazepam dosage required for endoscopy. *Can. Med. Ass. J.* **118**, 513–514.

Haldemann, G., Schmidt, E., Frey, P., Hossli, G. & Schaer, H. (1975) Wirkung von Ethrane auf die Kreislaufgarossen geriatrischen patienten. *Anaesthetist* **24**, 343–346.

Harper, K.W., Collier, P.S., Dundee, J.W., Elliot, P., Hobday, N.J. & Lowry, K.G. (1985) Age and nature of operation influence the pharmacokinetics of midazolam. *Br. J. Anaesth.* **57**, 866–871.

Helmers, H., Van Peer, A., Woestenborghs, R., Noorduin, H. & Heykants, J. (1984) Alfentanil kinetics in the elderly. *Clin. Pharmacol. Ther.* **36**, 239–243.

Herman, R.J., McAllister, C.B., Branch, R.A. & Wilkinson, G.R. (1985) Effects of age on meperidine disposition. *Clin. Pharmacol. Ther.* **37**, 19–24.

Homer, T.D. & Stanski, D.R. (1985) The effect of increasing age on thiopental disposition and anesthetic requirement. *Anesthesiology* **62**, 714–724.

Hudson, R.J., Stanski, D.R. & Burch, P.A. (1982) Comparative pharmacokinetics of methohexital and thiopental. *Anesthesiology* **57**, A240.

Kanto, J., Mäenpää, M., Mäntylä, R., Sellman, R. & Valovirta, E. (1979) Effect of age on the pharmacokinetics of diazepam given in conjunction with spinal anesthesia. *Anesthesiology* **51**, 154–159.

Kay, L.A. (1987) The need for autologous blood transfusion. *Br. Med. J.* **294**, 137–138.

Kortilla, K. & Tarkkanen, J. (1985) Comparison of diazepam and midazolam for sedation during local anaesthesia for bronchoscopy. *Br. J. Anaesth.* **57**, 581–586.

Kristensen, G., Guldager, H. & Gravensen, H. (1986) Prevention of perioperative hypothermia in abdominal surgery. *Acta Anaesth. Scand.* **30**, 314–316.

Lavery, G.G. Mirakhur, R.K., Clarke, R.S.J., Gibson, F.M. & Lowry, K.G. (1987) Does the choice of the neuromuscular blocking agent affect the cardiovascular response to intubation? *Acta Anaesth. Scand.* **31**, 239–243.

Lowry, K.G., Mirakhur, R.K., Lavery, C.G. & Clarke, R.S.J. (1985) Vecuronium and atracurium in the elderly: a clinical comparison with pancuronium. *Acta Anaesth. Scand.* **29**, 405–408.

Marsh, R.H.L., Chmielewski, A.T. & Goat, V.A. (1980) Recovery from pancuronium. A comparison between old and young patients. *Anaesthesia* **35**, 1193–1196.

Matteo, R.S., Backers, N.W. & McDaniel, D.D. (1985) Pharmacokinetics and pharmacodynamics of d-tubocurarine and metocurine in the elderly. *Anesth. Analg.* **64**, 23–28.

Matteo, R.S., Ornstein, E., Young, W.L., Schwartz, A.E., Port, M. & Chang, W.J. (1986) Pharmacokinetics of sufentanil in the elderly. *Anesth.Analg.* **65**, S94.

Moffitt, E.A., Barker, R.A., Glenn, J.J., Imrie, D.D., Del Campo, D., Landymore, R.W., Kinley, E. & Murphy, D.A. (1986) Myocardial metabolism and hemodynamic responses with isoflurane anesthesia for coronary artery surgery. *Anesth. Analg.* **65**, 53–61.

Muravchick, S., Owens, W.D. & Felts, J.A. (1979) Glycopyrrolate and cardiac arrhythmias in geriatric patients after reversal of neuromuscular blockade. *Can. Anaesth. Soc. J.* **26**, 22–25.

Oduah, M. (1969) Effectivitat und Wirkungsdauer von Thiopental beim Menschen in Abhängigkeit vom Alter. *Anaesthetist* **18**, 308–310.

O'Malley, K. (Ed.) (1984) *Clinical Pharmacology and Drug Treatment in the Elderly.* Churchill Livingstone, Edinburgh.

Owen, J.A., Sitar, D.S., Bergh, L., Brownell, L., Duke, P.C. & Mitenko, P.A. (1983) Age-related morphine kinetics. *Clin. Pharmacol. Ther.* **34**, 364–368.

Owens, W.D., Waldbaum, L.S. & Stephen, C.R. (1978) Cardiac arrhythmias following reversal of neuromuscular blocking agents in geriatric patients. *Anesth. Analg.* **57**, 186–190.

Pauca, A.L., Savage, R.T., Simpson, S. & Roy, R.C. (1984) Effect of pethidine, fentanyl and morphine on postoperative shivering. *Acta Anaesth. Scand.* **28**, 138–143.

Phillips, P.A., Rolls, B.J., Ledingham, J.G.G., Crowe, M.J. & Wollner, L. (1983) Reduced thirst in the elderly after 24 hours water deprivation. *Clin. Sci.* **64**, 61P–62P.

Reiz, S., Bålfors, E., Sørensen, M.B., Ariola, S., Friedman, A. & Truedsson, H. (1983) Isoflurane — a powerful coronary vasodilator in patients with coronary artery disease. *Anesthesiology* **59**, 91–97.

Roe, C.F., Goldberg, M.J., Blair, C.S. & Kinney, J.M. (1966) The influence of body temperature on early postoperative oxygen consumption. *Surgery* **60**, 85–91.

Roizen, M.F., Lampe, G.H., Sheiner, L.B., Alpert, R.A., Frazer, B.M., Chan, R.P. & Eger, E.I. 11 (1985) Aging increases hemodynamic responses to induction and incision. *Anesth. Analg.* **64**, 275.

Rydvall, A., Häggmark, S., Nyhman, H. & Reiz S. (1984) Effects of enflurane on coronary haemodynamics in patients with ischaemic heart disease. *Acta Anaesth. Scand.* **28**, 690–695.

Sheref, S.E. (1985) Pattern of CNS recovery following reversal of neuromuscular blockade. Comparison of atropine and glycopyrrolate. *Br. J. Anaesth.* **57**, 188–191.

Simpson, K.H., Smith, R.J. & Davies, L.F. (1985) A comparison of the effects of atropine and glycopyrrolate on cognitive function following general anaesthesia. *Br. J. Anaesth.* **57**, 821P.

Smith. D.S., Orkin, F.K., Gardner, S.M. & Zakeosian, G. (1979) Prolonged sedation in the elderly after intraoperative atropine administration. *Anesthesiology* **51**, 348–349.

Smith., R.J., Roberts, M., Raper, M., Rodgers, R.J. & Bennett S. (1985) Cognitive effects of general anaesthesia in young and elderly patients. *Br. J. Anaesth.* **57**, 352P.

Stephens, L.D., Ho, P.C., Holloway, A.M., Bourne, D.W.A. & Triggs, E.J. (1984) Pharmacokinetics of alcuronium in elderly patients undergoing total hip replacement or aortic reconstructive surgery. *Br. J. Anaesth.* **56**, 465–471.

Swales, J.D. (1987) Dangers in treating hyponatraemia. *Br. Med. J.* **294**, 261–262.

Takunnen, O. & Takunnen, H. (1982) Peak airway pressure as pointer to risk of postoperative deep venous thrombosis. *Lancet* **1**, 1066.

Tokics, L., Bismar, B. & Hedenstierna, G. (1986) Splanchnic blood flow during halothane-relaxant anaesthesia in elderly patients. *Acta Anaesth. Scand.* **30**, 556–561.

Tweedie, I.E., Baxter, J.N., Taylor, G.T., Keens, S.J. & Campbell, I.T. (1986) Intraoperative fluids — How much and of what? *Br. J. Anaesth.* **58**, 1329P.

Virtanen, R., Kanto, J., Iisalo, E., Iisalo, U.M., Salo, M. & Sjövall, S. (1982) Pharmacokinetic studies on atropine with special reference to age. *Acta Anaesth. Scand.* **26**, 297–300.

Walker, J., Shanks, C.A. & Triggs, E.J. (1980) Clinical pharmacokinetics of alcuronium chloride in man. *Eur. J. Clin. Pharmacokinet.* **17**, 449–457.

Wetherell, A. (1980) Some effects of atropine on short term memory. *Br. J. Clin. Pharmacol.* **10**, 627–628.

Further reading

Dodson, M.E. (1984) Anaesthesia in the elderly. In *Clinical Pharmacology and Drug Treatment in the Elderly* (Ed. K. O'Malley). Churchill Livingstone, Edinburgh, pp. 196–217.

Dodson, M.E. & Parkhouse, J. (1985) Anaesthesia in old age. In *Textbook of Geriatric Medicine and Gerontology*. (Ed. J.C. Brocklehurst). Churchill Livingstone, Edinburgh, pp. 944–957.

13 | The place of regional anaesthesia for the aged

J.A.W. WILDSMITH

Introduction

The last 10 to 15 years have seen a considerable increase in the interest in, and use of, regional anaesthetic techniques. There are a number of reasons for this, but a major factor has been advances in the surgery of conditions which are particularly common in the old. Many of the procedures are performed on parts of the body that are readily anaesthetized with regional blocks and the incidence and severity of intercurrent disease in old patients mean that the use of general anaesthesia may be a cause of concern to all (patient and surgeon, as well as anaesthetist) involved. The positive features of regional anaesthesia also mean that its use may contribute to a successful outcome in ways other than avoidance of general anaesthesia. However, the old may be more susceptible to some of the complications and problems of regional anaesthesia than are the young. The aim of this chapter is to examine the features of regional anaesthesia and indicate how they may affect the aged to their advantage and disadvantage. In addition, some of the general aspects of the management of regional anaesthesia in old patients will be considered.

Features of regional anaesthesia

Preservation of consciousness

Properly performed regional anaesthesia should not, in itself, impair consciousness. This is usually considered an advantage because the airway and its protective reflexes are maintained. In the unprepared patient the protection of the airway so produced can be a distinct benefit, but fear of being aware of surgery causes many patients to refuse a regional technique. This anxiety is less of a problem in the old, because they usually have a more phlegmatic approach and they often appreciate that the presence of intercurrent disease may increase the risk of general anaesthesia. Thus, aged patients will usually accept regional anaesthesia more readily than younger ones. A minor problem is that deafness, or the mental slowing that can accompany old age, may make it more difficult to communicate with these patients and to make them understand what is required of them during the performance of the block.

Whilst the latter point has to be remembered, the preservation of consciousness usually has the advantage that the patient retains the ability to communicate with the attendant staff. Thus, a diabetic patient can recognize and report the initial symptoms of hypoglycaemia. In addition, a patient's distress during transurethral prostatectomy may give early warning that bladder irrigation fluid has entered the circulation. This means that such complications may be dealt with before they become severe. However, when a patient is conscious during an operation it does cause problems. All theatre staff must avoid unguarded sights and sounds and there are some operations — a limb amputation is the most obvious — that no patient should be aware of. A further problem is that it is very difficult to lie still on a hard operating table for a long time. Considerable discomfort may develop in those parts of the body that are not affected by the block. Joints stiffen in the aged and their bony prominences are less well covered so they are more likely to suffer from such discomfort.

The management of the conscious patient is a skill just as important as that of block performance. Explanation and reassurance contribute much, but just as vital is the ability to select the appropriate premedicant, sedative, analgesic and even anaesthetic drugs to supplement the block. The factors governing the choice of such agents are considered below, but a most important principle is to appreciate that the injection of the local anaesthetic drug is not the end of the procedure for the anaesthetist.

Profound analgesia

Without doubt a most valuable feature of regional anaesthesia is the production of complete block of afferent impulses. This may simplify the anaesthetic management by preventing the marked cardiorespiratory stimulation that occurs during very painful procedures and can mean that the patient is returned to bed free of both pain and the risk of central respiratory depression from opioid therapy. Thereafter, there is a gradual return of sensation and a decreased requirement for analgesics even after a single injection local technique. Fewer doses of opioids also means fewer side-effects. A good example is the way that the use of a caudal block for haemorrhoidectomy produces better analgesia and an earlier return of bowel function (Berstock, 1979). After major surgery the continued use of an epidural will maintain both respiratory function (Spence & Smith, 1971) and gastric emptying (Nimmo et al., 1978) nearer to normal.

Prolonged lack of sensation can cause problems. Some patients find it distressing and in the aged in particular it may predispose to urinary retention and skin damage. Careful choice of technique will minimize these problems, but extra nursing care is essential in the patient with an extensive block of long duration.

Muscle relaxation

Most local anaesthetic techniques block motor as well as sensory nerves, so that quite profound muscle relaxation may be produced. The advantage is that this relaxation is produced with minimal effect on the muscles of respiration and without any concern about the adequacy of reversal or metabolism of neuromuscular blocking drugs. Epidural and spinal blocks that are extensive enough to permit abdominal surgery may affect the innervation of some respiratory muscles, but the adverse physiological effects are minimal (Bowler et al., 1986). After upper abdominal or thoracic surgery the beneficial effect of profound analgesia on freedom to cough can more than compensate for any adverse effect of motor weakness.

Some patients find the inability to move the blocked limb(s) distressing, but advance warning usually prevents undue anxiety. Of more concern, is that lack of muscle tone may allow the limb to be placed in a position that may damage joints. The prevalence of rheumatoid and osteoarthritic disease in the old means that 'hyperextension' injuries are particularly likely to occur.

Sympathetic block

Sympathetic nerves are also involved in the majority of regional techniques. The physiological derangements produced can be quite major, with the effect depending on the extent of the block, the dose of local anaesthetic used, the use of vasoconstrictor and the type of sedative or anaesthetic supplement used (Bowler et al., 1986). Young, fit subjects tolerate surprisingly extensive spinal or epidural block with minimal cardiovascular changes, but this is not true of the old. Even in the absence of overt disease, they have a reduced capacity for adapting to the peripheral and cardiac effects of sympathetic block. Significant disease (often associated in the aged with the actions of beta adreno-receptor blocking drugs on heart rate, diuretics on blood volume and antihypertensives on vasomotor tone) may further limit the patient's ability to compensate for decreased sympathetic activity.

Profound hypotension can thus result, but symphathetic block may have some advantages. A moderate degree of hypotension may, by decreasing preload, afterload and heart rate, have a beneficial action on cardiac function (Merlin, 1981) and also improve the surgical field by decreasing bleeding. As long as cardiac output is maintained at a reasonable level, either by careful choice of technique or use of vaso-active drugs, blood flow through the blocked area will be vigorous. This has even been shown to be the case after the insertion of arterial grafts (Cousin & Wright, 1971). Such an active lower limb blood flow may be one of the reasons why the incidence of thromboembolic disease is decreased when regional anaesthesia is used (Thorburn et al., 1980).

Symphathetic block will also affect the other systems. Much surgery in the aged is to the gastro-intestinal tract. Sympathetic block relaxes sphincters and increases bowel motility. Bowel incontinence would seem more likely, but seems no more common than during general anaesthesia. A more serious risk is rupture of an obstructed viscus and this is one reason (fluid imbalance and uncertainty about the extent of surgery being the others) why spinals and epidurals should not be used for abdominal emergencies. Other techniques may still have a place, and in the elective, prepared case the situation is very different (Aitkenhead, 1984). Sympathetic block shrinks the bowel (making surgical access easier), increases colonic blood flow, provides muscle relaxation without the need to give neostigmine and, if the block is continued after surgery, helps avoid opioid-induced ileus. Postoperative distension and anastomotic leakage should be minimized.

Sequelae, morbidity and mortality

Many of the features of regional anaesthesia that have been mentioned would seem to be to the patient's advantage and there is a growing body of evidence that the morbidity, and perhaps even the mortality, of surgery may be decreased by the wider use of regional techniques. Certainly the incidence of many of the traditional minor sequelae of general anaesthesia (nausea, vomiting, sore throat, etc.) may be minimized (Brown, 1987), although whether this is at the expense of an increased incidence of complications due to the block has yet to be properly quantified. The aged might be more prone to retention of urine after an epidural or to develop backache because of the difficulty of penetrating dense, aged ligaments.

Much has been made of the way regional anaesthesia decreases the 'stress' response. Major surgery performed under general anaesthesia has quite considerable metabolic and hormonal effects. By preventing noxious stimuli from reaching the central nervous system, regional anaesthesia can considerably modify this response (for a review, see Kehlet, 1984). Certainly a decrease in circulatory catecholamines can only be good for a patient with cardiac disease, but the precise significance of the changes (or lack of them) has yet to be explained.

Of more immediate relevance have been epidemiological studies of the outcome of certain types of surgery when performed under either general or regional anaesthesia. These have usually been conditions that are particularly common in the aged, such as hip fractures (McLaren et al., 1978), transurethral prostatectomy (McGowan & Smith, 1980) and limb amputation (Mann & Bissett, 1983). Some papers reported quite spectacular differences in mortality, with the advantage being with regional anaesthesia, but these major differences have not been confirmed (Valentin et al., 1986). However, there have been quite consistent reports of reduced early morbidity.

Postoperative hypoxaemia (McKenzie et al., 1980), anastomotic breakdown (Aitkenhead *et al.*, 1978), bronchopneumonia (McLaren, 1982), time to resumption of oral fluid intake (Mann & Bissett, 1983) and thromboembolic complications (Thorburn *et al.*, 1980) have all been shown to be decreased by regional anaesthesia compared with general anaesthesia. Hip replacement surgery is common in the old and causes a high incidence of the latter complication. A continous epidural can decrease this (Modig, 1982) by increasing mobility (better analgesia) and lower limb blood flow, and decreasing the stress response, the need for blood transfusion and platelet 'stickiness' — the last a direct pharmacological effect of local anaesthetic drugs.

Pharmacological considerations

The pharmacology of drugs in the aged is considered in general terms elsewhere (Chapter 8), but a few specific points about the drugs used during regional anaesthesia are worthy of re-emphasis.

Local anaesthetics

Certain local anaesthetic techniques require very large doses of drug. Given the very profound effects that these agents may have on the cardiovascular and central nervous system, it is understandable that there should be anxiety about the way that aged patients metabolize them. In Chapter 8 and in a comprehensive review (Tucker, 1986) Tucker concludes that old age (uncomplicated by disease) has a relatively minor effect on the kinetics of these drugs. Overt cardiovascular and liver disease produce much more significant changes. Two recent studies of the kinetics of lignocaine (Bowdle *et al.*, 1986) and bupivacaine (Veering *et al.*, 1987) after epidural injection have confirmed that peak plasma concentrations are unaffected by age. However, both studies showed that the clearance of the drugs was delayed in the older patients so that cumulation may occur with repeated doses. The risk would seem to be greater after lignocaine than bupivacaine because of the difference in duration of action.

Supplementary drugs

Of greater clinical relevance is the increased sensitivity to sedative drugs seen in the aged. For instance, midazolam is a very useful sedative drug during regional anaesthesia (McClure *et al.*, 1983), but its elimination half-life is prolonged even in patients over 50 years of age (Harper *et al.*, 1985). In older patients, doses of only 1–2 mg may be sufficient. Larger doses may have a very prolonged action and quite marked cardiorespiratory effects. Oxygenation is usually unaffected by regional anaesthesia, even in the aged (Muravchik & Johnson, 1986), but when sedative drugs are used it is wise to give additional oxygen to breathe.

Patient management

Preoperative factors

The anaesthetist considering a regional technique has to make several decisions. He must decide between it and general anaesthesia, and then pick from a number of local techniques that might be suitable. In old patients the presence of intercurrent disease will be a very significant factor in making these decisions. The influence of different disease states on the use of regional anaesthesia has been reviewed (Charlton, 1987) and these techniques have much to offer. However, a vital principle is that the chosen method must be one that the anaesthetist has sufficient experience of to use it in an unhealthy patient. A second, related principle is that the assessment and preparation of a patient who is to receive regional anaesthesia should be as rigorous as for a general anaesthetic. The aim of using a regional anaesthetic in these patients must be to improve their management, not to cut corners.

The other major decision to be made is which particular block should be used. Obviously the block and its duration must match the intended operation, and often the decision is simple. When a choice of two or more is possible, the anaesthetist must consider his own ability, the features of the possible techniques and relate all of these factors to the individual patient. In the lower half of the body, the choice is often between intradural and extradural block. In the aged, the former is perhaps to be preferred unless there is a need to continue the block postoperatively. Only a small dose of drug is needed, spinal abnormalities make it simpler and headache due to cerebrospinal fluid leakage is a less common problem in the old.

Technical problems

The anatomical distortion that is to be found in many old people, particularly curvature or rotation of the spine, can make the performance of techniques more difficult. Intervertebral spaces may be narrowed by such distortion, or by osteophytes, and deep structures may not bear the same relationship to standard superficial landmarks. The difficulties that these problems produce may be overcome by careful positioning of the patient to try to eliminate the distortion, or by a careful consideration of its nature and then inserting the needle at an angle that takes it into account. Finally, with a little flattery it is often possible encourage an aged patient to flex his or her spine to a degree that he or she had long thought impossible! However, even the most experienced practitioner must be prepared to admit that occasionally these anatomical problems are insurmountable. An alternative technique should always be in mind.

The increase in the rigidity of tissues that occurs with ageing can help as well as hinder a block technique. Needle advancement can be more difficult, especially through calcified ligaments, and catheters often seem less ready to advance into the epidural space than in the young, but differences between planes may be more easily appreciated. The reduced elasticity of tissues may be one reason why blocks are often more extensive. This is well recognized in regard to epidural (Bromage, 1987) and spinal (Cameron et al., 1981) blocks and may apply to other techniques as well. However, what is not so widely appreciated is that the *range* of block levels seen in older patients is as great as is seen in the young, so the fact that spread is, on average, slightly greater is of little predictive value.

The onset and effectiveness of regional blocks in the old seem to differ little from that seen in young patients. Because there may be greater spread, regression may be faster (Veering et al., 1987) since each nerve has been exposed to a lower concentration of drug, but this is of little clinical significance.

Sedative and anaesthetic supplements

A local anaesthetic block may be supplemented with many drugs given either as premedication or during the course of the procedure. An oral sedative, given in advance, may be all that is required, especially in the aged. Once a block has taken away the pain of an ischaemic limb, a chronically distended bladder or a diseased hip joint (common conditions in the old) the patient often starts to catch up on the considerable sleep deprivation that these may have caused. The greater sensitivity to parenteral sedative drugs has been referred to and the traditional opioids are perhaps more predictable in old patients. They certainly help control the discomforts that arise from lying on an operating table for any length of time. Chlormethiazole is also useful and the author finds an i.v. infusion after premedication with morphine a useful supplement to regional anaesthesia in old patients.

Whatever parenteral drugs are used, it must be recognized that recovery will be prolonged if large doses are needed to control the patient. Whether this is because the patient is very anxious, is particularly uncomfortable lying still or the surgery is very prolonged, the effect is the same. The solution is to use the inhalational route, although this does not imply the inevitable use of a conventional general anaesthetic since the drugs may be used to provide conscious sedation or light sleep as well. For very major surgery, the combination of a regional technique with a full general anaesthetic, including endotracheal intubation, still has much to offer. However, it is essential that the anaesthetist has experience of the management of this combination.

The choice of supplement will depend on the type and duration of surgery, the patient's medical status and level of anxiety and, not least, the skill, personality and experience of the anaesthetist. Every practitioner has his own favourite techniques, but two drugs that are most useful in the aged are nitrous oxide and ketamine. Spinal anaesthesia is widely used for the surgery of hip fractures, but a major problem is moving the patient into position without causing pain. The inhalation of a low concentration of nitrous oxide or the i.v. administration of small doses of ketamine are very useful in these circumstances.

Complications

One of the aims in using a regional anaesthetic in any patient is to try to reduce the risk of complications developing. Regional techniques have, of course, their own complications and in the main these are no more or less likely to occur in the aged. There are exceptions and some of these have been referred to. The risk of any patient being injured in some way while the block is effective must always be kept in mind, particularly when dealing with the aged. Skin and joints are much more prone to damage and the method of prevention is constant awareness and attention to detail. A ripple mattress should be used more readily than it would be in younger patients and it is advantageous to have one that is also heated. The vasodilatation produced by sympathetic block leads to an increased rate of heat loss and patients are then more prone to hypothermia (Vaughan *et al.*, 1981).

Hypotension

Undoubtedly the most frequent cause for concern during major regional techniques is hypotension due to sympathetic block. If an aged patient has arterial disease, such hypotension is more likely to have adverse effects and the frequency with which it occurs is increased. The reasons for the latter have been mentioned and hypotension is likely to be particularly severe once the block extends above T5 and the sympathetic drive to the heart is affected. The prevention and treatment of such hypotension is an area of some controversy at present, but one line of recommended action will be described.

Firstly, a reasonable attempt should be made to try to limit the amount of sympathetic block that is produced. Major peripheral blocks may be more appropriate than central techniques, but even if the latter are used they should be controlled as far as possible. For surgery to the lower half of the body, an isobaric spinal solution will, in this age group, usually produce an adequate block with little chance of spread to the upper thoracic dermatomes. If an epidural is more appropriate, then a small volume of a concentrated solution (i.e. 10 ml of 0.75% bupivacaine) injected at mid or low lumbar level will usually be satisfactory. In both cases, onset may be a little slower than with other methods, but in aged patients this may minimize the upset of any sympathetic block that does develop. The more gradual onset may allow the circulation more time to adapt or gives the anaesthetist time to deal with the problem.

Having decided on a method, then hypotension has to be anticipated, although it should be emphasized that not every patient with an extensive sympathetic block becomes hypotensive. Every patient should be placed in a slight (5°) head-down tilt to ensure venous return, and the latter also requires that blood volume *must* be adequate. This is *not* to advocate the infusion of large volumes of fluid before the institution of the block, but all fluid and blood losses must be recognized and corrected.

The practice of 'preloading' is often ineffective (Clark *et al.*, 1976) and is really illogical, because the cause of the hypotension is not hypovolaemia, but vasodilatation with or without a decrease in cardiac output. As well as being ineffective, preloading can lead to considerable problems in the aged. As the block wears off, the fluid will leave the circulation, usually to end up in the bladder and occasionally to cause acute retention of urine because bladder sensation may still be blocked. Worse still, the fluid may cause pulmonary oedema in patients with cardiac or renal disease. The needless infusion of fluid to treat hypotension due to sympathetic block is similarly to be deprecated.

It is more sensible to watch the patient carefully and to administer drugs which maintain the circulation by correcting the physiological alteration caused by the block. Some degree of hypotension is, in the majority of patients, advantageous, but it is wise to decide on a lower limit in advance. In young fit patients, a decrease in systolic pressure by up to one-third may be of little concern, but in older patients a more stringent limit may be preferable (e.g. one-quarter).

If the pressure is below that limit and there is a bradycardia (heart rate below 60), atropine (0.3 mg i.v.) may be sufficient to maintain the circulation. If the heart rate is above 60, then ephedrine (increments of 3-6 mg i.v.) is used, but if heart rate is above 85-90 it may be more appropriate to use methoxamine (increments of 1-2 mg i.v.) since it will not further increase heart rate and myocardial oxygen consumption. The response to these drugs is very variable and may be quite slow in developing in old patients. Often only one or two doses are required.

Overview

One of the major features of regional anaesthesia is that it may considerably simplify an anaesthetic procedure. A single injection of one drug may provide most, if not all, of the requirements for surgery. In old patients one benefit of this is that there is no anxiety about their ability to metabolize drugs (e.g. opioids and neuromuscular blocking agents) with potent effects on respiration. The counter argument is that the injection may not be so simple from a technical point of view and the effects of the block (especially on the circulation) may be more exaggerated.

This perhaps illustrates that, while there are no differences in kind

Table 13.1. Some factors affecting the use of regional anaesthesia in the aged. In general the effects of ageing itself are much less than those of any intercurrent disease.

Regional anaesthesia more readily accepted by the aged
Possible advantage must be balanced against risk of complication
Anatomical changes in old age increase technical difficulty and may modify
drug spread.
Peak concentration of local anaesthetic drugs unrelated to age, but clearance is
prolonged so there is a slightly increased risk of cumulation
Sensitivity to supplementary drugs (i.e. sedatives) is increased
Circulation more sensitive to effects of sympathetic block

---

between using regional anaesthesia in the old and the young, there are certainly differences in emphasis (Table 13.1). The point made earlier about not using these methods simply because there is some inconvenient medical or administrative contraindication to general anaesthesia bears repeating. The most distal block suited to the individual patient and particular operation is chosen, remembering that the patient must be carefully managed throughout. The anaesthetist may need to be very patient and give very explicit warnings of what is to happen when performing a block in aged patients who may be deaf or a little slow in understanding. Finally, no matter what anaesthetic technique is used in the aged, highly skilled care is essential.

References

Aitkenhead, A.R. (1984) Anaesthesia and bowel surgery. *Br. J. Anaesth.* **56**, 95.

Aitkenhead, A.R., Wishart, H.Y. & Peebles-Brown, D.A. (1978) High spinal nerve block for large bowel anastomosis: a retrospective study. *Br. J. Anaesth.* **50**, 177.

Berstock, D.A. (1979) Haemorrhoidectomy without tears. *Ann. R. Coll. Surg. Engl.* **61**, 51.

Bowdle, T.A., Freund, P.R. & Slattery, J.T. (1986) Age-dependent lidocaine pharmacokinetics during lumbar peridural anesthesia with lidocaine hydrocarbonate or lidocaine hydrochloride. *Reg. Anesth.* **11**, 123.

Bowler, G.M.R., Wildsmith, J.A.W. & Scott, D.B. (1986) Epidural administration of local anesthetics. In *Acute Pain Management. Clinics in Critical Care Medicine 8* (Eds M.J. Cousins & G.D. Phillips). Churchill Livingstone, Edinburgh, p. 187.

Bromage, P.R. (1978) *Epidural Analgesia.* Saunders, Philadelphia.

Brown, D.T. (1987) The features of regional anaesthesia. In *Principles and Practice of Regional Anaesthesia.* (Eds J.A.W. Wildsmith & E.N. Armitage). Churchill Livingstone, Edinburgh, p. 8.

Cameron, A.E., Arnold, R.W., Ghoris, M.W. & Jamieson, V. (1981) Spinal analgesia using bupivacaine 0.5% plain. Variations in the extent of block with patient age. *Anaesthesia* **36**, 318.

Charlton, J.E. (1987) The management of regional anaesthesia. In *Principles and Practice of Regional Anaesthesia* (Eds J.A.W. Wildsmith & E.N. Armitage) Churchill Livingstone, Edinburgh, p. 37.

Clark, R.B., Thomson, D.S. & Thomson, C.H. (1976) Prevention of spinal hypotension associated with Caesarean section. *Anesthesiology* **45**, 679.

Cousins, M.J. & Wright, C.J. (1971) Graft, muscle and skin blood flow after epidural block in vascular surgical procedures. *Surg. Gynec. Obstet.* **133**, 59.

Harper, K.W., Collier, P.S. Dundee, J.W., Elliott, P., Halliday, N.J. & Lowry, K.G. (1985) Age and operation influence the pharmacokinetics of midazolam. *Br. J. Anaesth.* **57**, 866.

Kehlet, H. (1984) Stress-free anaesthesia: regional anaesthesia. In *Regional Anaesthesia 1884–1984*. (Eds D.B. Scott, J.H. McClure & J.A.W. Wildsmith) ICM AB, Sodertalje, p. 159.

McClure, J.H., Brown, D.T. & Wildsmith, J.A.W. (1983) Comparison of the intravenous administration of midazolam and diazepam as sedation during spinal anaesthesia. *Br. J. Anaesth.* **55**, 1089.

McGowan, S.W. & Smith, G.F.N. (1980) Anaesthesia for transurethral prostatectomy: a comparison of spinal intradural analgesia with two methods of general anaesthesia. *Anaesthesia* **35**, 847.

McKenzie, P.J., Wishart, H.Y., Dewar, K.M.S., Gray, I. & Smith, G. (1980) Comparison of the effects of spinal anaesthesia and general anaesthesia on postoperative oxygenation and perioperative mortality. *Br. J. Anaesth.* **52**, 49.

McLaren, A.D., Stockwell, M.C. & Reid, V.T. (1978) Anaesthetic techniques for surgical correction of fractured neck of femur. A comparative study of spinal and general anaesthesia in the elderly. *Anaesthesia* **33**, 10.

McLaren, A.D. (1982) Mortality studies: a review. *Reg. Anesth.* **7**, S172.

Mann, R.A.M. & Bisset, W.I.K. (1983) Anaesthesia for lower limb amputation. A comparison of spinal analgesia and general anaesthesia in the elderly. *Anaesthesia* **38**, 1183.

Merin, R.G. (1981) Local and regional anesthetic techniques for the patient with ischemic heart disease. *Clev. Clin. Quart.* **48**, 72.

Modig, J. (1982) Thromboembolism and blood loss: continuous epidural block versus general anesthesia with controlled ventilation. *Reg. Anesth.* **7**, S84.

Muravchick, S. & Johnson, R. (1986) Oxygenation of peripheral tissues in young and elderly patients during spinal anesthesia. *Reg. Anesth.* **11**, 7.

Nimmo, W.S., Littlewod, D.G., Scott, D.B. & Prescott, L.F. (1978) Gastric emptying following hysterectomy with extradural analgesia. *Br. J. Anaesth.* **50**, 559.

Spence, A.A. & Smith, G. (1971) Postoperative analgesia and lung function: a comparison of morphine with extradural block. *Br. J. Anaesth.* **43**, 144.

Thorburn, J., Louden, J.R. & Vallance, R. (1980) Spinal and general anaesthesia in total hip replacement: frequency of deep vein thrombosis. *Br. J. Anaesth.* **52**, 1117.

Tucker, G.T. (1986) Pharmacokinetics of local anaesthetics. *Br. J. Anaesth.* **58**, 717.

Valentin, N., Lomholt, B., Jensen, J.S., Hejgaard, N. & Kremer, S. (1986) Spinal or general anaesthesia for surgery of the fractured hip. A prospective study of mortality in 578 patients. *Br. J. Anaesth.* **58**, 284.

Vaughan, M.S., Vaughan, R.W. & Cork, R.C. (1981) Postoperative hypothermia in adults: relationship of age, anaesthesia, and shivering to rewarming. *Anesth. Analg.* **60**, 746–751.

Veering, B.T., Burm, A.G.L., van Kleef, J.W. & Hennis, P.J. (1987) Epidural anaesthesia with bupivacaine: effects of age on neural blockade and pharmacokinetics. *Anesth. Analg.* **66**, 589–593.

14 | Postoperative complications in the aged

D.G. SEYMOUR & F.G. VAZ

Introduction

The aged postoperative patient is worthy of special attention for several reasons:

(i) The older the patient, the greater is the likelihood of coincidental medical disease. Much of the excess postoperative morbidity in the aged surgical patient has its roots in pre-existing medical problems.

(ii) For a given surgical problem, old people are more likely to present to surgeons and anaesthetists as emergencies than are younger adults. The time for preoperative assessment and stabilization is correspondingly shorter.

(iii) Medical and surgical postoperative problems may present atypically in the older patient. Thus, an anastomosis breakdown may occur with a minimum of abdominal signs, and surgical or medical sepsis may not induce pyrexia. Postoperative myocardial infarctions are often painless in the older patient.

(iv) Age-related changes in homeostatic mechanisms mean that the aged surgical patient tends to be less competent in dealing with the physiological stresses of surgery, fluid depletion, volume overload and hypoxia.

(v) Drug doses, including those of premedications, anaesthetic agents, postoperative analgesics and antibiotics, may need to be reduced in older patients. The incidence of drug side-effects tends to rise with age.

This chapter utilizes the growing world literature on the older postoperative patient, but draws particularly on the findings of two prospective studies of surgical patients aged 65 years and over. The first of these (the Dundee study) looked at preoperative risk factors and postoperative outcome in 258 general surgical patients (Seymour & Pringle, 1983). The more recent Cardiff study had a similar design but also included admissions for a fractured neck of femur (Vaz & Seymour, 1988). The commonest postoperative problems encountered in the Cardiff study are shown in Fig. 14.1.

Postoperative respiratory problems

Incidence

Depending on the criterion used, between 12% and 40% of patients aged 65 years and over develop a postoperative respiratory complication, a

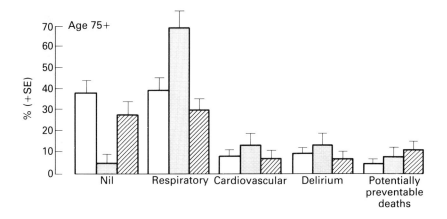

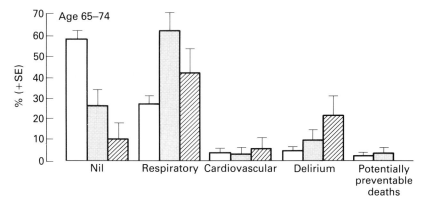

Fig. 14.1. Cardiff study, postoperative complications □ — Elective operations; ▦ — non-elective operations; ▨ — fractured femur operations. Data from a prospective study of 394 patients, aged 65 years and over, admitted to general surgical and trauma wards (Vaz & Seymour, 1987). Patients with a proximal femoral fracture have been analysed separately because they tend to be older and frailer than other surgical admissions. 'Elective' and 'non-elective' refer to types of admission.

respiratory morbidity rate which is two to three times that of younger adults. In the Dundee and Cardiff studies, a quarter of the potentially preventable postoperative deaths which occurred were due to respiratory problems.

In the Cardiff study an attempt was made to classify postoperative respiratory complications into *atelectasis* (defined as reduced basal breath sounds but with no productive cough and temperature below 38 °C) *pneumonia* (signs of consolidation, with sputum production and often with pyrexia) or *bronchitis* (a productive cough, rhonchi, but no consolidation). Using these criteria, postoperative atelectasis was diagnosed in 17% of patients, pneumonia in 8% and bronchitis in 24%. The peak incidence of respiratory complications was on the second and third postoperative days, and over 90% of respiratory complications occurred in the first postoperative week.

Some authors also describe *microatelectasis*, which shows itself as hypoxaemia in the absence of physical signs in the chest. In the aged, a degree of hypoxaemia is almost universal postoperatively (Helms *et al.*, 1979).

Diagnostic difficulties

It is well recognized that respiratory infections may develop insidiously in older patients. Thus, drowsiness or confusion may be the presenting signs, rather than fever or purulent sputum. In the first few postoperative days, regular chest examinations (particularly of the lung bases) are necessary in order to attempt to detect early pneumonia. Extra vigilance is needed in the case of high risk patients, as is described below.

Pathophysiology of postoperative chest infections

Changing theories of the pathophysiology of postoperative respiratory complications have led to new strategies in prevention and therapy. Older concepts viewed *retention of respiratory secretions* as the primary cause of postoperative respiratory morbidity. The secretions were thought to lead in turn to airways collapse, atelectasis and then pneumonia. While accepting that retention of secretions is an important phenomenon in some patients who develop respiratory complications, work in the last two decades has pointed to other mechanisms. Full details of the changing concepts can be found in a number of reviews (Peters, 1979; Tisi, 1979; Bartlett, 1980; Lewis, 1980) but the central conclusions of recent research are as follows. It is now thought that, in the majority of postoperative cases, *collapse of small airways* rather than retention of secretions is the primary event, with atelectasis and infection occurring secondarily. Attention has therefore shifted to those mechanisms which favour small airways collapse.

Basal airways tend to collapse in the presence of factors which cause the lung *closing volume* to rise, namely advanced aged, smoking and lung disease. Basal collapse is also favoured by factors causing the *functional residual capacity* to fall, i.e. general anaesthesia, the supine position, and incisions near the diaphragm. An important mechanism for keeping basal airways open is the periodic occurrence of *sustained maximal inspirations* (SMIs or sighs) six to eight times an hour. If SMIs are absent for as little as one hour, e.g. due to oversedation, then airways collapse can begin. Old patients are particularly susceptible to the effects of sedatives, and central respiratory control mechanisms may also become impaired with age. Both these factors favour the abolition of SMIs in the older patient.

Good postoperative pain control, e.g. by epidural analgesia or nicely judged doses of drugs, encourages adequate ventilation and reduces the chance of postoperative atelectasis in the old. However, excessive doses of analgesic drugs may have the opposite effect through oversedation.

Identifying the high risk patient

Risk factors which have been correlated with an above average rate of postoperative respiratory complications in the aged include preoperative lung disease, smoking, incisions near the diaphragm, immobility prior to surgery, poor peak flow rate, generalized sepsis and volume depletion (see Table 14.1). Postoperative respiratory complications also become more common with increasing age, probably because older patients tend to have more of the above risk factors. Men have more postoperative respiratory complications than women, but this seems to be attributable to sex differences in smoking history (Table 14.2).

Screening of preoperative aged surgical patients by means of pulmonary function tests is an attractive idea, but there is as yet too little published work in this area to enable detailed recommendations to be made. A succinct account of the subject as it relates to younger patients is given by Tisi (1979). Table 14.3, which is taken from Seymour (1986), lists a variety of 'normal values' of pulmonary function tests which have been used in the older patient, but much further study is required.

There is evidence that spinal (or epidural) anaesthesia is associated with less postoperative hypoxaemia than is general anaesthesia, but it is not clear whether or not this is clinically significant. The duration of anaesthesia was also positively correlated with postoperative respiratory morbidity in the studies in Dundee and Cardiff but this may be related more to the extent of surgical disease and operative trauma.

Table 14.1. Preoperative risk factors for postoperative respiratory complications in the old

Past or present lung disease
Smoking
Incisions near the diaphragm
Fluid/volume depletion
Emergency operation
Age over 75 years
Dyspnoea on minimal exercise (NYHA Grade 3 or 4)
ASA score 3 to 5
Body weight of 120% ideal or more
Peak flow $<250 \text{ l min}^{-1}$
FEV_1/FVC <70%
Male sex (probably due to higher incidence of smoking)

(From Seymour (1986); Vaz & Seymour, 1987.)

Table 14.2. History of smoking in a group of general surgical patients aged 65 years and over (Dundee study)

	Men (%)	Women (%)
Never smoked	8	61
Smoked now or within last year	57	23
Not smoked for one year	5	11
Not smoked for five years	30	5

Table 14.3. Provisional 'abnormal values' for preoperative pulmonary function tests. The valves listed are provisional and should not be regarded as a reason for witholding surgery (from Seymour, 1986)

Pulmonary function test	Studies in old general surgical patients	Studies in general surgical patietns of all ages
FVC	<75% predicted*	<70% predicted[†]
FEV_1	<2 l in thoracotomies in the over-60s[§]	<2 standard deviations below mean[¶]
FEV_1/FVC	? <80%**	<65%[†]
Peak flow	? <270 l min^{-1} (males) ? <250 l min^{-1} (females)	
MEFR	<200 l min^{-1} **	<300 l min^{-1} (under 40) <200 l min^{-1} (over 40)
Arterial carbon dioxide		>45 mm (6.0 kPa)**

*Noviant *et al.* (1976)
[†]Latimer *et al.* (1971)
[§]Boushy *et al.* (1971)
[¶]Schlenker & Hubay *et al.* (1973)
**Stein *et al.* (1962)

Prevention of postoperative respiratory complications

In the *minority* of patients, where retention of secretions is the primary cause of postoperative respiratory problems, 'raising the sputum' by *expiratory* manoeuvres, gentle chest percussion and suction is likely to be beneficial. Secretions that are obtained can be cultured to enable correct antibiotic therapy should subsequent infection develop. Attention should be paid to inhalations: warm, dry gases make secretions more tenacious, while high concentrations of oxygen cause both ciliary paralysis and absorption collapse of alveoli.

In the *majority* of patients, where airways collapse is a primary postoperative respiratory event, the emphasis should be on *inspiratory* rather than expiratory augmentation. Devices such as the incentive spirometer may have a place (Craven *et al.*, 1974; Bartlett, 1980; Hedley-Whyte *et al.*, 1976). As well as being supported by theory, inspiratory strategies also tend to be less painful than the 'classical' techniques of deep expiration, coughing, and percussion. Murray (1979) has suggested that if expiratory techniques fail to produce more than 30 ml of sputum at a time, they should be abandoned in favour of inspiratory procedures.

General measures that should reduce postoperative respiratory complications include early mobilization, avoidance of oversedation, and adequate analgesia. The simulation of sustained maximal respirations during anaesthesia will also encourage basal airways to re-expand. Treatment of bronchospasm is a logical therapy and respiratory stimulants may be of use in some cases, but there appear to be no formal trials of these therapies in the aged. The banning of preoperative smoking is a worthy objective, but at least six weeks of abstinence may be necessary before clinical effects are seen on postoperative respiratory morbidity.

Postoperative cardiovascular problems

Postoperative *myocardial infarction* occurs in 1–3% of patients over 65 following general surgery, usually in the first three postoperative days. Over half of these infarctions occur without chest pain, presenting instead as dyspnoea, hypotension, delirium, or electrocardiogram (ECG) changes. Studies of large numbers of middle-aged and old surgical patients have detected correlations between postoperative myocardial infarctions and several risk factors, including a recent (less than three months) preoperative infarction (Topkins & Artusio, 1964; Tarhan *et al.*, 1972; Steen *et al.*, 1978; Salem *et al.*, 1980), age (see Seymour, 1986, pp. 89–91), unstable angina (Miller *et al.*, 1979), intraoperative hypotension (Mauney *et al.*, 1970; Goldman *et al.*, 1978; Steen *et al.*, 1978), and possibly intraoperative hypertension (Steen *et al.*, 1978). Unfortunately, when dealing with an individual patient, it is difficult to predict the risk of infarction, possibly because a critical coronary artery stenosis may not reveal itself until tested by the stresses of anaesthesia and surgery.

Postoperative *cardiac failure* (in the absence of a myocardial infarction) occurs in 5–10% of general surgical patients aged 65 years and over. The risk of this complication is at its highest when there is evidence of limited cardiac reserve prior to surgery, e.g. in patients with evidence of cardiac failure on preoperative examination or chest X-ray. A history of dyspnoea on exertion may also be obtained but is less reliable in the older patient who may not experience symptoms because his or her habitual level of activity is very low. The authors routinely enquire about exercise tolerance and activity level, and the latter is often the more informative. Other preoperative risk factors which correlate with post-operative cardiovascular complications are listed in Table 14.4.

Unfortunately, despite a careful history and examination, the first clinical indication that cardiac reserve is limited may be when acute heart failure develops during or after an operation. For this reason, some centres advocate a direct measurement of cardiorespiratory function in high risk patients, even when they are undergoing non-cardiac operation. This usually involves Swan-Ganz catheters, arterial cannulas, and a bedside computer, and is thus both labour-intensive, invasive and expensive. However, the reported results are good and deserve further validation (Babu *et al.*, 1980; Del Guercio & Cohn, 1980). The major claim of these studies is that they allow precise and continuous information about left ventricular function, so that 'fine tuning' can be achieved by a manipulation of preload, afterload and inotropic therapy.

A number of other preoperative risk factors appear to be associated with an increased incidence of postoperative cardiac failure (Seymour, 1986, pp. 89–95). These include age (but in some studies only),

Table 14.4. Preoperative risk factors for postoperative cardiac complications in the over-65s*

Preoperative risk factor	Postoperative CVS complications — increase in relative risk		
	Myocardial infarction	Cardiac deaths	All CVS complications
Acute heart failure	? 12×	10–15×	
NYHA Grade 3	2–4×	2–4×	2–4×
Controlled heart failure or stable angina		1.5–2×	2–3×
Myocardial infarction within three months	5–8×[†]	5–8×[†]	
Myocardial infarction three to six months before	2–4×[†]	2–4×[†]	
Age over 70 years (probably due to age-associated heart disease)	2–4×	2–12×	2–3×
Emergency admission		4× in cardiac surgery	2×

*Based on Seymour (1986) pp. 89–106
[†]Relative to patients with infarctions more than six months old
CVS — cardiovascular system.

emergency operations (Goldman *et al.*, 1977; Waters *et al.*, 1981; Seymour & Pringle, 1983), poor mobility or exercise tolerance prior to operation, recent myocardial infarction, cor pulmonale (Skinner & Pearce, 1964) and, to a lesser extent, other types of heart disease (Seymour, 1986, pp. 96–100). Surprisingly, however, the few studies on old patients with preoperative hypertension have failed to find a correlation with postoperative cardiovascular complications (Walker & MacDessi, 1966; Goldman & Caldera, 1979; Seymour, 1986, p. 98). Of the *intraoperative* factors that have been studied, intraoperative hypotension has been most closely correlated with postoperative cardiac complications and death (Walker & MacDessi, 1966; Kraas *et al.*, 1977; Goldman *et al.*, 1978), and intraoperative hypotension and hypoxia have also been implicated as important triggers for arrhythmias (Vanik & Davis, 1968).

For the foreseeable future, most of our aged patients are not going to undergo surgery with a Swan-Ganz catheter in situ, or have a computerized system to monitor their cardiorespiratory status. What sort of measures can be taken to ensure that cardiac risk is kept to a minimum? A practical strategy is to assume that a degree of cardiac risk is present in the aged, even when history and examination are normal. The reduction of homeostatic function with ageing means that hypotension, hypertensive episodes, tachycardia, hypoxia, fluid/volume depletion or overload are much more poorly tolerated. The effect of individual anaesthetic agents on the ageing myocardium is an important consideration, but there is little published work on this subject.

Early detection of cardiac complications which develop is of obvious importance. The atypical presentation of myocardial infarction in the older surgical (and non-surgical, for that matter) patient has already been referred to. As the risk of postoperative infarction is highest in the first 72 h postoperatively, there is much to be said for routine ECGs during this time, and at other times if dyspnoea, hypotension, tachycardia or confusion develop. As over 50% of fit old people have abnormalities on their ECGs, a preoperative ECG for comparison is highly desirable (Seymour et al., 1983). Like myocardial infarction, cardiac failure may be difficult to detect in the older patient, where ankle oedema from postural causes is common, and where basal lung crepitations are often found. Here a comparison with a preoperative chest X-ray is particularly useful (Seymour et al., 1982).

Postoperative mental status

The most dramatic change in mental status which may develop in the aged postoperative patient is an acute confusional state, or delirium (see Fig. 14.1). As in non-surgical situations, the great majority of cases of delirium seen in the aged are due to acute physical illness (particularly infection), metabolic upset, or drugs (particularly those with an anticholinergic or sedative action). It is a matter of urgency that the underlying cause or causes of the delirium are diagnosed and treated. Symptomatic treatment with sedatives is likely to be counterproductive, and may be disastrous in hypoxic patients.

The type of delirium most commonly encountered on the surgical wards has been termed *interval delirium* by Lipowski (1980a), and usually occurs between the second and seventh postoperative day. Anaesthetists, however, also encounter *emergence delirium*, as the patient recovers from anaesthesia. Emergence delirium can occur in all age groups, and may even be commoner in the young than in the old. It appears to be closely related to the anticholinergic effects of many anaesthetic and analgesic agents. Finally it should not be forgotten that delirium due to *withdrawal* from alcohol, benzodiazepines and other psychoactive agents can occur at any age.

Postoperative central nervous system problems

Postoperative strokes occurred in around 1% of the general surgical patients aged over 65 years in the Dundee and Cardiff studies, and the reported incidence in the literature is between 0.4% and 3.3% (Seymour, 1986, p. 226). It is likely, however, that less obvious neurological deficits, such as a transient asymmetry in tendon reflexes, could go unnoticed, so the true incidence of cerebrovascular events might be higher than these estimates.

As a postoperative stroke is a relatively uncommon event following general surgery, the limited clinical data so far available makes it difficult to predict those patients who are at particular risk. At present there is no clear-cut evidence that a previous history of cerebrovascular disease predisposes a general surgical patient to a postoperative stroke, although this appears to be the case in operations involving open heart surgery. Similarly, there is no indication that an *asymptomatic* carotid bruit discovered in the preoperative period presages postoperative cerebral ischaemia (Corman, 1979). The incidence of postoperative stroke appears to rise with age, but in a group of general surgical patients over 80 years old the incidence was only 3.3% (Corman, 1979). The timing of postoperative strokes has received little attention, but in the Cardiff study three out of six occurred in the first week, and five out of six in the first 10 days.

In healthy young individuals, autoregulation tends to maintain a constant cerebral blood flow when systemic arterial pressure lies between 60 and 180 mmHg. In older patients with arterial disease or hypertension, however, this range may be much narrower and thus there is a sound theoretical reason for attempting to avoid extremes of hypo- or hypertension during the surgical period. Careful positioning of the neck of patients during anaesthesia has also been stressed by many anaesthetists, as the age-related problems of atheroma, rigid arteries and cervical spondylosis favour vertebral and carotid artery occlusion.

Renal function and fluid/electrolyte balance in the postoperative period

Even in fit old people, the glomerular filtration rate tends to fall by about 1% per year after the age of 35, (Seymour & Seymour, 1988), and with age the kidney may also become progressively more sensitive to toxic or hypotensive insults. There is also evidence from physiological studies that the older kidney takes longer to excrete an acid or alkali load, and the ability to concentrate or dilute urine also appears to be reduced with age. For all these reasons, fluid and electrolyte balance needs to be maintained within tighter limits in the aged. On the one hand, volume depletion is likely to lead to renal insufficiency, while on the other, excessive amounts of salt and water are more likely to precipitate left ventricular failure than in the young because of age-related falls in renal and vascular capacity.

The risk of postoperative acute renal failure in general surgical patients aged over 65 years appears to be between 1% and 3% (Seymour, 1986, p. 194), although it is the experience of the authors that for every case of frank renal failure that develops there are two to three others where transient renal insufficiency occurs (as witnessed by a doubling of urea levels for a week or more). In special circumstances, such as operations on the abdominal aorta, open heart surgery, and operations on jaundiced patients, the incidence of renal failure tends to be higher.

Avoidance or treatment of volume depletion in the aged should prevent many of these cases of renal failure, but the clinical assessment of salt and water depletion may be very difficult for reasons listed in Table 14.5. Even when surgery is taking place on an elective basis, it cannot necessarily be assumed that salt and water depletion are absent. Many older patients in the general population habitually have a low fluid intake, often in a vain attempt to reduce symptoms of frequency or nocturia. Postural oedema in the ankles is common and is often inappropriately treated by diuretics. These may precipitate urgency of micturition, which leads to further voluntary fluid restriction. Sepsis before or after surgery may also precipitate volume depletion: pyrexia leads to excessive water loss, while malaise and possibly delirium reduce fluid intake.

The interaction of drugs and renal function also deserves special comment. Some drugs are nephrotoxic and may precipitate acute interstitial nephritis and acute renal failure. Examples include many antibiotics, cimetidine, phenytoin, frusemide and thiazide diuretics. Diuretics may also have an indirect effect on renal function through volume depletion. Non-steroidal anti-inflammatory drugs may precipitate acute renal failure, but often have a more insidious action, reducing glomerular filtration by perhaps one-fifth in many aged patients. Other drugs do not directly damage the kidney, but tend to accumulate where glomerular filtration is impaired, as it often is in the aged. The classical example is digoxin which rarely needs to be given in a maintenance dose of more than 0.125 mg in patients over 65, and which may be effective in even lower doses. Aminoglycosides such as gentamicin may accumulate

Table 14.5. Clinical signs of salt and water depletion in the old and the young*

'Textbook signs'	Problems of interpretation in the aged
Cardiovascular	
Postural hypotension	Common even in fit aged
Supine hypotension	May be masked by pre-existing systolic hypertension
Tachycardia	Response of heart rate to stress may be impaired
Poor peripheral perfusion	Valid, but a late sign
Reduced central venous pressure (CVP)	CVP may not reflect left heart function if heart or lung disease present
Reduced pulmonary wedge pressure	Usually valid but invasive
Absent peripheral oedema	Local causes of oedema common
Tissue changes	
Dry tongue	Unreliable sign
Reduced tongue volume	Hard to quantify
Reduced skin turgor	Loss of skin elasticity with age
Sunken eyes	Valid, but very late sign
Oliguria	May be less marked as impaired renal concentrating ability is common
Drowsiness, apathy, stupor	Non-specific signs

*Based on Seymour (1986), Table 6.3

in the presence of renal impairment, and are themselves nephrotoxic.

Prevention of postoperative renal insufficiency primarily involves avoidance of fluid and electrolyte depletion. However, specific measures which have been advocated in addition include preoperative mannitol and/or fluid loading prior to vascular surgery, and the administration of bile salts to jaundiced patients. The latter therapy has received relatively little attention and probably deserves to be better known. Since the beginning of the century it has been recognized that acute tubular necrosis is a commoner outcome of surgery in patients with obstructive jaundice than in those in whom jaundice was absent. It has been suggested that the renal damage is due to the absorption of bacterial endotoxins from the gut, a process which appears to be inhibited by the presence of bile salts. Recently, two regimens involving oral bile salts (in addition to mannitol) prior to operation have been used with apparent success in patients with obstructive jaundice:

(i) (After Evans *et al.*, 1982)
  (a) Forty-eight hours before surgery: give oral sodium taurocholate, 1 g three times daily up to time of operation.
  (b) Fourteen hours before surgery: give fluid load of 1000 ml of dextrose/saline intravenously.
  (c) Two hours before induction of anaesthesia: give 200 ml of 10% mannitol intravenously to run over 2 h.
  (d) With the premedication: give gentamicin (80 mg i.m. or i.v.), cephradine (500 mg i.m. or i.v.) and metronidazole (500 mg i.v. or rectally). Continue these antibiotics for five days, monitoring gentamicin doses and adjusting them depending on blood levels and renal function. For body weights under 60 kg, 60 mg of gentamicin rather than 80 mg is recommended as the initial dose.

(ii) (After Cahill, 1983)
  (a) Forty-eight hours before surgery: give oral sodium deoxycholate, 500 mg three times daily up to time of operation.
  (b) Two hours before induction of anaesthesia: give infusion of 540 ml of 10% mannitol intravenously.
  (c) Intraoperatively: give prophylactic broad spectrum antibiotics intravenously and administer for 48 h.

Postoperative venous thromboembolism

Following general surgery

The work of Kakkar *et al.* (1969, 1975) has shown the probable events leading to thromboembolism after general surgery. The primary event appears to be immobility of the calf muscles which results in local venous thrombosis. In a proportion of cases, the thrombosis extends above the knee and then the risks of subsequent pulmonary embolism are much higher. The risk of deep venous thrombosis (DVT) and pulmonary embolism increases with age, but is also correlated with malignancy, obesity, prolonged immobility, the extent and duration of surgery and the presence of cardiac and respiratory disease. As might be expected, patients with a previous history of venous thromboembolism are at particular risk.

It is well known that the clinical signs and symptoms of DVT and pulmonary embolism are unreliable. For instance, the work of Kakkar has indicated that about 50% of patients thought to have DVT on clinical grounds will have normal phlebograms, and that 50% of patients with abnormal phlebograms will have no clinical signs. When the technique of ^{125}I-fibrinogen scanning is used it has been reported that the rate of venous thromboembolism following general surgery is 20% for patients aged 40 to 60 years, around 40% for the age-group 61 to 70, and 60% for those over 71 (Borow & Goldson 1981).

Special problems following orthopaedic surgery

Surgery on the hip or in the pelvis involves a risk of venous thrombosis which is greater than that seen in general surgical patients. This is because operative procedures may cause direct trauma to femoral and iliac vessels, initiating venous thrombosis at these sites. The resulting thromboses, being proximal, are particularly likely to lead to massive pulmonary emboli. Thus in many published series, pulmonary embolism is the leading cause of death postoperatively in old gynaecological and orthopaedic patients, while respiratory and cardiac causes head the table after general surgery. In addition, the approach to prevention needs to be different in general and orthopaedic surgical patients.

Prevention of venous thromboembolism

General methods of prevention which are applicable to all old surgical and medical patients revolve around early mobilization. In middle-aged and old general surgical patients, there is evidence that low doses of heparin (5000 u s.c. 2 h before surgery and 8 to 12 hourly thereafter) can reduce the number of deep venous thromboses, and probably the number of pulmonary emboli that develop. However, in patients undergoing hip surgery, prophylactic doses of s.c. heparin on their own appear to be ineffective in preventing DVT, although they may delay the onset of DVT (Sikorski *et al.*, 1981). Other recommended measures of prevention include new dosage regimens of heparin and warfarin, novel types of heparin, dextran, aspirin, and/or physical methods such as antiembolism stockings, intermittent calf compression, or electrical contraction of leg muscles (Seymour, 1986, pp. 289-293). Of particular interest to the anaesthetist is the evidence that thromboembolic complications are less common when hip or prostate surgery is carried out using regional rather than general anaesthesia. This apparent anti-thrombotic effect has been reviewed by Kehlet (1984a,b) and is thought to result from the ability of low spinal or epidural anaesthesia to increase blood flow in the veins of the lower limb. Thoracic epidural anaesthesia has not been demonstrated to have an anti-thrombotic effect.

Postoperative mortality

Even in frail old people, a death which is directly attributable to the anaesthetic is now a rarity (Lunn & Mushin, 1982). In the experience of the authors, the commonest causes of postoperative deaths in aged general and orthopaedic patients are medical complications, the effects of the underlying surgical disease, and surgical complications, in that order. Of the medical causes of postoperative death, respiratory, cardiac and thromboembolic causes have featured prominently in reports published over the last two decades. While anaesthesia may contribute to the postoperative medical problems which develop, it is probably much less important than the presence of pre-existing medical diseases.

In the Dundee and Cardiff studies, the crude mortality rates after general surgery in patients aged 65 and over were 12% and 5.4% respectively. The Cardiff study (see Fig. 14.1) also contain a group of patients undergoing emergency surgery for a fractured femur, and here the crude mortality rate was almost 13%. In the old general surgical patients in these two studies, the death rates were high but in half of the Dundee cases and a third of the Cardiff cases death was due to underlying surgical disease (usually a malignancy) which had progressed beyond the stage of cure by the time of presentation. This led Seymour & Pringle (1982) to propose a method of classifying operative and non-operative deaths which attempted to separate those cases which were potentially viable from those which were not. This proposed classification is shown in Table 14.6.

Future developments

Our understanding of the mechanisms leading to postoperative complications in aged patients is still at a very rudimentary level, and much research remains to be done. This is an area where anaesthetists can make a major contribution, particularly in relation to cardiorespiratory function and cerebral status in the operative and early postoperative period. The action of individual anaesthetic agents in the aged has also been little studied, and the long standing debate about the relative merits of general and regional anaesthesia has only recently stimulated properly randomized studies (Berggren et al., 1987; Davis et al., 1987). Large surveys of aged surgical patients have their place, but there is also much to be said for research projects which concentrate on well defined

Table 14.6. Proposed classification of surgical mortality (Seymour & Pringle, 1982)

Non-viable

Here it was judged that death could not have been prevented by surgical intervention, or a modification of surgical procedure, or an alteration in preoperative, intraoperative, or postoperative care.

This group was subdivided into those with:

(1) Advanced malignancy with surgery performed for diagnostic or palliative reasons.
(2) Advanced malignancy, with no surgery performed.
(3) No malignancy, but underlying disease not amenable to surgical intervention — myocardial infarction presenting as abdominal pain, massive bowel infarction, or stroke complicating a surgical illness.

Potentially viable

The potentially viable group comprised patients dying in the surgical unit who did not fall into the non-viable category. This group was subdivided into:

(1) Postoperative deaths due to a surgical complication.
(2) Postoperative deaths due to a medical complication.
(3) Non-operative deaths, where surgery offered a chance of cure, however small — for instance, ruptured aneurysm or peritonitis in a moribund patient.

In addition

Record the number of patients who leave the unit alive, but who are known to have residual malignancy at the time of discharge.

groups of patients who are at particular risk. A good example of the latter is the patient with a fractured neck of femur who often has a variety or preoperative medical illnesses in addition to the problems of trauma and surgery. In such situations, the medical and anaesthetic skills of the anaesthetist may be the crucial factor in the postoperative outcome of the individual patient. In addition, the anaesthetist is well placed to make systematic observations, which will lead to a better postoperative outcome for such patients in the future.

References

Babu, S.C. Sharma, P.V.P., Raciti, A., Mayr, C.H., Elrabie, N.A., Clauss, R.H., Stahl, W.M. & Del Guercio, L.R.M. (1980) Monitor-guided responses. Operability with safety is increased in patients with peripheral vascular diseases. *Arch. Surg.* **115**, 1384–1386.

Bartlett, R.H. (1980) Pulmonary pathophysiology in surgical patients. *Surg. Clin. North Am.* **60**, 1323–1338.

Beggren, D. *et al.* (1987) Post-operative confusion after anaesthesia in elderly patients with femoral neck fractures. *Anaesth. Analg.* **66**, 497–504.

Borow, M. & Goldson, H. (1981) Post-operative venous thrombosis. Evaluation of five methods of treatment. *Am. J. Surg.* **141**, 245–251.

Boushy, S.F. *et al.* (1971) Clinical course relevant to pre-operative and post-operative pulmonary function in patients with bronchogenic carcinoma. *Chest*, **59**, 383–391.

Cahill, C.J. (1983) Prevention of post-operative renal failure in patients with obstructive jaundice — the role of bile salts. *Br. J. Surg.* **70**, 590–595.

Corman, L.C. (1979) The pre-operative patient with an asymptomatic cervical bruit. *Med. Clin. North Am.* **63**, 1335–1340.

Craven, J.L., Evans, G.A., Davenport, P.J. & Williams, R.H.P. (1974) The evaluation of the incentive spirometer in the management of post-operative pulmonary complications. *Br. J. Surg.* **61**, 793–797.

Davis, F.M. *et al.* (1987) Prospective, multi-centre trail of mortality following general or spinal anaesthesia for hip-fracture surgery in the elderly. *Br. J. Anaesth.* **59**, 1080–1088.

Del Guercio, L.R.M. & Cohn, J.D. (1980) Monitoring operative risk in the elderly. *JAMA* **243**, 1350–1355.

Evans, H.J.R., Torrealba, V., Hudd, C., Knight, M. (1982) The effect of pre-operative bile salt administration on post-operative renal function in patients with obstructive jaundice. *Br. J. Surg.* **69**, 706–708.

Goldman L. & Caldera D.L. (1979) Risks of general anaesthesia and elective operation in the hypertensive patient. *Anesthesiology* **50**, 285–292.

Goldman L., Caldera, D.L, Nussbaum, S.R., Southwick, F.S., Krogstad, D., Murray, B., Burke, D.S., O'Malley, T.A., Goroll, A.H., Caplan, C.H., Nolan, J., Carabello, B. & Slater, E.E. (1977) Multifactorial index of cardiac risk in noncardiac surgical procedures. *New Engl. J. Med.* **297**, 845–850.

Goldman, L. Caldera, D.L., Southwick, F.S, Nussbaum, S.R., Murray, B., O'Malley, T.A., Goroll, A.H., Caplan, C.H., Nolan, J., Burke, D.S., Krogstad, D., Carabello, B. & Slater, E.E. (1978) Cardiac risk factors and complications in non-cardiac surgery. *Medicine* **57**, 357–370.

Hedley-Whyte, J., Burgess, G.E., Feeley, T.W. & Miller, M.G. (1976) *Applied Physiology of Respiratory Care.* Little, Brown & Co., Boston.

Helms, U., Weihrauch, H., Jakabitz, K., Steen, L. & Conrad, I. (1978) Die postoperativen Veränderungen der Blutgase nach unkomplizierten Oberbaucheingriffen bei hochbetagten Menschen *Prakt Anaesth.* **13**, 275–283.

Kakkar, V.V., Howe, C.T., Flanc, C. & Clarke, M.B.(1969) Natural history of postoperative deep-vein thrombosis. *Lancet* **2**, 230–233.

Kakkar, V.V., Corrigan, T.P. & Fossard, D.P. (1975) Prevention of fatal post-operative pulmonary embolism by low doses of heparin. An international multi-centre trial. *Lancet* **2**, 45–51.

Kehlet, H. (1984a) Does regional anaesthesia reduce post-operative morbidity? *Intensive Care Med.* **10**, 165–167.

Kehlet, H. (1984b) Influence of regional anaesthesia on post-operative morbidity. *Ann. Chir. Gynaecol.* **73**, 171–176.

Kraas V.E., Schwermann, R., Gogler, H., Beger, H.G. & Bettner, R. (1977) Risiko und Verlauf von abdominalen Operationen im Alter. *Zentralbl. Chir.* **102**, 297–304.

Latimer, R.G. *et al.* (1971) Ventilatory patterns and pulmonary complications after upper abdominal surgery determined by pre-operative and post-operative computerised spirometry and blood gas samples. *Am. J. Surg.* **122**, 622–632.

Lewis, F.R. (1980) Management of atelectasis and pneumonia. *Surg. Clin. North Am.* **60**, 1391–1401.

Lipowski, Z.J. (1980a) *Delirium. Acute Brain Failure in Man.* Thomas, Springfield, Illinois.

Lipowski, Z.J. (1980b) Delirium updated. *Compr. Psychiatry* **21**, 190–196.

Lunn, J.N. & Mushin, W.W. (1982) *Mortality Associated with Anaesthesia.* Nuffield Provincial Hospitals Trust, London.

Mauney, F.M., Ebert, P.A. & Sabiston, D.C. (1970) Post-operative myocardial infarction: a study of predisposing factors, diagnosis and mortality in a high risk group of surgical patients. *Ann. Surg.* **172**, 497–503.

Miller, R., Silvay, G. & Lumb, P.D. (1979) Anesthesia, surgery and myocardial infarction. A review. *Anesthes. Rev.* **6**, 14–20.

Murray, J.F. (1979) The ketchup-bottle method. *New Engl. J. Med.* **300**, 1155–1157.

Noviant, Y. *et al.* (1976) Etude de quelques éléments d'évaluation du risque respiratoire post-operatoire chez le subject agé. *Anesth. Anagl. Reanim.* **33**, 285–295.

Peters, R.M. (1979) Pulmonary physiologic studies of the perioperative period. *Chest* **76**, 576–584.

Salem, D.N, Homans, D.C. & Isner, J.M. (1980) Management of cardiac disease in the general surgical patient. *Curr. Probl. Cardiol.* **5**, 1–41.

Schlenker, J.D. & Hubay, C.A. (1973) The pathogenesis of post-operative atelectasis. *Arch. Surg.* **107**, 846–850.

Seymour, D.G. (1986) *Medical Assessment of the Elderly Surgical Patient.* Croom Helm, London.

Seymour, D.G. & Pringle, R. (1982) A new method of auditing surgical mortality rates: application to a group of elderly general surgical patients. *Br. Med. J.* **284**, 1539–1542.

Seymour, D.G. & Pringle, R. (1983) Post-operative complications in the elderly surgical patient. *Gerontology* **29**, 262–270.

Seymour, D.G. & Seymour R.M. (1988) Physiology of ageing. In *Practical in Geriatric Medicine* (Eds M.S.J. Pathy & P. Finucane). Springer-Verlag, London.

Seymour, D.G. & Vaz, F.G. (1987) Aspects of surgery in the elderly: pre-operative medical assessment. *Br. J. Hosp. Med.* **37**, 102–112.

Seymour, D.G., Pringle, R. & Shaw, J.W. (1982) The role of the routine pre-operative chest X-ray in the elderly general surgical patient. *Postgrad. Med. J.* **58**, 741–745.

Seymour, D.G., Pringle, R. & MacLennan, W.J. (1983) The role of the routine pre-operative electrocardiogram in the elderly surgical patient. *Age Ageing* **12**, 97–104.

Sikorski, J.M., Hampson, W.G. & Staddon, G.E. (1981) The natural history and aetiology of deep vein thrombosis after total hip replacement. *J. Bone Joint Surg.* **63–B**, 171–177.

Skinner, J.F. & Pearce, M.L. (1964) Surgical risk in the cardiac patient. *J. Chron. Dis.* **17**, 57–72.

Steen, P.A., Tinker, J.H. & Tarhan, S. (1978) Myocardial reinfarction after anaesthesia and surgery. *JAMA* **239**, 2566–2570.

Stein, M. *et al.* (1962) Pulmonary evaluation of surgical patients. *J. Am. Med. Ass.* **181**, 765–770.

Tarhan, S., Moffitt, E.A., Taylor, W.F., Giulani, E.R. (1972) Myocardial infarction after general anaesthesia. *JAMA* **220**, 1451–1454.

Tisi, G.M. (1979) Pre-operative evaluation of pulmonary function. *Am. Rev. Respir. Dis.* **119**, 293–310.

Topkins, M.J. & Artusio, J.F. (1964) Myocardial infarction and surgery. A five year study. *Anesth Analg.* **43**, 716–720.

Vanik, P.E. & Davis, H.S. (1968) Cardiac arrthythmias during halothane anaesthesia. *Anesth Analg.* **47**, 299–307.

Vaz, F.G. & Seymour, D.G. (1988) To be published.

Walker, R.L., & MacDessi, B.J. (1966) Myocardial abnormalities following geriatric surgery. *Med. J. Aust.* **1**, 783–786.

Waters, J., Wilkinson, C., Golman, M., Schoeppel, S., Linde, H.W. & Brunner, E.A. (1981) Evaluation of cardiac risk in noncardiac surgical patients. *Anesthesiology* **55**, A343.

15 | Intensive care for the aged

R.B. HOPKINSON

Introduction

The mean potential life expectation of both men and women is at present 85 years, varying between 70 and 100 years. As the mean age of the population rises so will the demand of the aged population for medical resources, including intensive care. Clearly all who are critically ill should not automatically be admitted to an intensive therapy unit (ITU). A necessary condition for admission is that the patient will benefit from such care. Patients who are near death, and for whom there is no known therapy, should not be deemed recoverable.

It is recommended that a patient should be admitted only after individual consideration and not because he or she belongs to any particular diagnostic category. No authority has recommended that there should be a limit to the application of intensive therapy to the aged.

Is there, however, any need to develop and apply special selection criteria to the age? In one study (Thibault et al., 1980) it was concluded that 'the aged and chronically ill have become principal consumers of intensive care'. Is this a rational allocation of a scarce resource, and should we consider whether such policies are diverting valuable services from the more deserving? Furthermore, should the financial burden of provision of such care influence the manner in which intensive therapy is provided for the aged?

How large is the problem?

The majority of data available is from the USA; the National Health Service provides few facilities for the collection of statistics on intensive therapy. There is some evidence that the numbers of aged patients being admitted to intensive care units is increasing (Thibault et al., 1980; Campion et al., 1981). However, an analysis of three years' admissions to the ITU of East Birmingham Hospital shows approximately 6% of aged patients admitted (Table 15.1). This appears to be as elsewhere though it will depend on the age of the surrounding population. An ITU survival rate of around 80% for all ages is unexceptional, with no increasing mortality with age (Fig. 15.1). Seventeen per cent of these patients were ventilated, half of whom died. The relatively small numbers involved limit the conclusions that can be drawn.

Table 15.1. 1983–1985 Patients aged >74 years admitted to the ITU, East Birmingham Hospital (yearly statistics)

	1983	1984	1985	Total
Total patients	775	625	782	2182
Patients aged >74 years (%)	39	40	48	127 (6)
Male	21	18	23	62
Died (%)	7 (18)	7 (17)	8 (17)	22 (17)
Ventilated (%)	6 (15)	9 (22)	10 (21)	25 (20)
Ventilated patients who died	4	4	3	11

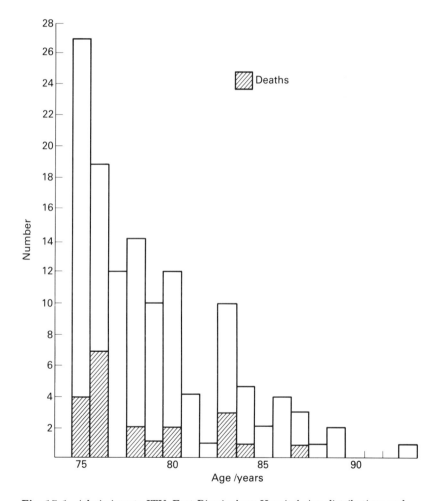

Fig. 15.1. Admissions to ITU, East Birmingham Hospital. Age distributions and mortality for the aged, 1983–85.

Selection of patients

Until recently there have been little data available on the benefits, outcome and costs of intensive therapy, let alone intensive therapy for the aged. Over recent years scoring systems such as APACHE II (Acute Physiology and Chronic Health Evaluation) have been developed, enabling some groups, notably in the USA, to undertake multi-institutional prognostic studies of survival from intensive care (Knaus et al., 1985). The diversity of disease and the varying nature of ITUs has limited the ability to compare outcomes. APACHE II scores 12 acute variables plus chronic health and age points in order to stratify patients prognositically by risk before treatment (Fig. 15.2). Different treatment regimens may then be compared.

Our considerations must go beyond survival in the intensive therapy unit or even the hospital. Other measures, such as the Sickness Impact Profile (Bergner et al., 1981) and Uniscale (Spitzer et al., 1981), are being used to assess quality of life following discharge from hospital. The former (Fig. 15.3) assesses specific physical, emotional and social health-related disabilities, while the latter (Fig. 15.4) obtains a subjective estimation of the patient's quality of life.

Does provision of intensive therapy for the elderly provide any special problems? Certainly in *medical* intensive care there is evidence to demonstrate that age significantly influences survival in hospital and mortality after discharge (Thibault, 1984) (Tables 15.2 and 15.3).

A study of 2693 admissions for medical intensive care and coronary care is revealing (Campion et al., 1981). Twenty-one per cent of these admissions were 75 years old or more, an age group that composed only 5% of the catchment population.

Once admitted to ITU, major interventions were commoner in the aged (32%), while the figure for the 55 to 64 year old group was 22%. The in-hospital mortality doubled between these groups, from 8% to 16%, mainly attributable in this survey to an increase in myocardial infarction case mortality rates.

Interestingly, intubation with ventilation, while associated with a consistently high in-hospital mortality at all age groups, varied little (47–49%), and there was no increase in mean length of stay, or hospital charges. However, a sharp decline with age in the ratio of mean hospital charges of survivors to non-survivors, suggests that there was selective allocation of resources to the younger patients.

However, a recent study of mixed medical and surgical ITU patients demonstrated that only acute health score predicts in-hospital mortality, while only age predicts post-discharge mortality (Sage et al., 1986).

Cullen et al. (1976) made a number of studies of survival after critical surgical illness. They concluded that survival was poorest in the older (>65) age group, but that age did not differentiate degree of recovery or quality of life. A subsequent review after five years confirmed these

Fig. 15.2. (*opposite*) An adaption of APACHE II (Knaus et al., 1985) for use on the ITU, East Birmingham Hospital.

	High abnormal range				0	Low abnormal range			
	4	3	2	1	0	1	2	3	4
Core temperature/°C	≥41	39–40.9		38.5–38.9	36–38.4	34–35.9	32–33.9	30–31.9	≤29.9
Mean blood pressure/mmHg	≥160	130–159	110–129	–	70–109	–	50–69	–	≤49
Heart rate/min⁻¹	≥180	140–179	110–139	–	70–109	–	55–69	40–54	≤39
Respiratory rate/min⁻¹	≥50	35–49	–	25–34	12–24	10–11	6–9	–	≤5
% inspired O₂/PaO₂/kPa	≥5.0	4.0–4.99	2.1–3.99	–	<2.09	–	–	–	–
Arterial H⁺	≥71	57–71	48–56	–	32–47	26–31	–	20–25	≤19
Creatinine/μmol l⁻¹	≥600	300–599	180–299	130–179	50–129	–	49	–	–
Sodium/mmol l⁻¹	≥180	160–179	155–159	150–154	130–153	–	120–129	111–119	≤110
Potassium/mmol l⁻¹	≥7.0	6.0–6.9	–	5.5–5.9	3.5–5.4	3.0–3.4	2.5–2.9		<2.5
Haemoglobin/g d l⁻¹	≥18.0	–	15.0–17.9	14.0–14.9	9.0–13.9	–	6.1–8.9	–	≤6.0
White cell count (× 10⁹ l⁻¹)	≥40.0	–	20.0–39.9	15.0–19.9	3.0–14.9	–	1.0–2.9	–	<1.0

Glasgow coma score (GCS):
Score = 15 minus actual GCS

(a) Total acute physiology score (APS):
   Sum of the 12 individual variable points

(b) Age points: assign points to age as follows:

Age/years	Points
≤44	0
45–54	2
55–64	3
65–74	5
≥75	6

(c) Chronic health points. If the patient has a history of severe organ system insufficiency or is immuno-compromised assign points as follows: a) for non-operative or emergency post-operative patients — 5 points
   b) for elective post-operative patients   — 2 points

DEFINITIONS
Organ insufficiency or immuno-compromised state must have been evident prior to this hospital admission and conform to the following criteria:
Liver: Biopsy proven cirrhosis and documented portal hypertension; episodes of past upper GI bleeding attributed to portal hypertension; or prior episodes of hepatic failure/encephalopathy/coma.
Cardiovascular: New York Heart Association Class IV.
Respiratory: Chronic restrictive, obstructive or vascular disease resulting in severe exercise restriction, i.e. unable to climb stairs or perform household duties; or documented chronic hypoxia, hypercapnia, secondary polycythaemia, severe pulmonary hypertension (40 mmHg), or respiratory dependency.
Renal: Receiving chronic dialysis.
Immuno-compromised: The patient has received therapy that suppresses resistance to infection, e.g. immuno-suppression, chemotherapy, radiation, long term or recent high dose steroids, or has a disease that is sufficiently advanced to suppress resistance to infection, e.g. leukaemia, lymphoma, AIDS.

APACHE II score   Sum of (a) + (b) + (c)

(a) APS points _____   (b) Age points _____

(c) Chronic Health Points _____   TOTAL APACHE II _____

Dimension	Items describing behaviour related to:
Independent categories	Sleep and rest Eating Work Home management Recreation and pastimes
I. Physical	Ambulation Mobility Body care and movement
II. Psychosocial	Social interaction Alertness behaviour Emotional behaviour Communication

Fig. 15.3. Assessment criteria used for the Sickness Impact Profile.

QUALITY OF LIFE UNISCALE   Study no. _____
                                 Rater's profession/occupation _____

Please mark with an X the appropriate place within the bar to indicate your rating of this person's quality of life during the past week. Lowest quality applies to someone completely dependent physically on others, seriously impaired mentally, unaware of surroundings and in a hopeless position. Highest quality applies to someone physically and mentally independent, communicating well with others, able to do most of the things enjoyed, pulling own weight, with a hopeful yet realistic attitude.

Lowest quality [   ] Highest quality

How confident are you that your rating of this quality of life is accurate?
Please ring the appropriate category.

Absolutely confident 1   Very confident 2   Quite confident 3

Not very confident 4   Very doubtful 5   Not at all confident 6

Fig. 15.4. The Uniscale Analogue.

---

results, without the decreased survival noted in the older group of patients (Cullen *et al.*, 1984).

A study of the functional outcome of medical patients demonstrated that severe pre-admission limitation of activity correlated with a high in-hospital mortality (Goldstein *et al.*, 1986). Shroeder *et al.* (1981), studying the outcome of high cost patients, identified patients over 64 years of age and medical, as opposed to surgical admission, as factors associated with poor survival.

There is certainly a distinction to be made between surgical patients, who are more likely to have self-limiting problems, and the medical population who tend to have more generalized and less reversible problems. It is these who are more likely to develop multiple organ failure and die. Draper *et al.* (1983) suggested that survival becomes unprecedented, when failure persists in three or more organ systems for over two days.

Sage *et al.* (1986) reported that ITU survivors suffered far less disability than patients with chronic physical or mental conditions.

Table 15.2. Outcome of medical intensive care mortality by decade

Age	Number	ICU mortality (%)	Hospital mortality (%)
0–19	52	5.8	7.7
20–29	354	4.4	4.8
30–39	375	5.9	8.5
40–49	687	3.6	5.8
50–59	1298	6.3	9.6
60–69	1705	8.4	14.0
70–79	1443	9.7	16.8
80–89	662	13.0	21.8
90+	104	12.5	26.9

Table 15.3. ICU outcomes: follow-up mortality by age

Age	Number	Post-hospital mortality
0–19	38	5.3
20–29	236	4.2
30–39	237	7.6
40–49	474	7.0
50–59	842	7.8
60–69	1015	12.7
70–79	831	19.5
80–89	389	23.6
90+	62	29.0

Moreover, the patient's assessment of his or her quality of life may differ from that of society. Older patients are more accepting of physical limitation and they do not suffer the 'psychosocial' stigma of illness that might be imposed upon the disabled middle-aged patient. Life, unattractive to an observer, may be perfectly satisfactory to the owner. Such patients are no more likely to make more use of hospital facilities than the rest of the population.

In Campion's study (1981) the majority of patients after discharge did not return to their pre-hospitalization level of activity, but again the aged group did not differ from the younger cohorts. This again may reflect 'gatekeeping decisions' by medical staff, which we must consider.

A retrospective Scandinavian review has confirmed many of these points. Reviewing 143 patients aged over 70 years who spent more than 48 h in intensive care, Grenrot *et al.* (1986) concluded that the cost of care and the mortality increased with age. However, nearly half of the patients were discharged home and the risks of long-term institutional care were small. The mortality for patients suffering cardiovascular and malignant disease was particularly high.

What is the influence of physician assessment, 'gate keeping', on patient selection? Rodman *et al.* (1978) examined whether the clinical acumen of experienced critical care physicians might be a better discriminator of high risk cases. They concluded that 'the sensitivity of clinical judgement, in accurately predicting survival, was not good enough to determine the allocation of resources', even at two and seven days following admission.

Perkins *et al.* (1986) confirmed the low predictive accuracy of medical decision for adult patients. They noted that those who were predicted to die but lived were generally much younger than the other patients in the group. This reinforces our belief that 'prognostic uncertainly is important in determining resource expenditures for the critically ill' (Detsky *et al.*, 1981).

Each intensive care patient is a unique clinical problem requiring their own individual therapeutic regimens. There are significant and exaggerated differences among patients with similar nominal diagnoses. It is therefore not possible to arbitrarily exclude those over a given age or those with a specific pre-existing disability.

In 1982 Chassin reviewed costs and outcomes in medical intensive care. While a number of variables, including age, were independently associated with survival, the study 'did not identify a subgroup of patients with a survival rate low enough to justify systematic exclusion from intensive care'. The most important practical problem would in any case be the decision as to what level of expected survival would justify exclusion from intensive care. Would survival have to be unprecedented or is 5% or 10% low enough? What of the views of relatives, and of course the patients themselves?

There are conclusions that we can suggest. Firstly, practical experience and many, but not all, studies would suggest 'the older the patient the greater the risk of dying'. Secondly, only on rare occasions, when advanced age is combined with a poor chronic health condition, a severe acute illness, or an untreatable disease, will we be able to identify, at the time of admission, patients whose hospital survival, given the current state of medical practice, is unprecedented. Only when survival is unprecedented can intensive therapy be denied.

Physiological changes in the aged

Aging results in many physiological changes which are of major practical relevance to the care they will receive before and during an ITU admission. The ubiquitous diagram of reported deteriorations in physiological functions indicates changes that may occur (Fig. 1.1).

Changes in *respiratory function* make the aged more prone to chest infection, and it is difficult to distinguish changes in *cardiovascular function* attributable to age from those of disease.

Failure of *autonomic function* in the aged is not uncommon. Postural hypotension is caused by impaired baroreceptor reflexes. The old are therefore particularly vulnerable to the effects of loss of circulating volume and raised intrathoracic pressure, because of inability to compensate with vasoconstriction.

Decline in *renal function* is well documented and explained by a falling glomerular filtration rate. Therapeutic doses of drugs, such as gentamicin, have to be determined with these factors in mind.

Impaired thermoregulatory reflexes, with a diminished sensitivity to cold, will contribute to the occurrence of hypothermia.

Pharmacological differences in old age

There are significant pharmacokinetic and pharmacodynamic changes in the aged that should influence therapeutic management in the ITU. These are particularly important, for sedative and analgesic regimens will affect the action of vasoactive drugs (Chapter 8).

The plasma half-life of diazepam is four times greater in the 80 year old than the 20 year old, even though there is no difference in plasma clearance. The beta elimination half-life of desmethyldiazepam, the active metabolite of diazepam, is 51–120 h. This makes control of sedation difficult and is liable to produce prolonged recovery. If infused through a peripheral vein, thrombophlebitis is common, unless a form of the drug prepared in lipid emulsion is used. Renal impairment will cause retention of drugs that are conjugated and excreted as glucuronides and reduced dosage will be required, e.g. lorazepam.

Midazolam is achieving deserved popularity as a sedative in the ITU as it has a shorter half-life (2–4 h) than diazepam and its metabolites. There is some evidence to suggest that its action may be prolonged in some cases, notably in patients with renal failure. Supplementation of a benzodiazepine with a narcotic, providing antitussive and analgesic effects, may avoid some of the problems of using benzodiazepines alone. Diazepam and morphine are popular, while infusion of a fixed combination of alfentanil and midazolam has been recommended (O'Dea & Hopkinson, 1987).

Several studies of benzodiazepines and narcotics have suggested that the ageing brain is more sensitive to their effects. This would agree with clinical experience. As there is considerable variation in individual requirements, careful i.v. titration, preferably by continuous infusion, can be best achieved with close supervision in the environs of an ITU. When prolonged administration is anticipated the central venous route is reliable and avoids the problems of thrombophlebitis and intermittent obstruction of cannulae.

The potential for drug dependence with narcotics and benzodiazepines should be acknowledged. A far greater practical problem of management of the aged in the ITU is that many drugs will cause delirium. These include anticonvulsants, antihistamines including H2 blockers, antihypertensives including methyl dopa, and beta blockers. The vicious cycle of sedate–delirium, delirium–sedate is difficult to avoid.

Sedation or analgesia by inhalation has been used in the past.

Nitrous oxide has enjoyed a vogue but recurring concern about its effects on the bone marrow require use 'with care and circumspection' (Gillman, 1987). It may be that in the future inhalational agents that undergo little biodegradation, such as isoflurane, may be used. Propofol is currently undergoing evaluation as a form of i.v. sedation in ITU (Grounds *et al.*, 1987). Any introduction is likely to be very cautious following past experience with the withdrawal of etomidate for long-term use by infusion (Newman *et al.*, 1987).

Aged heart muscle shows increased sensitivity to digoxin *in vitro*, while other studies have demonstrated a decreased sensitivity to other inotropes.

ITU patients will manifest a wide range of response to many drugs, and the aged are likely to be at the extremes. As a rule, short acting drugs, with rapid recovery, are best administered by continuous i.v. infusion, and their effects frequently assessed. The aim should always be to administer the lowest dose compatible with the desired end-point. This entails frequent adjustment of infusion rate to search for the minimum possible rate of infusion.

Disease states

Medical illness

Multiple pathology is very common in the aged with, often undiagnosed, chronic disease. Diagnosis may be confused by concurrent drug therapy producing iatrogenic disease.

It is not difficult to miss the diagnosis of a myocardial infarction or a perforated viscus in the elderly patient who has experienced little or no pain.

An acute confusional state is just as likely to be caused by pneumonia, urinary tract infection or myocardial infarction, as by an acute cerebral event or drug overdosage.

We should not forget endocrine disturbance. Patients with hypothermia, possibly associated with hypothyroidism, present from time to time on most ITUs.

In addition, loss of vision and hearing can impair communication already compromised by senility and cerebrovascular disease. Acute confusional states can be precipitated by any of these factors, the illness itself, drugs, and of course the hospital or ITU environment. Daylight, clocks that are easily read, pictures, radio and television if appropriate, and familiar objects and visitors should all be encouraged to ameliorate this condition. Visitors should be encouraged to talk to elderly patients even if there is no response. It is vital that nursing staff should have the time for a regular 'chat' with the patient beyond that necessitated by the performance of procedures.

Such problems are an important reason to restrict the stay of the aged in ITU to a minimum.

Trauma

Although, because of reduced exposure, the incidence of injury in the old is lower than other age groups, trauma is nevertheless the fifth most significant cause of death for patients over 65 years old. These older patients are more likely to die of their injuries and, as trauma is seen as being eminently amenable to treatment, such patients are likely to be admitted to ITUs.

Survival after trauma is related to the severity of the injury, the type of trauma, the organ systems injured and any complications that may develop. Pre-existing disease does not seem to increase mortality in the severely injured aged. Pre-hospital intubation, hypovolaemia, multiple injuries including significant head injury and five days' ventilation, together, have been found to correlate with a 100% mortality (Oresko-vich *et al.*, 1984).

It has been suggested that such aged patients can be managed with survival rates that are similar to those of other age groups (Horst *et al.*, 1986). Others disagree (Lauwers *et al.*, 1986). In both studies, sepsis and resulting multiorgan failure were harbingers of death. It seems that aggressive restoration of red cell mass during resuscitation might be particularly beneficial in the old as higher oxygen delivery correlates with survival.

The aged patient has a reduced cerebral reserve and is therefore much less able to withstand even minor head injury. Head injury in the old also differs in its presentation, occurring as often in women as men. Falls are the main cause, compounded in men by alcohol intoxication. Concurrent medical disorders, e.g. hemiparesis, may obscure a head injury or the head injury mask a medical disorder.

For patients who remain in coma for at least 6 h , the chance of death increases by 3.6% for every year of age above 35. By 75 years the chance of death or being left in a vegetative state is almost 100% (Galbraith, 1987). It follows that the aged head injury requires extra vigilance and immediate investigation should deterioration occur. In cases of persisting coma, survival is unlikely and careful thought should be given to the nature of further treatment, particularly in the ITU setting.

The prognosis from non-traumatic coma would not appear to be influenced by age (Levy *et al.*, 1981).

Renal failure

Age is a weak determinant of risk of dying from renal failure in some series and in others has no effect at all (Cameron, 1986).

Surgical illness

That the mortality from a variety of surgical procedures increases with increasing age is illustrated in Fig. 15.5. A significant proportion of these

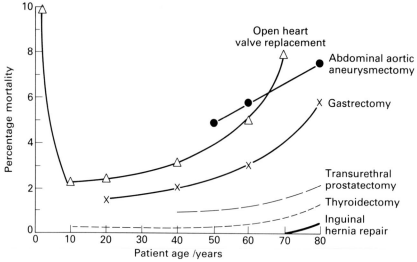

Fig. 15.5. The relationship of mortality to age for several surgical procedures. (From Polk, 1978.)

surgical cases will require careful monitoring postoperatively, while some will need significant active intervention. There are certain diseases more likely to require intervention than others, particularly in the aged, and they deserve special consideration.

A study of the outcome of surgery in 500 patients over 80 years of age (Djokovic & Hedley-White, 1979) showed a hospital mortality of 6%. Six of seven perioperative deaths were caused by mesenteric infarction, with myocardial infarction being the leading cause of postoperative death. In this series 24% of patients undergoing upper abdominal surgery and 57% after thoracic surgery 'required' controlled ventilation for more than one day postoperatively.

While these figures for artificial ventilation may seem high, they nevertheless demonstrate a need for intensive care of the postsurgical aged patient.

Abdominal surgery

Complications of abdominal surgery are likely to figure in the statistics of most ITUs. Twenty-five per cent of our aged patients were admitted by general surgeons, over a quarter required controlled ventilation, and 20% died in the ITU.

The mortality from acute rental failure in association with gastro-intestinal surgery is particularly high, especially when bowel rather than the stomach is involved (Cameron, 1986).

Intestinal malignancy

Colorectal carcinoma is the second most common malignancy in the UK and its incidence increases with age.

In a study of patients undergoing surgery for excision of obstructing colorectal carcinoma, the mortality doubled in those over 70 years old (40%). Cardiorespiratory complications accounted for over half of this mortality, though fatal technical complications occurred in nearly 20% (Waldron & Donovan, 1986). It was also observed that emergency procedures for colorectal surgery were tolerated poorly when compared with elective operations (Waldron *et al.*, 1986).

Intestinal ischaemia

Ischaemic disease of the intestinal tract is very much a disease of the old (Fig. 15.6). Classically described as an embolic complication of rheumatic heart disease, this cause is now less common but should always be suspected in patients with atrial fibrillation. Atheromatous disease of the visceral arteries is thought to be an important aetiology. Interestingly, at post-mortem, no reason is found for intestinal necrosis in one-third of the cases.

Major infarction can be present with little pain and result in late diagnosis. Acutely ill patients will be presented to the ITU for resuscitation and management of peritonitis of unknown cause, before surgical exploration. They will often be desperately ill with a paralytic

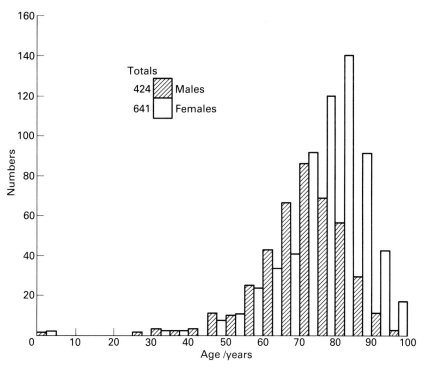

Fig. 15.6. Deaths from intestinal ischaemia in England and Wales, 1982, from Registrar General's data. (From Marston, 1985.)

ileus, distension and perhaps severe pain. They will be hypotensive, tachycardic, cyanosed and tachypnoeic, with poor urinary output; blood gas analysis will commonly demonstrate a non-respiratory (metabolic) acidosis.

These features are produced by a combination of fluid loss into the infarcted intestine, and septicaemia from resulting bacterial invasion. Effective fluid and antibiotic therapy are essential, and some authorities recommend heparinization (Marston, 1985).

The mortality of this condition, particularly of non-occlusive mid-gut infarction, remains high and the postoperative course is likely to be stormy. Re-operation 24 h postoperatively to assess the condition of the remaining intestine, regardless of the condition of the patient, has been advised (Marston, 1985). Parenteral nutrition may well be required because of prolonged ileus, and to cope with the losses from high intestinal fistulae that may develop.

With mesenteric infarction, resuscitation and surgical management must be bold to have any hope of success, and can best be conducted within an ITU.

Vascular surgery

Most general ITUs will have to care for patients who have undergone operation on the aorta, either elective or emergency. The latter are particularly liable to require intensive care as they have a perioperative mortality of around 50%. Additional risk factors are pre-existing cardiac and renal disease. These are more likely in the aged, though age alone should not contraindicate surgery as very old patients can survive (Campbell *et al.*, 1986). Some units have reported a decline in mortality from acute renal failure following aortic surgery, while others have failed to demonstrate any improvement over 10 to 20 years. Of nine patients who underwent emergency aneurysm surgery between 1983 and 1985 in East Birmingham Hospital, six required a period of controlled ventilation and four died. Preoperative hypotension, a large operative blood loss and volume of blood transfused were other risk factors.

Thoracic surgery

Breyer (1981) concluded that (i) thoracic surgery carried significantly less risk than intra-abdominal surgery for the over-70s, and (ii) no patient should be denied such surgery on the grounds of age. Non-fatal major complications, primarily cardiac and respiratory in nature, occurred in 18% of their patients. Major complications included the need for prolonged respiratory support and for multiple aspiration bronchoscopies. The hospital mortality in this series was 3% though other series report rates of 14–20%. One-third of these patients were aged 75 years or more.

Of approximately 1000 thoracotomies performed in the survey period at East Birmingham, 32 aged patients required ITU care. Only two were artificially ventilated and both died. This again illustrates 'gatekeeping' decisions taken preoperatively.

Interventions

Monitoring

It follows that having decided that the aged patient is suffering from a recoverable complaint that warrants intensive therapy, there can be little logic then in limiting the use of monitoring techniques if they are indicated. Electrocardiographic monitoring, urinary catheterization and measurement, and the measurement of core–peripheral temperature gradient should be used routinely.

Early use of invasive monitoring can be justified if it helps diagnosis, or enables more accurate treatment that may shorten ITU stay. The aged are likely to have cardiovascular disease with limited reserves and powers of compensatory vasoconstriction. This can make assessment of the haemodynamic state and the management of therapy difficult, and leave the patient particularly vulnerable to iatrogenic complications.

Arterial cannulation allows continuous observation of blood pressure while enabling frequent, pain-free blood sampling as necessary. This is especially useful during critical illness in the aged when therapeutic manoeuvres, such as tracheal intubation, may precipitate abrupt changes in blood pressure. Beat by beat observation will enable careful titration of vasoactive drugs and assessment of fluid therapy in this group where safety margins are particularly limited. Frequent blood gas analysis is also possible to assess respiratory and metabolic function. Cannulation of radial or dorsalis pedis vessels has few complications; the advantages of the technique will benefit the majority of aged patients admitted to the ITU.

Central venous cannulation for pressure measurement, or for fluid administration, can be justified if it prevents renal failure from unrecognized hypovolaemia, or pulmonary oedema and respiratory failure from overtransfusion. It will also provide a convenient path for the administration of fluids and drugs. In the aged, skeletal abnormality, notably kyphoscoliosis and neck rigidity, may make cannulation technically difficult. The consequences of complications such as pneumothorax will be dire, so that careful consideration should be given to the route used. The high internal jugular route on the right side gives direct access to the right atrium, is well away from the pleura and thoracic duct, and is readily accessible. For long-term cannulation, subclavian lines are easier to look after but a cephalic vein cut-down in the deltopectoral groove may be preferable to avoid pneumothorax or bleeding in patients with coagulation abnormalities.

Table 15.4. Uses of balloon flotation catheters

---

1 Measurement of central venous, right ventricular, pulmonary artery and pulmonary artery wedge pressures
2 Measurement of cardiac output by thermodilution technique enabling derivation of other cardiovascular parameters, notably systemic vascular resistance
3 Measurement of mixed venous oxygen saturation by intermittent or continuous techniques
4 Determination of right ventricular ejection fraction
5 Insertion of cardiac pacing wire
6 Pulmonary angiography
7 Pulmonary microvascular sampling
8 Transseptal left heart catheterization

The use of balloon flotation catheters should be specific (Table 15.4). Many of the dangers of the technique are those associated with central venous cannulation. The aged may be more prone to some of the commoner complications, e.g. bacteraemia, catheter site infection, pulmonary infarction and arrythmias. However, the greater likelihood of ischaemic heart disease increases the probability of a mismatch of right and left ventricular function, indicating the need for measurement of pulmonary artery wedge pressure (PAWP). This will be especially true in shock states when a precise assessment of myocardial function is required, and then measurement of cardiac output will assist in the choice and titration of vasoactive drugs.

Where there is a possibility of complete heart block developing, a balloon flotation catheter with an extra channel for a pacing wire can be used. Measurement of mixed venous oxygen saturation may be of value in assessing septic states.

The major risks are sepsis, dysrhythmia and pulmonary artery rupture. In the aged, the presence of sepsis may be difficult to diagnose. Death has been recorded from dysrhythmia and pulmonary artery rupture. The occurrence of these complications is rare and it would be hard to establish any increased risk in the aged; one might speculate that more brittle vessels might put them at greater risk from pulmonary artery rupture.

While we have used arterial and CVP monitoring widely over the last three years, we have only used pulmonary artery catheters in four patients in this age group. The use of invasive monitoring is likely to increase as there is little logic, once the patient is committed to intensive therapy, in witholding such methods. Nevertheless, extra care and discretion are necessary in their use.

Pacemakers will be indicated in cases of complete heart block, when cardiological advice should be sought. If transvenous pacemaking is not available locally, and chronotropic agents such as isoprenaline have failed, then oesophageal pacing may be indicated. There may also be the occasional need for aortic balloon pump support. This will usually be associated with cardiopulmonary bypass surgery, carried out at specialist centres.

Artificial ventilation

Older patients requiring respiratory support have a higher overall and in-hospital mortality rate, adjusted for severity of illness, than do a comparable group of younger patients (McLean *et al.*, 1985). Old survivors were not limited to low risk groups and their quality of life was considered satisfactory. Readmissions and those who suffered combined respiratory and renal failure did poorly. Numbers were, however, small.

There are no reasonable exclusion criteria that can be applied to the aged requiring respiratory support.

When using intermittent positive pressure ventilation with aged patients, care should be taken not to cause a precipitate fall in blood pressure. Hypovolaemia should be corrected, before intubation if possible. Use of a low dose of inotrope, particularly dopamine, may be justified to help maintain blood pressure and urinary output, especially if positive end expiratory pressure is being used to improve oxygenation. What would be regarded as an inadequate Pao_2 for a 20 year old, may be the norm for the 80 year old. Careful thought therefore needs to be given to what is an acceptable level of oxygenation, in order to avoid unnecessary and potentially dangerous therapy. The risks of pulmonary barotrauma oxygen toxicity are considerable.

Abrupt changes in acid-base status are to be avoided. Rapid reduction in carbon dioxide levels in patients suffering respiratory failure may cause a fall in cardiac output and blood pressure, while hypocarbia can reduce cerebrovascular blood flow. It may be undesirable to correct a degree of non-respiratory acidosis because this will shift the oxygen dissociation curve to the right, reducing oxygen supply to tissues. Rapid correction of respiratory acidosis will cause a fall in serum potassium level which could be dangerous in the presence of pre-existing hypokalaemia, which may be associated with hypophosphataemia (see below). The consequence of administering bicarbonate may be severe non-respiratory alkalosis later. A slow rate of change, with frequent assessment by blood gas analysis, is required because of tardy aged homeostasis.

Intermittent mandatory ventilation (IMV)

Use of IMV is now commonplace in most ITUs. The advantages of the technique are (i) reduced intrathoracic pressure with spontaneous breaths and resulting improved cardiac output and (ii) decreased need for neuromuscular blocking agents and sedation. These are especially desirable for the aged but one must make allowance for their decreased respiratory response to hypoxia and hypercarbia (Kronenberg & Drage, 1973).

Care of the airway

Minitracheotomy (Lewis *et al.*, 1986) is being increasingly adopted for the treatment of sputum retention. This technique offers improved access to the trachea for suction, while preserving glottic function, and may avoid the need for repeated fibre-optic bronchoscopy or formal tracheal intubation.

Should tracheal intubation be required, the nasal route, when possible, will be preferred being better tolerated by most patients. Because of neuromuscular or chronic airways disease, weaning may be prolonged. Tracheostomy should be an early consideration, particularly if the endotracheal tube is causing the patient discomfort.

Nutrition

Because of poor social circumstances and lack of attention, the old are more likely to present with protein-calorie malnutrition, infestations and bedsores which can be due to neglect. Nursing and medical staff should pay special attention to pressure areas, for once bedsores develop their progress is hard to arrest. The skin will be thin with poor subcutaneous support and will bruise easily. In difficult cases, especially if the patient is obese, specially designed beds may be helpful.

Recent evidence suggests that 10% of aged patients admitted acutely to hospital may have evidence of undernutrition (McEvoy et al 1983), and it is estimated that 12% of males and 8% of females over 80 years of age are malnourished.

In addition, up to 50% of patients may show signs of malnutrition during their hospital stay.

Exton-Smith (1980) has divided the causes of malnutrition in the old into two groups: those due to social and environmental factors, and those due to internal disorders. The former may be noticed incidentally during ITU admission, while the latter may be related to a primary, perhaps as yet undiagnosed condition.

Lean body mass

Progressive loss of body protein is a major feature of ageing throughout adult life. This affects muscle more than other tissues, protein content falling by 45% from the age of 25 to 75 years. There is no evidence to suggest that this is due to lack of protein in the average diet. There is, however, data to show that some older people may require more protein than do young adults in order to maintain nitrogen balance, especially if suffering from chronic disease. As caloric intake declines with age, this suggests that an increasingly larger percentage of dietary intake should be protein rather than calorie based (Exton-Smith, 1980).

As lean body mass decreases with age, there is a corresponding increase in body fat. Total body water declines in parallel with lean body mass and may account for much of the weight loss seen in very old patients, particularly females. Thirst and osmoregulatory mechanisms are disturbed, making the aged especially vulnerable to fluid shifts, particularly in the extracellular and vascular compartments. Excessive diuretic therapy, immobility and infection can rapidly lead to dehydration and haemoconcentration, especially if fluid intake is inadequate, or inadequately supervised.

Basal metabolic rate

Basal metabolic rate declines, with a fall in energy consumption from 2700 kcal (11 MJ) at 20–34 years to 2100 kcal (9 MJ) at 75–90 years. These figures were derived for a male American population and it is estimated that women require 500 kcal less; they are in broad agreement with the current recommended daily intakes for people in the UK (1979) (Beaumont & James, 1985).

It is also possible to derive basal energy expenditure from the Harris-Benedict formula which involves an adjustment for age and sex. Recent work (Van Lanschot *et al.*, 1986) has demonstrated a poor correlation between basal and total energy expenditure measured by indirect calorimetry, unless a correction factor was introduced to adjust for the patient's clinical condition.

Vitamin deficiencies

Vitamin deficiencies, while rare in the young, are more common in old age due to low dietary intake and physical disease.

Vitamin B complex deficiency may be manifest as cheilosis, angular stomatitis, glossitis and nasolabial seborrhoea. Deficiencies of riboflavin, nicotinamide and possibly pyridoxine have been reported. Neurological disorders, such as peripheral neuropathy and Wernicke's encephalopathy, may occur due to thiamine deficiency. The latter is normally associated with alcoholism and persistent vomiting. Acute confusional states can also be associated with thiamine deficiency.

When other causes are absent, acute cardiovascular beriberi should be suspected in malnourished old people with cardiac failure. It should be treated with large doses of thiamine.

Megaloblastic anaemia may be associated with folate or vitamin B_{12} deficiency, though the former is the most common because of inadequate dietary intake. Barbiturates and anticonvulsants interfere with folate metabolism and in epileptic patients can be responsible for folate deficiency. Folate deficiency may also cause confusion, depression, apathy and intellectual impairment.

Clinical features of vitamin B_{12} deficiency include glossitis, subacute combined degeneration of the spinal cord, peripheral neuropathy and mental changes.

Scurvy is still seen in the aged, especially men, and manifest as swelling and bleeding of the gums, weakness, anaemia and extensive haemorrhages in the skin of legs and arms ('sheet' haemorrhages).

Similar manifestations may occur with vitamin K deficiency. This may occur in the malnourished old who are given broad-spectrum antibiotics that interfere with the bacterial synthesis of the vitamin in the intestine.

Electrolytes and trace elements

Many aged patients in ITUs have low serum potassium levels. These may represent a chronic total body potassium depletion, which should be actively treated and monitored with frequent determination of serum levels.

There are cases in the American and English literature of hypophosphataemia, causing or being associated with acute respiratory failure and acidosis (Varsano et al., 1983; Storm, 1984). Phosphate is present in fat emulsions or may be administered separately as the potassium salt, which may contribute to the correction of an accompanying hypokalaemia (Kingston & Al-Siba'I, 1985). Hypomagnesaemia and hypocalcaemia can often be present with hypophosphataemia. Hypomagnesaemia should be corrected with magnesium sulphate since cardiac arrhythmia, neuromuscular problems and hypocalcaemia have been attributed to its deficiency.

It is important to consider the potential drug–nutrition interactions that may occur in the old. Chronic disease results in chronic medication which, in turn, increases the potential for interaction. Aspirin may cause ascorbic acid depletion, absorption of fat-soluble vitamins may be impaired by mineral oil laxatives, and prolonged diuretic therapy may result in depletion of key elements such as potassium, magnesium and zinc. Alcohol abuse in the aged may be as high as 10% with its well recognized effect on thiamine and other B complex vitamins. Whether or not the patient is receiving parenteral or enteral nutrition, one should be alert to the manifestations of nutritional disturbances which, even if not the prime cause of ITU admission, may contribute to morbidity or prolong stay.

Enteral routes of nutritional supplementation should be used whenever possible. Fine-bore nasogastric feeding, duodenal and jejeunal tubes are alternatives to a feeding gastrostomy or jejeunostomy. While not as frequent as with parenteral feeding, enteral nutrition does have its complications. Tubes may be displaced and the feeds aspirated, or the patient overloaded with nutrient containing fluid or electrolytes. The old, with less power of adaption, ageing anatomy, and declining organ function will be particularly prone to such problems. Hormonal imbalance and metabolic disturbance, diabetes, uraemia and myxoedema, may further compound these difficulties. The stress response, such as one would expect in the critically ill patient, produces disturbances of carbohydrate, fat and protein metabolism. Patients may have an increased oxygen consumption and be prone to fluid overload.

Perioperative nutrition

During short-term starvation, glycogen stores are consumed and proteolysis and lipolysis begin. This leads to a reduction of muscle mass with resulting weakness and impaired expectoration, exposing the patient to increased risk of developing hypostatic pneumonia. If preceded by pre-admission malnutrition, protein-sparing mechanisms will have reduced urinary nitrogen losses to a minimum, with a parallel decline in basal metabolic rate by as much as 40%. In one study a weight loss in excess of 20% was associated with a postoperative mortality of 33%, but others disagree. Is there a case therefore for perioperative parenteral nutrition? Muggia-Sullam & Fischer (1983) have reviewed the putative indications for nutritional supplementation.

Pancreatitis

Alcoholism and chronic malnutrition are associated with pancreatitis, which itself may cause periods of prolonged paralytic ileus, particularly while a pseudocyst or abscess evolve. While there is little evidence that parenteral nutrition has any direct effect on the acute phase of the disease, it is generally regarded as necessary to feed the patient until surgery is possible.

Gastrointestinal-cutaneous fistulae

Parenteral nutrition has been shown by some to increase the rate of spontaneous closure of fistulae and may decrease the mortality from this condition.

Inflammatory bowel disease

Perioperative parenteral nutrition may reduce postoperative complications and the extent of surgery.

Cancer surgery

The evidence regarding the value of preoperative nutrition in aged patients is conflicting. Some studies do show benefit while others question the effect of parenteral nutrition on tumour growth.

There is a little evidence to show that perioperative parenteral nutrition will reduce morbidity or mortality other than in specific circumstances. While parenteral nutrition may be indicated in individual and possibly extreme cases, neither laboratory nor clinical measurement is currently capable of reliably identifying such patients.

Such conclusions are not to be taken as an excuse to neglect the correction of preoperative fluid, electrolyte and protein (albumin) deficiencies when present.

Initial weight reduction following surgery is likely to result from water loss, but protein losses will commence after the first week. If nutritional support is required, it would seem sensible to start earlier rather than later and should be considered towards the end of the first postoperative week.

Parenteral nutrition

Tables have been produced in an attempt to quantify the reduction in energy needs of the elderly population. These are of little help in assessing the needs of individuals, some of whom may be sedentary, while others may be as active as they were at 40 years of age. Many dietary surveys have suggested a wide variance in the intake of most nutrients by old people. These factors summate, to make the assessment of malnutrition and of calorie and nitrogen requirements in the ITU doubly difficult.

If parenteral nutrition is indicated, strict fluid balance with an allowance for insensible losses is mandatory. Administration of glucose-containing solutions should be monitored with frequent measurement of blood glucose. With proper training and supervision, bedside monitoring will be satisfactory. Insulin infusion may be necessary but rapidly increasing requirements may indicate the development of a hyperosmolar state from excessive glucose administration. This is less likely if part of the calorie requirement is provided by fat emulsion.

Excessive provision of carbohydrate calories may increase carbon dioxide production, which will prevent weaning from ventilation. This can be measured. In the aged, calorie requirements in excess of 2000 kcal will be unusual.

Twenty-four hourly urinary collection for determination of urea and electrolyte excretion will enable nitrogen losses to be calculated. Adjustment must always be made for changes in serum urea. Nitrogen-containing solutions, with appropriate electrolyte content, can then be administered within the volume dictated by losses.

Immunology

Immune function may be compromised, both because the patient is old and also because of concurrent protein-calorie malnutrition.

Age-associated immune deficiency may have a causative role in the pathogenesis of disease or attenuate the response of the body to the disease process. If this is the case, correction of immune deficiencies might have a place in treatment of the critically ill. This is only possible if antibody deficiency is present.

Organized lymphoid tissue, the spleen and the lymph nodes, undergo regressive changes with age, while there is a parallel increase of diffuse lymphoid tissue throughout the body. This results in a striking increase in the number of lymphoid follicles found in the bone marrow, salivary glands and lung parenchyma.

T cells are derived from lymphoid precursor cells that migrate via the thymic subcapsular cortex, where they become thymocytes, and thence to the peripheral lymphoid tissues. They initiate cell-mediated immunity, those immune reactions transferred by cells and not by serum. This is important in host defence against virus, fungal and mycobacterial attack, and also plays an active role in delayed hypersensitivity, graft rejection, graft-versus-host disease, and cancer rejection. In the aged, there is a physiological involution of the thymus and decrease in T-cell numbers, though this is not dramatic. If, as has been hypothesized, a thymic hormone stimulates T-cell responses, then this too might compromise the immune response in the elderly. Cell-mediated immunity can be assessed by the delayed hypersensitivity skin response to recall antigens. A reduction in their responses has been found to correlate with severe sepsis by some, although this is not invariably so.

Some serum antibody levels decline with advancing age, but levels of serum immunoproteins show no fall. The age-related pattern of childhood diseases would suggest that secondary humoral immune responsiveness remains intact with age. There is evidence of disordered immune control in the elderly, in that autoantibodies are detectable with increased frequency, but the incidence of true autoimmune diseases is less than in middle age.

There is an increased incidence of cancer with advancing age. However, the assumption that this develops principally as the result of an individual's weakened immune system has proved to be an oversimplification of the very complex tumour–host relationship.

Malnutrition, vitamin deficiency, diabetes and anaemia, all age-associated conditions, can affect the immune system and are capable of correction. It is difficult to discern cause and effect but no causal relationship has been established between malnutrition, immune function and any decreased host resistance to infection. It is important that the practitioner be aware of such problems when treating the aged in ITU. Although at present immunology has little specific to offer in either the diagnostic or therapeutic fields, the contribution of impaired immunity caused by some diseases and drugs requires recognition.

Resuscitation

In the ITU, the drive to sustain life can conflict with the other fundamental objective. of medicine, the relief of suffering. This is particularly so with the application of cardiopulmonary resuscitation (CPR). Should CPR be considered in every patient because they are deemed worthy of ITU admission? If not, when should CPR be witheld? Is age a criterion for application (or non-application) of CPR?

Bedell *et al.* (1983) discussed the latter point in their comprehensive, prospective review of nearly 300 patients, resuscitated in a university teaching hospital. They disagreed with other investigators in concluding that it is the underlying disease, not the year of birth, that influences survival.

Only 14% of their patients were discharged from hospital, while pneumonia, hypotension, renal failure, cancer and a restricted pre-admission life-style were associated with high in-hospital mortality. No patient with oliguria, acute stroke, sepsis, metastatic cancer, or pneumonia survived. These conclusions were broadly supported by Gulati *et al.* (1983), who found that resuscitation was more successful in patients with ventricular fibrillation. Whatever the age of the ITU population, it is apparent that a poor outcome from CPR can be expected of resuscitation.

By contrast, many units adopt 'Do Not Resuscitate' orders. In one series of over 7000 ITU admissions, 39% of all deaths were preceded by such instructions (Zimmerman *et al.*, 1986). Over half such orders were for patients older than 65 years and 40% had severe failing health before admission. The patients' diagnosis had a significant impact on when the order was written. This was earlier for patients with intracranial haemorrhage or cardiac arrest, and later for those suffering respiratory arrest or septicaemia. Ninety-four per cent died in hospital with most (74%) dying in the ITU. These patients also received a disproportionately large amount of ITU resources.

Such decisions will also be accompanied by other changes of management, e.g. limitations on the use of other therapy such as blood transfusion, vasoactive drugs, artificial ventilation or dialysis. It may be that decisions on the latter two points are often left too late, i.e. until such therapy has been initiated, when withdrawal becomes more difficult. It is then particularly important to involve the patient or close relatives in such decisions, for their views, or perceived views, will be paramount. Since adequate discussion takes time and thought, such decisions must be taken in advance of crisis, and of course they must be clearly documented. Futhermore, in an ITU, such decisions cannot be regarded as immutable, for a change in condition may warrant a change in response.

The ethics of intensive care

In the UK, beds in ITUs comprise only about 1% of the acute total. The figure for the USA is 15%. Even there, albeit reluctantly, it is recognized that health care has to be rationed.

We must also ask whether intensive care is prolonging life which is already of a quality that the patient considers unacceptable. Will it give such a limited period of survival that the burden exceeds the benefit? Could witholding of intensive therapy be considered, or come to be considered, negligent?

The following four principles of medical ethics are worth considering in the ITU setting. (Beauchamp & Childress, 1983). They are particularly applicable to the aged.

(i) Beneficence: what is the probability that life of reasonable quality and duration will be restored?

(ii) Non-maleficence: how much stress, hazard and indignity are likely to be associated with treatment?

(iii) Patient autonomy: informed of this balance of probabilities what is, or might be, the patient's preference?

(iv) Justice: does the expected benefit to the individual justify the cost in community resources?

The potential reversibility of the critical illness has been frequently discussed. It is often impossible to evaluate the likely outcome of treatment, until the patient has undergone a period of observation in ITU. The very admission of the patient then becomes a decision to treat, and it is far more difficult then to withdraw therapy already under way.

For the aged, considerations of duration and quality will differ from younger groups. The older patient will be more accepting of a degree of disability that would be socially crippling for the younger patient. In the event of illness of acute onset, the aged may welcome even a few extra weeks to arrange their affairs and be with family.

Most patients who are critically ill remember little of their stay in an ITU. Stress will be born by the relatives who will also recognize the indignity. It is for doctors to recognize and acknowledge the many hazards that accompany a period of intensive therapy.

One important sub-group in the East Birimingham ITU is comprised of those coming for postoperative monitoring. The level of intervention required in this group is small. Are the benefits of intensive care here marginal? Are we unjustifiably exposing elderly patients to the psychological tensions and social deprivations of the ITU and perhaps to the hazards of invasive monitoring?

It is essential that patients, or relatives on their behalf, are allowed to exercise autonomy as an older person would perceive it. As the understanding of the public of such matters increases, more patients will wish to express their own preferences on treatment. They may have strong views as to whether 'extraordinary' as opposed to 'ordinary' means are used to support their lives. 'Ordinary' has been defined as interventions which offer a reasonable hope of benefit, and which can be obtained and used without excessive expense, pain, or other inconvenience.

There are two aspects of justice: justice for the individual, and justice to the community. One recent paper, when considering the Medicare reimbursements to hospitals in the USA for provision of intensive care, even comments on the hospitals' 'loss per discharge' and 'loss per death' (Bellamy et al., 1987). The appropriate ground for the distribution of the medical commons is ill health, not social worth, individual merit, lottery or age! Yet there is uneven distribution of facilities, and skill, even in affluent communities. The individual has a prima-facie 'right to life'.

A 'right'

> '*A vital interest grounded in the nature of man and recognised by competent authority as capable of being enjoyed and protected.*'

> (Dunstan, 1985)

Duties attach to rights. The basing of decisions on outcome prediction has been termed 'consequentialism'. Duties are distinctive principles of action which are morally obligatory regardless of consequences. Two principles of duty should define the framework of patient care. Firstly, the prime loyalty of medical staff is to their patients. Secondly, the conduct of therapy should accord as much as possible with the patient's own wishes and values, while recognizing that circumstances may impair the decision-making abilities of patient and family. The duty of the doctor is to protect the patient in the enjoyment of his right. But there is no performative duty, no duty to cause either life or death to happen. The physician is sandwiched between the two protective duties, of the 'right' to live and of the 'right' to die.

Patients who cannot recover tend to stay longer in the ITU and cost more than the survivors. Continued support is usually justified on the grounds of uncertain prognosis. Decisions to discontinue intensive care are therefore very important, so as to abort 'the vicious cycle of commitment'.

While there are a number of prognostic criteria available, unfortunately they are not absolute, and there are many patients alive today who have thwarted a prognostician's doom.

It is likely that intensive therapy can only influence outcome in a limited subset of patients. Even the technology may be of less importance than the organization of care (Knaus *et al.*, 1986). Jennett (1984) suggests five non-Us for ITU which, though applying to all age groups, are particularly important for the older patient:

Do not use the ITU
Unnecessarily; if the end could be achieved by simpler means.
Unsuccessfully; because the condition is beyond influence.
Unsafely; because the risks outweigh the benefits.
Unkindly; because quality of life afterwards is unacceptable.
Unwisely; because resources are diverted from more useful activities.

Epitome

> 'The success of intensive care is not, therefore, to be measured only by the statistics of survival, as though each death were a medical failure. It is to be measured by the quality of life preserved or restored; and by the quality of the dying of those

whose interest is to die; and by the quality of human
relationships involved in each death.'

(Dunstan, 1985)

Acknowledgement

I thank Dr R.A. Thompson, Consultant Immunologist, Director of the
Regional Immunology Laboratory, East Birmingham Hospital for his
help with the section on Immunology.

References

Beauchamp, T.L. & Childress, J.F. (1983) *Principles of Biomedical Ethics*, 2nd Edn.
Oxford University Press, New York.

Beaumont, D.M. & James, O.F.W. (1985) Aspects of nutrition in the elderly. In *Clinics in
Gastroenterology 14* (Ed. O.F.W. James) **4**, 811–27; *Gastrointestinal Disorders in the
Elderly*. Saunders, Philadelphia.

Bedell, S.E. *et al.* (1983) Survival after cardiopulmonary resuscitation in the hospital. *New
Engl. J. Med.* **309**, 569–576.

Bergner, M. *et al.* (1981) The Sickness Impact Profile: Development and final revision of a
health status measure. *Med. Care* **XIX**, 787–805.

Bellamy P.E. *et al.* (1987) Admitting elderly patients to the ICU: dilemmas and solutions.
Geriatrics **42**, 61–68.

Breyer R.H. *et al.* (1981) Thoracotomy in patients over age seventy years. *J. Thorac.
Cardiovasc. Surg.* **81**, 187–193.

Cameron, J.S. (1986) Acute renal failure in the intensive care unit today. *Intensive Care
Med.* **12**, 64–70.

Campbell, W.B. *et al.* ((1986) The mortality of abdominal aortic aneurysm. *Ann R. Coll.
Surg. Engl.* **68**, 276–278.

Campion, E.W. *et al.* (1981) Medical intensive care for the elderly. *J. Am. Med. Ass.* **246**,
2052–2056.

Chassin, M.R. (1982) Cost and outcomes of medical intensive care. *Med. Care* **XX**,
165–179.

Cullen, D.J. *et al.* (1976) Survival, hospitalization charges and follow-up results in critically
ill patients. *New Engl. J. Med.* **294**, 982–987.

Cullen, D.J. *et al.* (1984) Results, charges, and benefits of intensive care for critically ill
patients: Update 1983. *Crit. Care Med.* **12**, 102–106.

Detsky, A.S. *et al.* (1981) Prognosis, survival, and the expenditure of hospital resources for
patients in an intensive-care unit. *New Engl. J. Med.* **305**, 667–672.

Djokovic, J. L. & Hedley-Whyte, J. (1979) Prediction of outcome of surgery and anesthesia
in patients over 80. *J. Am. Med. Ass.* **242**, 2301–2306.

Draper, E.A. *et al.* (1983) Prognosis from combined organ system failure. *Abstract Crit.
Care Med.* **11**, 236.

Dunstan, G.R. (1985) Hard questions in intensive care. *Anaesthesia* **40**, 479–482.

Exton-Smith, A.N. (1980) Nutritional status: diagnoses of prevention of malnutrition. In
Metabolic and Nutritional Disorders in the Elderly (Eds A.N. Exton-Smith & F.I.
Caird). John Wright, Bristol, pp. 66–76.

Galbraith, S. (1987) Head injuries in the elderly. *Br. Med. J.* **294**, 325.

Gillman, M.A. (1987) Haematological changes caused by nitrous oxide. Editorial, *Br. J.
Anaesth.* **59**, 143–145.

Goldstein, R.L. *et al.* (1986) Functional outcomes following medical intensive care. *Crit.
Care Med.* **14**, 783–788.

Grenrot, C. *et al.* (1986) Intensive care of the elderly — a retrospective study. *Acta
Anaesth. Scand.* **30**, 703–708.

Grounds, R.M. *et al.* (1987) Propofol for sedation in the intensive care unit: preliminary
report. *Br. Med. J.* **294**, 397–400.

Gulati, R.S. *et al.* (1983) Cardiopulmonary resuscitation of old people. *Lancet* **2**, 267–269.

Horst, H.M. *et al.* (1986) Factors influencing survival of elderly trauma patients. *Crit. Care Med.* **14**, 681–684.

Jennett, B. (1984) Inappropriate use of intensive care. *Br. Med. J.* **289**, 1709–1711.

Kingston, M. & Al-Siba'I, M.B. (1985) Treatment of severe hypophosphataemia. *Crit. Care Med.* **13**, 16–18.

Knaus, W.A. *et al.* (1985) APACHE II: A severity of disease classification system. *Crit. Care Med.* **13**, 818–829.

Knaus, W.A. *et al.* (1986) An evaluation of outcome from intensive care in major medical centres. *Ann. Intern. Med.* **104**, 410–418.

Kronenberg R.S. & Drage, C.S. (1973) Attenuation of the ventilatory and heart rate responses to hypoxia and hypercapnia with aging in normal men. *J. Clin. Invest.* **52**, 1812–1819.

Lauwers, L.F. *et al.* (1986) A retrospective study of 130 consecutive multiple trauma patients in an intensive care unit. *Intensive Care Med.* **12**, 296–301.

Levy, D.E. *et al.* (1981) Prognosis in nontraumatic coma. *Ann. Intern. Med.* **94**, 293–301.

Lewis, G.A. *et al.* (1986) Minitracheotomy. A report of its use in intensive therapy. *Anaesthesia* **41**, 931–935.

Marston, A. (1985) Ischaemia. In *Clinics in Gastroenterology 14* (Ed. O.F.W. James) **4**, 847–62. *Gastrointestinal Disorders in the Elderly*. Saunders, Philadelphia.

McEvoy, A.W. *et al.* (1983) Bacterial contamination of the small intestine is an important cause of occult malabsorption in the elderly. *Br. Med. J.* **ii**, 789–793.

McLean, R.F. *et al.* (1985) Outcome of respiratory intensive care for the elderly. *Crit. Care Med.* **13**, 625–629.

Muggia-Sullam, M. & Fischer, J.E. (1983) Current concepts of indications for preoperative parenteral nutrition. In *Clinics in Anesthesiology 1* (Ed. J.F. Biebuyck) **3**, 579–98. Saunders, Philadelphia.

Newman, L.H. *et al.* (1987) Propofol for sedation in the intensive care unti. Correspondence, *Br. Med. J.* **294**, 970.

O'Dea, J. & Hopkinson, R.B. (1987) Alfentanil–midazolam infusion. *Care Crit. Ill* **3**, 20–21.

Oreskovich, M.R. *et al.* (1984) Geriatric trauma: Injury patterns and outcome. *J. Trauma* **24**, 565–569.

Perkins, H.S. *et al.* (1986) Providers as predictors: Using outcome prediction in intensive care. *Crit. Care Med.* **14**, 105–110.

Polk, H.C. (1987) The mathematics of clinical judgement. In *Basic Surgery*, 3rd edn (Eds B. Gardner *et al.*). Appleton-Century-Crofts, Noswalk.

Rodman, G.H. *et al.* (1978) How accurate is clinical judgement? *Crit. Care Med.* **6**, 127 (abstract).

Sage, W.M. *et al.* (1986) Is intensive care worth it? An assessment of input and outcome for the critically ill. *Crit. Care Med.* **14**, 777–782.

Shroeder, S.A. *et al.* (1981) Survival of adult high-cost patients. *J. Am. Med. Ass.* **245**, 1446–1449.

Spitzer, W.O. *et al.* (1981) Measuring the quality of life of cancer patients: A concise QL-index for use by physicians *J. Chronic Dis.* **34**, 585.

Storm, T.L. (1984) Severe hypophosphataemia during recovery from acute respiratory acidosis. *Br. Med. J.* **289**, 456–457.

Thibault, G.E. (1984) The medical intensive care unit. In *Major Issues in Critical Care Medicine* (Eds J.E. Parrillo & S.M. Ayres) Williams & Wilkins, London, pp. 9–15.

Thibault, G.E. *et al.* (1980) Medical intensive care: Indications, interventions, and outcomes. *New Engl. J. Med.* **302**, 938–942.

Van Lanschot, J.J.B. *et al.* (1986) Calculation versus measurement of total energy expenditure. *Crit. Care Med.* **14**, 981–985.

Varsano, S. *et al.* (1983) Hypophosphatemia as a reversible cause of refractory ventilatory failure. *Crit. Care Med.* **11**, 908–909.

Waldron, R.P. & Donvan, I.A. (1986) Mortality in patients with obstructing colorectal cancer. *Ann. R. Coll. Surg. Engl.* **68**, 219–221.

Waldron, R.P. *et al.* (1986) Emergency presentation and mortality from colorectal cancer in the elderly. *Br. J. Surg.* **73**, 214–216.

Zimmerman, J.E. *et al.* (1986) The use and implications of do not resuscitate orders in intensive care units. *J. Am. Med. Ass.* **255**, 351–356.

16 | Chronic pain in the aged

P.J.D. EVANS

Introduction

The management of chronic pain has become an area of increasing interest during the past 20 years. No doubt the general improvement in the quality of life has led to expectations of a decrease in the degree of discomfort that should be tolerated. We live in a society with a mean age that is rising (Central Statistical Office, 1981). Since chronic pain is frequently associated with the ageing process, it is likely that demand for the relief of this condition will increase and a complimentary increase in facilities will be required.

Chronic pain is described as pain that persists beyond the usual course of an acute disease or a reasonable time for an injury to heal, and recurs at intervals for months or years (Bonnica, 1985). It is a popular concept to think that chronic pain is a modern problem but there are many references in history to the condition (Todd, 1985). However, it may be that changes in society and improvement in the standard of living may make it a more urgent problem.

Inspection of the patients attending any pain clinic will indicate that a wide range of conditions are treated (Table 16.1). Many affect patients of all ages, although a number of specific problems are commonly observed in those over 50 years of age (Table 16.2). Most pain clinics see more female than male patients. It is difficult adequately to explain this sex difference, although frequent suggestions would hint at biological as well as psychological factors (Table 16.3).

During the past 10 years there has been a significant shift in the emphasis in the way patients with chronic pain have been treated. Traditional concepts in management have required pain to be considered in a largely physical sense, and consequently treatment has been directed towards the interruption of pain pathways or towards the suppression of pain appreciation through drug therapy. Chronic pain is very much a perceptual experience and frequently does not respond to this model of management. If therapy is to be effective, it is likely that a 'whole person' approach is required and allowance must be made for the physical, emotional and reactive components of the condition. Single modality treatment is often ineffectual.

In many old patients chronic pain develops because it is the final insult in terms of disease on an otherwise downhill course. For others it is a cry for help. Both these factors suggest that the way that society treats the old may contribute to the continuation of symptoms. Patients with little family support, or with few friends or who have been widowed may be at particular risk. The physician is often incapable of offering suitable resources for these patients. It has been suggested that better deployment of social workers, occupational therapists, physiotherapists and other paramedical therapists would provide greater amelioration of symptoms than can be achieved through traditional means. Scott (1982), in her article on the continuing problem of pain, argues that it is the 'quality of life' that is important rather than the absolute reduction in pain and that sometimes an aggressive approach to management can increase symptoms rather than relieve them.

Table 16.1. Typical incidence of non-malignant pain

Pain condition	%	Sex ratio (M : F)	Mean duration (years)
Low back pain	26.2	1 : 1.7	8.8
Postherpetic neuralgia	10.8	1 : 1.6	2.6
Post-trauma neuralgia	8.6	1 : 1.2	4.8
Atypical facial pain	5.9	1 : 2.0	4.3
Intercostal neuralgia	5.2	1 : 1.5	4.3
Trigeminal neuralgia	4.6	1 : 2.4	9.3
Perineal neuralgia	3.9	1 : 1.9	6.8
Abdominal neuralgia	3.7	1 : 1.2	5.6
Stump pain	3.0	1 : 0.4	12.5
Osteoarthritic hip	2.8	1 : 1.2	4.3
Sympathetic dystrophy	2.4	1 : 1.1	4.2
Coccydynia	2.3	1 : 4.2	5.7
Cervical spondylosis	2.1	1 : 1.5	5.9
All other conditions	18.5		

(Data collected from 1115 patients attending the Oxford Regional Pain Relief Unit.)

Table 16.2. Chronic pain problems seen in aged patients

Postherpetic neuralgia
Cancer related pain
Osteoarthritis and rheumatic pain
Trigeminal neuralgia
Thalamic syndrome
Stump pain
Perineal neuralgia
Claudication
Deafferentation pain

Table 16.3. Factors predisposing to chronic pain in women

Physical	Emotional
Osteoporosis	Depression
Postural effects of pregnancy	Loss of drive
Hormone changes	Loss of children
Menopause	Unemployment
Genetic difference	Marital disharmony

Clearly from the foregoing discussion the primary aim in management is to bring about a reduction in the level of symptoms rather than attempt to produce an absolute cure. This poses two major problems. Pain is a perceptual experience so how can it be accurately measured, and where treatment is offered how can its efficacy be judged, when it may be necessary to include in the measurement such factors as the patient's ability to cope better or to improve their mobility.

In the past, too much reliance has been placed on empiricism and the anecdotal collation of particular cases. Wild claims have been made for the efficacy of specific treatments when clearly such success is not reproducible (Rees, 1975; Schreuder, 1982).

Measurement

It is often suggested that poverty and increasing age predispose to chronic pain and that the aged are less able to tolerate persistent discomfort. This is not confirmed from studies (Larson & Marcer, 1984) although it is possible that, while the tolerance for cutaneous pain increases, that for deep 'muscle' pain decreases (Woodrow et al., 1972). Whatever the mechanisms, in practice adequate measurement of pain in the old is more difficult. Apart from obvious factors such as senility and confusion, the impact of systemic diseases can reduce any patient's abilities to co-operate. There is little in the literature to confirm the other oft held notion that the aged are less sensitive to acute pain.

The primary objectives in pain measurement in any patient concern the need to assess the severity of the initial symptoms, to measure the response to initial and continued treatment, and to gauge some outcome statistic to validate the treatment amongst the whole patient group.

Pain intensity

The nature of pain is such that all measurements tend to be subjective and are either obtained by self-analysis by the patient or with the use of trained observers. The latter tend to reduce the positive bias observed in chronic patients who, as the result of a study, have an unusual amount of attention lavished upon them. Standard scales of severity and relief are commonly used and these should be combinations of verbal rating and visual analogue types. Where a number of scales are used, cross-correlation will help to improve the validity of the measures obtained, even when the results are contrary to expectation (Evans et al., 1982). These types of measurement are extremely useful in testing the response to single doses of drugs such as new analgesics but have limited roles in other respects. In many chronic states it is possible that responses will not be observed for a considerable period of time. For example, patients undergoing acupuncture treatment may take several weeks to respond. In other situations, e.g. migraine, the natural history of the pain waxes and wanes, making sequential analysis difficult. Thus, it is necessary to include other tests, such as global measures, tablet counts, frequency of demands for pain relief, and mood and activity scales. In addition, it is of value to record the temporal aspects of pain. The McGill pain questionnaire has proved to be a useful tool in this respect as it is reliable and quick to complete (Melzack, 1983). These types of analysis are extremely important where physical therapies are in use. Often it may be impossible to produce acceptable control groups, e.g. acupuncture, or ethically acceptable to have a placebo group, e.g. percutaneous cordotomy, and it is then paramount that accurate recordings of patients' responses are observed.

Where treatment includes a number of modalities given concurrently, then outcome measures have a place. These at least will show trends in the responses for large numbers of patients and may go some way to suppress individual bias. End-points with regard to treatment can be set and the percentages of patients achieving these goals can be recorded (Evans, 1985). In the aged, the quality of life indices will obviously be relevant. Frequently the only outcome in response to treatment is the observation that a greater range of movement or activity is achieved before pain supervenes.

General management

From the foregoing it will be appreciated that there are two essential elements in the composition of a patient's pain: the primary physical disorder, such as the arthritic process or the expanding malignant tumour, and the emotional reaction to the problem, i.e. the amount of distress that is caused. This has over the years occasioned two almost opposing schools of management: the peripheral 'attack', where pain is treated by such physical methods as injections or drug therapy, and the central 'attack', where pain is controlled by psychological methods (Crue, 1985). However, this 'either/or' type of management is rarely effective and it is only where an integrated approach is used, combining all modalities, that worthwhile results are obtained. A wide variety of treatments are available (Table 16.4).

Physical methods

A graded approach is to be advocated. Simple physical forms of treatment, such as physiotherapy, acupuncture, exercises, manipulation or heat therapy, should be employed first. A finite course of treatment should be offered and realistic goals or end-points set. For many patients, repetition of treatment after an interval is worth considering. It is not unusual for patients to obtain increased mobility and increased self-esteem as a result of these treatments rather than obvious reductions in pain.

Table 16.4. Treatment modalities for chronic pain

	Treatment modalities	
Physical	Psychological	Pharmacological
Simple non-invasive	Counselling	Analgesics — NSAIDs
Simple invasive	Relaxation	Narcotic analgesics
Injections	Hypnosis	Sedatives
Nerve destruction	Group therapy	Antidepressants
Empirical methods	Operant conditioning	Antiepileptics
Cryotherapy	Biofeedback	Steroids
Radiofrequency lesion	Goal setting	Adrenergic blockers
	Psychotherapy	Topical creams
		Antiemetics

Acupuncture is a most useful method of treatment in the older patient. It is accepted well, avoids the risks of other forms of treatment and is particularly suited to arthritic conditions. It is suggested that there is a significant placebo effect and patients' beliefs about the treatment can influence the outcome. This may explain why the initial high response (60–70%) to a course of treatment is not sustained (Richardson & Vincent, 1986). However, animal evidence would suggest that partial analgesia can be achieved (Melzack, 1984). There are no predictors indicating who will do well but, whichever method of acupuncture is employed, if no progress is observed after three or four treatments then it is unlikely that long-term gain will be obtained. By contrast, the use of transcutaneous electrical nerve stimulation (TENS) should be capable of producing a reduction in pain at the first session. The best results are observed where considerable time and effort is taken to educate the patients and locate the best dermatomal positions. It does not work particularly well for intermittent movement related pain or the hyperaesthesia associated with many reflex sympathetic dystrophies. Many aged patients suffer practical difficulties which limit the benefit, e.g. lack of assistance for placement of pads and difficulties in adjusting the fine controls. In addition, most studies report a fall off with time, the peak effect is within six months and few patients after one year are still using the machine regularly (Woolf, 1984).

Many patients are offered injections either for assistance in diagnosis or as definitive treatment. The range is great, from simple trigger point injections to epidurals and plexus blocks. In the majority, local anaesthetics with or without depot steroid drugs will be used, although in cancer related pain neurolytic blocks may well be considered. The two principal considerations affecting aged patients are drug toxicity and the production of side-effects. The inappropriate use of high concentrations or large volumes of local anaesthetics may put patients at risk rather than provide benefit. For example, it has yet to be adequately explained why prolonged pain relief can be obtained after simple local anaesthetic injections unless it is a placebo response. Therefore the use of large doses of local anaesthetic, as in the case of hip block for osteoarthritic pain, has to be questioned (Edmonds-Seal, 1982). Likewise, careful consideration must be given to the types of solution used for epidural injections. Studies have shown that for the relief of back pain many factors are contributory to the results obtained (Yates, 1978). Since the tolerance of aged patients to local anaesthetics is low, it would seem prudent in most cases to use normal saline as both the carrier and the volume component for epidural blocks.

The development of side-effects following local anaesthetic injections is uncommon. However, where blocks containing steroid preparations are used the risks are increased. There are no reports to date relating to specific hazards from peripheral injections of steroids but neither are there adequate data confirming any efficacy. Where benefit is achieved, it is reasonable to continue treatment at intervals using the minimum effective dosage. Studies have demonstrated some degree of adrenocortical suppression following epidural steroid administration (Jacobs *et al.*, 1983) and it is inadvisable to repeat blocks at intervals of less than one month in this group of patients. This suppression may be produced by leakage of steroid into the cerebrospinal fluid, with the subsequent rostral spread to the cerebral ventricles inducing effects on the pituitary–hypothalamic axis.

Some patients after epidural steroid injections do experience short-term feelings of malaise, although the injection of depot steroids into other tissues is unlikely to produce similar systemic reactions.

Psychological techniques

Symptom control is the goal of every pain therapist, yet there are many conditions in which good pain relief can be difficult to achieve. The pain on movement in the arthritic patient is a typical example where drugs and injections can be of limited value. Yet even where good pain control can be obtained, fear, anxiety and lack of understanding may well ensure that the aged patient remains distressed. Physical disabilities can prevent patients moving about freely and they may become trapped in their homes. They may become lonely, depressed and highly dependent on others. Frequently the support they require is not forthcoming and in these situations the level of pain may well increase.

Clearly these types of difficulty cannot be resolved by physical methods and it is necessary to rely on supportive techniques or psychological care for patients. Gross psychological disease is uncommon but where overt depression is observed it should be treated. Frequently a small night-time dose of an antidepressant is adequate, particularly if the drug has sedative properties. Compounds such as mianserin, dothiepin and clomipramine are suitable, although there is an increased incidence of side-effects in this age group. Dementia can cause patients to appear in extreme pain and the screaming patient can be distressing both to staff and relatives. The best relief can be obtained through good nursing practice and the use of simple analgesics and sedatives. Aggressive techniques, such as anaesthetic blocks, produce bad results, are technically difficult to perform and frequently bring increased distress to relatives.

For the majority, the best assistance is achieved through behaviour modification, relaxation techniques, hypnosis and group therapy (Fulton, 1985). This type of approach has a number of advantages. It provides a focal point for patients to attend, introduces them to others in similar difficulties and helps foster a group spirit. It enables patients to be relieved of fears and anxieties and encourages them to be more positive about life. The frequent visits to the hospital, although expensive of services in the short term, can reduce the long-term dependency on hospital care. The patient is taught to accept the pain, to alter their activity to give them greater mobility before pain occurs and to learn how to relieve muscular spasm.

Drug therapy

Drugs are frequently used and misused in attempts to manage chronic non-malignant pain. Aged patients are very susceptible to side-effects and often cause problems in maintenance and control. Analgesics remain the principal agents of choice. These are usually the simple or non-steroidal anti-inflammatory drugs (NSAIDs); however, narcotic analgesics are increasingly being prescribed. Indifference to their use and tolerance are observed with all analgesics. Gastric irritation remains a major complication with all NSAIDs. Many patients take large quantities and frequently there is duplication in medication. It is naive and optimistic to believe that the continuous use of such drugs has a significant impact on the level of pain and the prudent approach is to withdraw as many as possible of these analgesic compounds. This can be done by substituting courses of physical therapy, such as physiotherapy, ultrasound and hydrotherapy. Subsequently NSAIDs can be administered in short courses to get over particular episodes of increased pain where there is evidence of a peripheral (tissue) component or active inflammation is observed (raised ESR, etc.). Patients may resist such strong attempts to alter medication and it may be necessary to provide a buffer with a simple analgesic such as paracetamol which is both cheap and an effective pain killer.

A limited number of patients may prove refractory to this kind of management. For them, positive consideration should be given to the use of narcotic analgesics. They should meet certain criteria (Table 16.5).

If the pain is opiate sensitive and the patient is happy to receive the medication, then a twice daily regimen of sustained-release morphine can be used. A larger morning dose will correlate well with increased activity during the day. Although dependence on the drug is inevitable,

Advanced disease	**Table 16.5.** Criteria for opiate
Movement related pain	therapy in chronic non-malignant pain
Failure of all other reasonable therapy	
Proven response to opiates	
Insight into the role of the drug	
Informed consent	
Regular pattern of administration	

the improved analgesia and the increased quality of life justify the use. However, strict prevention of side-effects such as nausea and constipation is essential if patient co-operation is to be maintained. Alternative medications include methadone and, where suitable, oxycodone suppositories for night-time use.

Anxiolytics and night sedatives are often requested by patients. Low doses of benzodiazepines may have a role in the management of the agitated aged patient but the shorter acting compounds are preferred to drugs such as lorazepam as it is easier to modify the amount needed and reduce the incidence of 'hang over' effects. Unfortunately they have no analgesic properties and for many patients they only increase the level of confusion. It is frequently better to prescribe such drugs as night sedation. In practice patients who suffer interrupted patterns of sleep are less able to tolerate pain.

Postherpetic neuralgia

Of the many conditions that present in the old, postherpetic neuralgia is the condition most refractory to treatment. The mechanism of pain production is ill understood. Two quite distinct types of pain are observed: a superficial hypersensitivity, often in a dermatomal distribution and closely aligned to the area of partial or complete anaesthesia, and a second deep-seated pain, frequently severe and often vague in distribution. It is usually the latter pain that is difficult to contain. The nature of the pain implies different conducting mechanisms and demonstrates that the consequences of the viral infection are widespread on the nervous system.

It appears that zoster is the unmasking of a latent virus that has been present since the primary varicella infection in early life. The reason that it presents late has been attributed to reductions in antibody titres with increasing age. This correlates well with the high incidence of the condition in the aged, those with malignant disease and those on immunosuppressive drugs. It has also been stated that local trauma, surgery and radiotherapy can be trigger factors. The term zoster is derived from the Greek word for girdle and aptly describes the dermatomal distribution of the disease. It is probable that the virus attacks sensory nerve fibres, cells in the dorsal root ganglion and cells in the dorsal horn area of the grey matter.

Zoster infections are rarely seen in childhood but the condition is common with advancing years (Hope-Simpson, 1975). The principal sites of attack are the head and neck and thoracic regions. Pain is a severe complication of the condition and when symptoms persist beyond two months the term postherpetic neuralgia is used. As the incidence of zoster increases, so does the incidence of the protracted pain of postherpetic neuralgia (Table 16.6). It is uncommon in those under 50 years of age and is more common in women (Burney & Peeters-Asdourian, 1985).

Table 16.6. Incidence of postherpetic neuralgia

Age (years)	Incidence (%)
20–29	1
30–39	8
40–49	7
50–59	18
60–69	37
70–79	45

Management of the problem can be split into three phases: care for the initial viral infection, care for the intermediate phase up to six months, and late management. It is not proposed to discuss therapy for the initial period, although it should be stressed that the condition is often very painful and that powerful analgesics should be supplied readily. The introduction of antiviral agents such as acyclovir and idoxuridine have had a major impact on terminating the acute attack but it is too soon to know if the incidence of postherpetic neuralgia will fall in parallel.

There is a common belief that if active treatment can be undertaken in the intermediate phase then the problem can be aborted. There is little controlled evidence to support this contention but, clearly, aggressive early treatment does at least offer the patient the hope and possibility of an early remission. Two distinct types of treatment have been advanced. The use of steroids has been advocated to minimize changes in the nerves and the use of sympathetic blocks has also been advocated to relieve the deafferentation element of the condition.

The steroid of choice is methyl prednisolone and this can be administered peripherally into the tissues in combination with a local anaesthetic or, for large areas such as the trunk, epidural administration has been advised. Studies have suggested that where this treatment is given within six months of the onset, improvement in pain levels can be expected. Repetition of the injection on at least one occasion is worthwhile even when no initial improvement is seen. Sympathetic blocks, either lumbar, thoracic or stellate, have a much more limited role. The same time requirement applies but it is usual to perform the injections with local anaesthetic and not with neurolytic substances. Repetition is essential and the interval should not be greater than one week. In view of the morbidity of the blocks, the most practical is the stellate injection for the relief of head and neck pain (Loesser, 1986).

Sadly, many patients present late for management. They are burdened by persistent pain and their resistance and morale is often low. As two differing types of pain exist, it is frequently necessary to employ several modes of treatment. A vast array of treatments have been offered and the range merely reflects the failure to understand the nature of the condition. No one treatment is outstanding and it may well be necessary to offer the complete range to provide relief.

It is always important to direct part of the treatment towards the area of superficial discomfort in an attempt to relieve hypersensitivity. Local anaesthetic sprays and ointments are of value in this respect. They can be applied frequently, are relatively non-toxic and have the additional attribute of massage. Many compounds are available, and if nothing else at least the patients can feel that they are doing something positive for their condition. Vibration and percussion are also of some value as many patients are less distressed by heavy pressure than by light touch. TENS electrodes placed around the periphery of the lesions can also work in a similar fashion. Recently the ionophoretic use of neurotoxins such as vincristine has been advocated as a method of selectively inhibiting conduction in sensory nerve fibres but early studies are not promising: only 27% were showing improvement after six weeks (Layman *et al.*, 1986).

Systemic support is usually achieved by attempting to reduce nerve excitability. Carbamazepine in low dosage (300 mg per day) should be tried and a similarly small dose of clomipramine (10 mg) may help sleep patterns and reactive depression. Alternative compounds include clonazepam, sodium valproate and flupenthixol. Postherpetic neuralgia is an opiate insensitive pain but it is worth assessing responsiveness in individual patients and if a positive result is obtained then the evening use of buprenorphine, to avoid ambulatory side-effects, should be tried. Unfortunately, almost 50% of the patients receiving this drug will find it unacceptable and for these a short-acting opiate such as dextromoramide is of value for peak pain.

Although it is intriguing to believe that if complete denervation can be achieved by techniques such as neurolysis then pain will subside, in reality this is not the case. The results from this approach are uniformly bad and the potential side-effects in otherwise healthy individuals are great. This is a reflection of the viral damage occurring in the cord which always remains proximal to any nerve destruction short of cordotomy.

Other neuralgias

There are four interesting neuralgias more commonly observed in the old. Two are the consequences of vascular disease — thalamic syndrome and post-amputation stump pain — and two are of unknown aetiology — trigeminal neuralgia and perineal neuralgia. All cause intense pain.

Thalamic syndrome

This diffuse pain invariably affects one half of the body and in more than 80% of cases occurs following cerebrovascular haemorrhage or occlusion. It presents within two weeks to two years of the injury. Typically the pain is ill defined, not related to dermatomes and affects primarily skin muscle and bone. The pain may have a spreading character and there may often be a focus on one part of the body from where the pain emanates. The characteristics are typically autonomic, with hypersensitivity and burning sensations. The condition derives its name from the belief that damage to the internal capsule is the causative factor.

As for postherpetic neuralgia, there is no effective treatment. Peripheral nerve blocks and rhizotomy have no place. Sympathetic denervation has been advocated on the basis that blocking sympathetic outflow reduces the input coming from peripheral somatic receptors but the results are highly variable (Pagni, 1984). It is probable that more effective results can be achieved by nerve stimulation, either peripherally using TENS or centrally by dorsal column stimulation. However, for many patients the only help that can be derived is through medication. Attempts have been made to alter the chemical balance within the central nervous system and a number of novel compounds have been explored. Drugs such as bromocriptine, baclofen, cinnarazine and naloxone have been tried, as well as the more traditional antidepressant and antiepileptic compounds. None are particularly meritorious but this type of empirical approach in the long term may offer solutions. Ironically opiates are particularly ineffective, less than 10% of patients given i.v. morphine showed any reduction in pain and in a number pain was in fact increased (Evans, personal data).

Stump pain

Although it is traditional to group all post-amputation pain under the general heading of stump pain, there are in reality two clear problems. The first concerns peripheral injury changes in the nerve at the site of amputation and is frequently associated with neuromata, whilst the second — phantom limb pain — is a form of deafferentation injury. In many patients there may be components from both causes.

Stump pain is usually associated with localized tenderness and hypersensitivity near to the nerve ending and can lead to considerable difficulty in the use of prostheses. A combined approach to treatment is often effective. Simple treatments such as TENS therapy, percussion and massage can provide temporary benefit. Likewise, local anaesthetic injections of bupivacaine into the trigger zone can provide more sustained relief. When the relief remains inadequate, permanent benefit may be achieved by producing a neurolytic injury with phenol or producing a cryosurgical injury (Evans, 1981a). The latter is to be preferred. Unfortunately, both carry the risk of producing an increase in the pain by damaging otherwise healthy tissue. It is always difficult to obtain a precise location for the trigger point. Many surgical techniques have been developed to try to reduce the incidence of stump pain and they are to a degree successful but if pain starts to return further operations are rarely successful.

Phantom limb pain by definition is the persistence of sensation, usually painful, of a limb that has been removed. Most amputees will suffer some phantom sensations in the immediate postoperative period but a minority will develop painful sensations, often burning or hyperaesthetic in character , which increase in severity with time. The aged are more predisposed to this problem. It is a form of deafferentation syndrome and like many of these neuralgias is difficult to treat. The problem may well be associated with a significant psychological overlay. The pain is often extreme and many patients resort to narcotic analgesics in an attempt to control symptoms (Evans, 1981b). The use of all the centrally active drugs, such as the anticonvulsants, the antiepileptics and the phenothiazines, should be explored and the patient should be offered both hypnosis therapy and psychotherapy as concurrent management (Katz, 1985). In those patients where the burning element of the pain can be relieved by local anaesthetic injections, chemical sympathectomy should be attempted. In the past, cordotomy and sensory rhyzolysis have been undertaken to relieve pain and whilst the initial results are often very good, studies have shown that within two years over 50% of patients have suffered a recurrence of pain.

Trigeminal neuralgia

This is a well described but uncommon condition which affects branches of the fifth cranial nerve. It is more common in the old, affects women more often than men and more frequently presents in the lower two divisions of the nerve. The pain is intermittent, often lancinating and can be provoked by such simple activities as talking, smiling or chewing food. The spasms of pain are extreme — hence the old name 'tic doloreux' — and are very disabling and distressing for the patient. The management of the condition is clear. Carbamazepine in doses up to 1200 mg per day should produce a marked reduction in pain. Provided drug side-effects are not a problem, then this is the standard treatment of choice. The drug dose can be adjusted according to the severity of pain. For those in whom this is unacceptable, the most promising form of treatment is microvascular decompression of the trigeminal nerve root. In over 90% of patients so treated, a minor vascular abnormality causing pressure on the nerve root can be observed. Padding the vessel away from the nerve produces relief of symptoms without causing any permanent nerve injury (Janetta, 1976). In those patients declining carbamazepine treatment or unsuitable for surgery the possibility of a radiofrequency destruction of the gasserian ganglion exists. This will produce anaesthesia in the treated side of the face but relapses of pain will occur in as many as 20% of patients (Pawl, 1979). Many other forms of treatment have been suggested but their value is limited in comparison to the three so far described. Cryoanalgesia remains the most promising. It has proved easy to freeze branches of the nerve, and periods of analgesia in excess of the period of nerve destruction have been observed. (Barnard, Lloyd and Glynn 1978). The recent innovation of a Gausserian block with glycerin to produce pain relief without anaesthesia has not proved outstanding and is not now widely practised.

Perineal neuralgia

This unusual condition, often thought to have a strong psychological overlay, is more frequently observed in the aged. It predominantly affects women but isolated cases in males are also observed. In the majority there may be a surgical trigger such as a pelvic floor repair or an anorectal procedure but in others spontaneous pain occurs. The pain is posture related, always causing discomfort on sitting and frequently relieved by standing or walking. Another unusual characteristic is that sleep is never disturbed by pain. A variety of symptoms are reported. These frequently include, burning vulval and vaginal pain, hyperaesthesia, tenesmus and general feelings of pelvic pressure. Natural activities such as urination and defecation do not usually influence either the severity or frequency of symptoms. A diagnostic caudal block provides limited information, as over 50% of patients will not get temporary pain inhibition. For those that do, peripheral measures such as TENS or further injections of local anaesthetics are advised. For the remainder, general measures such as acupuncture and medication are advocated. Low dose clomipramine and carbamazepine in combination can be dramatically effective. Second-line drugs include clonazepam and sodium valproate. Analgesic drugs, by contrast, have little place; the pain is typically insensitive to opiates.

Most patients, by the time that they attend the pain clinic, will have a strong emotional overlay and it may well be necessary to treat symptoms of acute anxiety or hysterical conversion. Because of these factors the condition can produce major disruption to domestic and family life and it is not unusual for extremes of behaviour to be observed. In these cases prolonged counselling, constructive support and firm control of patients' activities is required to induce behavioural changes.

Degenerative joint disease

One of the particularly sad aspects of chronic pain therapy is the management of patients with degenerative joint disease. Osteoarthritis is the commonest of all rheumatic diseases and causes symptoms in a large proportion of aged people (Wood, 1976). In contrast, the incidence of chronic back pain tends to diminish in the old.

Most patients seek and gain help by attending departments of rheumatology or orthopaedic surgery. It is only those few that prove refractory to traditional therapy who appear in pain relief clinics. Needless to say, they are the extremes of rheumatological disease. They usually have multiple joint symptoms, are severely crippled and often have marked joint deformity. They present a pathetic group, greatly dependent on others. Their pain is invariably movement related and because of this many suffer the indignity of being confined to a bed or a wheelchair. The mechanism of pain, progressive joint and capsule destruction, with secondary chemical irritation by kinins and prostagalandins, is no different to other forms of arthritis and is triggered by pressure and abnormal load bearing. However, in this sub-group quite clearly the limitations of drug therapy can be observed. It has already been stated that peripherally acting analgesics and NSAIDs have a ceiling effect and only a limited response can be observed. In most cases it is better to replace the many analgesics with a very basic compound such as paracetamol and then reintroduce NSAIDs for short courses (7–10 days) to overcome particularly severe episodes of pain. In this manner the value of NSAIDs may still be observed and the patient will suffer fewer side-effects whilst still having some analgesic support.

Secondary depression is a feature of prolonged suffering and one of the difficult decisions when treating patients with degenerative joint disease is knowing when to provide active treatment for this problem. There are no absolute indications but signs such as early morning waking, prolonged crying bouts, loneliness and persistent melancholia should be taken seriously. The choice of agents for the aged is limited but compounds such as fluvoxamine and mianserin have proved to be particularly suitable.

It has already been stressed that a variety of measures are often required. Simple physical techniques such as heat, exercises, wax bathes and hydrotherapy are encouraged and abundant use is made of acupuncture even though these techniques may have been used before. The latter technique is particularly useful as needling can easily be applied for multiple joint involvement. Unfortunately, the use of TENS is much more restricted. Often patients do not have adequate dexterity to easily handle the machines or they may find physical difficulty in adequately placing electrodes on the skin surface.

The use of local anaesthetic injections with or without the use of depot steroids is often undervalued in these patients. Certainly the frequent use of steroids is to be deprecated; however, the occasional injection of a trigger site over a joint or a ligament with a mixture of methyl prednisolone and bupivacaine can be very beneficial. On occasions, the benefit is sustained but even when relief is temporary the psychological value to the patient is high. Unfortunately, the use of such injections in load bearing joints such as the hip is extremely harmful and is strongly condemned.

Where pain is primarily spinal in origin and not eased by simple methods then consideration can be given to techniques such as epidural and facet joint injection of steroids. There is an extensive literature on the subject and, although it is frequently reported that little long-term benefit is derived, the injections are frequently given (Benzon, 1986). Much of the argument on the subject concerns the specific actions of the steroids when administered. As yet this is not adequately explained but in one of the few properly controlled studies on their use it was clearly shown that in patients receiving epidural injections, significantly better results were observed in those receiving steroids than in those receiving normal saline or local anaesthetic injections alone (Yates, 1978). There are few convincing studies on the benefit of facet joint rhyzolysis and it is likely that simple injections into the joints are as effective as are attempts at radiofrequency lesion generator destruction of nerves to the joints.

There is little doubt that these patients need care and sympathy for their many complaints but often resources are inadequate to provide this support and even where they are available it is unlikely that an out-standing improvement in pain will occur. This concern for their welfare has prompted many physicians to assess the value of narcotic analgesics in these patients. The most acceptable agent appears to be sustained-release morphine (MST) given twice daily. Of 27 patients treated with morphine, 10–20 mg in the morning and 10 mg at night, 10 (37%) reported improvement in pain whilst 14 (52%) reported improvement in well being (Evans, unpublished data). The risks of addiction and tolerance are exaggerated and the more common problems of respiratory depression and sedation are not observed on these low doses. In the very old, dysphoria and confusion may be noted but in all cases stopping the drug resolves the problem.

The pain of cancer

With the increasing age of the populace and death occurring from a number of causes, a relatively high incidence of cancer related pain will present. The more common conditions in the aged include pancreatic carcinoma, large bowel malignancy, head and neck tumours and, in men, bladder and prostatic cancer. Carcinoma of the lung is also prominent, especially as there is an increasing incidence in women. All these tumours have a tendency to cause pain and the principal reasons are soft tissue enlargement, nerve compression and the appearance of skeletal deposits. Treatment is also responsible for the appearance of pain and in one study approximately one-third suffered pain as a secondary feature, chronic postoperative pain being the most common (Foley et al., 1978).

The incidence of pain associated with cancer is always difficult to predict. A number of tumours, e.g. ovary and prostate, may have pain as an early symptom whilst others, e.g. cervical cancer, will have pain as a late feature. However, most studies have shown that as many as 60% of terminally ill patients will suffer severe pain and 30% of patients will die without adequate relief of symptoms (Stjernsward, 1985).

Management can be separated into three overlapping areas:
  (i) the patient,
  (ii) the disease,
  (iii) the symptom.

Most seriously ill patients fear death but cancers seem to provoke excessive dread and often the illness gives rise to feelings of helplessness and loss of personal control. This is particularly apparent if the tumour is aggressive and attempts at treatment are unsuccessful. The patients will feel hopeless and may well become markedly depressed. Anxiety is frequent in patients with cancer and they will become distressed not only about their future but about their family needs and financial support. All these features will be enhanced if unrelieved pain is an associated factor, or physical limitations and debility resulting from the disease prevent normal social activity and contacts with family and friends.

Clearly the cancer patient has a great number of needs which require careful evaluation. The advent of hospices and home care teams has had significant effect on helping these patients to cope. With this type of help, patients are given an enormous degree of support. Their symptoms of pain are normally well managed, they feel secure and often develop a sense of belonging in response to the love and understanding of the staff. All this helps patients to gain acceptance of their condition and gives them the self-esteem that is often denied them in large institutions. Frequently it is the very trivial problems that cause patients great distress and provoke exacerbations in pain.

By the time the cancer patient is referred to the pain relief clinic, active treatment for the disease has usually been concluded. However, further radiotherapy, chemotherapy and surgery should not be ignored. Sometimes, if the tumour spreads to a new area, it may be possible to reintroduce therapy. Of late there has been a revival in surgery for advanced bone disease, not as an attempt to treat the condition but to provide support to maintain mobility and to relieve overt nerve root pressure. Inevitably the most difficult decision to make is when such heroic attempts should cease. This is always an individual decision but certainly the degree of additional suffering that may be caused, the potential improvements in the quality of life that may be achieved, and the morale and hopes of the patient are important considerations.

Pain remains the most significant symptom associated with malignancy and the one that causes the most distress and fear. Part of this fear is the realization by patients that the symptom is difficult to control and the increases in pain may herald advancement of the disease. Thus, simple non-invasive pain measures such as acupuncture and TENS are not particularly effective. The principal measures are the use of analgesics and the use of nerve destructive procedures. None will solve all pain problems but there are certain types of pain that are better suited to particular therapies.

Analgesics

Traditionally an 'analgesic ladder' is used. The weakest and most simple analgesics are used first and as pain is increased so is the strength of the analgesics. A typical classification is shown in Table 16.7.

Table 16.7. Classification of analgesics

Weak/non-opiate	Weak opiate	Strong opiate
Aspirin	Codeine	Morphine
Paracetamol	Dextropropoxyphene	Diamorphine
NSAID	Pentazocine	Methadone
Nefopam	Oxycodone	Dextromoramide
Meptazinol		Dipipanone
		Buprenorphine
		Nalbuphine

In general, all weak analgesics have ceiling effects and increased use does not equate with increased efficacy. With the exception of mixed agonist/antagonist compounds such as buprenorphine and nalbuphine, the strong analgesics are pure agonists and the only limitation on their use is the development of side-effects.

Even when patients require strong analgesics it is sensible to continue the use of non-steroidal or aspirin-like compounds. Their action is peripheral and they are more effective than the opiates at controlling soft tissue and inflammatory components of pain.

Morphine remains the principal strong analgesic and has replaced many of the more traditional cocktail mixtures which were unnecessarily rigid in their recipes and produced excessive sedation. It is now formulated as a slow-release compound (MST) and this has resolved many of the difficulties of oral morphine solutions. The tablets can be taken twice daily and provide good 24 h coverage. There is no limit on the dose required and the only constraints are the development of pain relief or the production of excessive sedation. Although there is no evidence to suggest that sustained-release morphine tablets provide a better quality of analgesia than four hourly administered morphine solutions, there is evidence to confirm the improved sleep patterns in these patients (Hanks *et al.*, 1987).

The tablets are available in 10, 30, 60 and 100 mg sizes which enable infinite variations in dosage to be obtained. When commencing therapy, early instability can be buffered by using a short-acting potent opiate such as dextromoramide 5 mg or by commencing patients on oral morphine solution until titration is complete. The former drug can also be used for the occasional episodes of breakthrough pain without significantly interfering with the background pain relief of the morphine. For those patients unable to swallow tablets, oral solutions of morphine are available but these have to be administered four hourly and it is usually necessary to supplement the drug at night. Diamorphine in tablet or liquid form is also used for maintenance. It has little to recommend its continuation. Pharmacologically it is a pro-drug for morphine and clinically it is difficult to distinguish the two compounds in spite of the exaggerated claims made of lower side-effects, less sedation and improved pain relief made for diamorphine (Twycross & Lack, 1984). Only when the drugs are given by the spinal route can differences be observed. It is then noted that the duration of analgesia with diamorphine after a single injection is significantly shorter than that for morphine (Evans *et al.*, 1987).

For those patients intolerant to morphine, a number of other compounds are available. Dipipanone and methadone have proved popular. But they need to be given regularly. Methadone poses special problems. It has a long half-life and the dose has to be built up slowly over a period of one week. During this time the quality of pain control may be less than adequate.

The mixed agonist/antagonist compounds, such as buprenorphine and nalbuphine, are gaining popularity and can be used as second-line drugs if morphine is not tolerated. On occasions, patients may be found taking these compounds in conjunction with morphine. Although there is no specific contraindication to this practice, there is little to recommend it as it probably leads to a lessening of analgesic effect.

The new analgesics were introduced in an attempt to reduce the incidence of side-effects associated with opiates. This is not always the case and when it does occur there is usually a reduction in the quality of analgesia. With buprenorphine only half of the patients taking the drug sublingually will gain adequate pain relief and of those a further 50% may stop the drug because of unacceptable side-effects. In contrast, over 90% of patients will obtain some analgesia following morphine administration.

Parenteral administration of opiates is usually unnecessary until patients become debilitated. However, increasing use is being made of continuous infusion pumps. They are particularly suited to home-care nursing and it is one of the situations where the use of diamorphine is a distinct advantage. The drug is dispensed in powder form and consequently it is possible to produce small volume, high concentration solutions which are ideal for the battery powered portable pumps. A once daily change of the syringe is sufficient and when this method is combined with the use of a short-acting oral opiate, high quality pain relief is achieved. There is a subjective impression that the incidence of side-effects with this approach is less than that following oral morphine and certainly when large daily doses of opiate are required it is an appropriate method.

Whichever analgesic is used to relieve severe pain it is essential that early consideration is given to the potential side-effects. Patients fear taking opiates because they believe the many myths attributed to these drugs and because they believe it signals the end of their lives. Thus, concern for this problem and adequate explanation of the action of narcotic analgesics is an important part of management. Constipation, nausea, vomiting and sedation are the immediate problems and they must be treated early if the patient is to continue with narcotic analgesics.

Nausea and vomiting

Provided the dose is increased slowly these side-effects are short lived and although transient nausea can be observed in patients on oral morphine immediately following each dose this is usually well tolerated. For those who prove refractory, a once or twice daily dose of haloperidol 1.5 mg is usually effective. Persistent vomiting in patients taking opiates should be investigated as it is more probably due to physiological mechanisms such as bowel obstruction or uraemia than due to side-effects of a specific drug.

Constipation

This is a most disabling problem for patients and must be managed from the commencement of opiate therapy. It is preferable to give a combination of a mild laxative such as sennoside or lactulose, as well as a faecal softener such as docusate sodium. Where possible they should be encouraged to have a varied diet.

Sedation and respiratory depression

It is inevitable that some degree of sedation will occur with opiate administration but with correct drug management the quality of life for patients should not be impaired. Respiratory depression is overstressed and is not clinically a problem. Usually the stimulus of severe pain is sufficient to maintain adequate respiratory drive. Only on rare occasions, when somatic pain inadequately controlled with opiates has subsequently been relieved by intrathecal neurolysis, has this problem been reported (Hanks et al., 1980) and then reduction in the analgesic dose has relieved the problem.

Tolerance

Tolerance is a feature observed with many kinds of drugs but particularly opiates. It will occur, but the risk should not be over-emphasized. It is noted that the longer the duration of drug administration the longer will be the periods between drug increases and the smaller will be the increments.

Spinal opiates

Unfortunately, one of the problems with prolonged opiate administration has been the gradual escalation in dose. In the last eight years considerable interest has been attracted by spinal opiates. The implication has been that giving the narcotic analgesic epidurally or intrathecally a better quality of analgesia can be achieved with a much smaller dose. This has yet to be adequately confirmed. After single administrations, prolonged episodes of analgesia are observed; however, after repeated administration, tachyphylaxis rapidly occurs and to an extent this negates the benefit of this approach. In many of the published studies from those committed to this approach the dose of morphine at the time of change-over has been relatively small, so it has been difficult to assess true benefit; in other studies this method has been used to treat opiate insensitive pain with anticipated poor results (Editorial, 1986).

A variety of implantable systems are now available and whilst there is little doubt that they can deliver opiates at constant low rates it is also abundantly clear that much greater understanding of the pharmacology of both the drugs, the route and the dura is required before this method can be strongly recommended.

Destructive methods for pain relief

In 1955 Maher pioneered the use of intrathecal neurolysis as an absolute method of pain relief for patients with the pain of cancer. Since that time a number of techniques have been developed (Table 16.8) and although a variety of neurolytic solutions have been used the principal agents remain alcohol and phenol.

Although neurolysis appears to offer a quality of pain relief unobtainable by other means, it suffers a number of serious disadvantages (Table 16.9).

Table 16.8. Neurolytic techniques

Technique	Agent	Condition
Intrathecal block	Absolute alcohol 5% Phenol in glycerin	Peripheral somatic pain
Coeliac axis block	60% Alcohol	Pancreatic pain Stomach or other pain Visceral tumour
Epidural block	8-10% Phenol in water	Sacral pain, generalized somatic pain
Pituitary injection	Absolute alcohol	Metastatic bone pain

Table 16.9. Limitations of neurolysis

Non selective of nerve fibres
Permanent
Unpredictable in effect
Serious side-effects
Liability to deafferentation pain

All neurolytic agents will coagulate protein and hence do not show selectivity for particular types of nerve fibre. It has been advocated that certain 'weaker' solutions will have less effect on motor fibres but this is not confirmed by clinical practice. In consequence it is often necessary to restrict the use of the technique to sites where motor activity is of a lesser importance. Furthermore, there is an incidence of between 10% and 24% of incontinence when blocks are performed in the lower thoracic or lumbar areas.

Although pain relief can be dramatic when it occurs, it is often unpredictable. Frequently only a brief effect is observed and, where analgesia is sustained, many studies report that in spite of persisting anaesthesia, pain relief may only last about three months (Katz, 1974). The technique is of no value for head and neck pain or for that around orifices but is particularly effective for invasive tumours of the neck and thorax. Sadly, not all patients can accept the disassociative sensory loss and complain bitterly of rigidity and wooden feelings in superficial tissues akin to a deafferentation syndrome. In others, inadequate destruction may cause a neuritis which itself can produce intense burning pain.

Thus, it is clear that whilst this technique has a place in relieving the pain of cancer the effective role is severely limited by the significant and serious side-effects.

For some patients with peripheral and unilateral pain it may be possible to offer a percutaneous cordotomy. Whilst this technique has a mortality of 1%, it can provide more refined pain relief without having to resort to complete denervation (Lipton, 1984)

Ironically the most imprecise technique, that of infiltration of alcohol into the coeliac plexus is often the most rewarding and effective of all the neurolytic methods used. The technique is particularly suited to relieving pancreatic pain but it has also been beneficial in relieving stomach and colonic pain.

In summary, whilst a variety of methods can be adopted for the control of cancer pain, morphine and its analogues remain the principal agents of choice in the treatment of severe and advanced pain.

References

Barnard, J.D.W., Lloyd, J.W. & Glynn, C.J. (1978) Cryosurgery in the management of intractable facial pain. *Br. J. Oral Surg.* **16**, 135–142.

Benzon, H.T. (1986) Epidural injections for low back pain and lumbo sacral radiculopathy. *Pain* **24**, 277–297.

Bonica, J.J. (1985) Introduction. In *Evaluation and Treatment of Chronic Pain* (Ed. G.M. Arnoff). Urban & Schwarzenberg, Baltimore, p. xxxi.

Burney, R.G., Peeters-Asdourian, C. (1985) Herpetic neuralgia. *Semin. Anaesth.* **4** (No. 4), 275–280.

Central Statistical Office (1981) *Social Trends No 11.* HMSO, London.

Crue, B.L. (1985) Foreword. In *Evaluation and Treatment of Chronic Pain* (Ed. G.M. Arnoff). Urban & Schwarzenberg, Baltimore.

Editorial (1986) Spinal opiates revisited. *Lancet* **1**, 655–656.

Edmonds-Seal, J. (1982) Regional hip blockade in osteoarthritis. *Anaesthesia* **37**, 147–152.

Evans, P.J.D. (1981a) Cryoanalgesia. *Anaesthesia* **36,** 1003–1013.

Evans, P.J.D. (1981b) Narcotic addiction in patients with chronic pain. *Anaesthesia* **36**, 597–602.

Evans, P.J.D., McQuay, H.J., Rolfe, M., Bullingham, R.E.S. & Moore, R.A. (1982) Zomepirac, placebo and paracetamol/dextropropoxyphene combination compared in orthopaedic postoperative pain. *Br. J. Anaesth.* **54**, 927–934.

Evans, P.J.D. (1985) Simple rating system for assessing treatment outcome in chronic pain patients. In *Advances in Pain Research and Therapy,* Vol. 9 (Eds H.L. Fields., R. Dubner & F. Cervero) Raven Press, New York.

Evans, P.J.D. Kotob, H.I.M. & Rubin, A.P. (1987) Clinical efficacy of Intrathecal morphine versus diamorphine. *Pain Suppl.* **4**, p. S70.

Foley, K., Rogers, A. & Houde, R. (1978) Pain in patients with cancer *Proc. Am. Soc. Cancer Res.* **19**, 357–362.

Fulton, W.M. (1985) Psychological strategies and techniques in pain management. *Semin. Anaesth.* **4** (No.3).

Hanks, G.W., Twycross, R.G. & Lloyd, J.W. (1980) Unexpected complication of successful nerve block. *Anaesthesia* **36**, 37–39 (Eds H.L. Fields *et al.*). Raven Press, New York.

Hanks, G.W., Twycross, R.G. & Bliss, J.M. (1987) Controlled release morphine tablets a double blind study. *Anaesthesia* **42**, 840–845.

Hope-Simpson, R.E. (1975) Post Herpetic Neuralgia. *J. R. Coll. Gen. Pract.* **25**, 571–575.

Jacobs, S., Pullan, P.T., Potter, J.M. & Shenfield, G.M. (1983) Adrenal suppression following extradural steroids *Anaesthesia* **38**, 953–956.

Janetta, P.J. (1976) Microsurgical approach to the trigeminal nerve for Tic Douloureux. *Prog. Neurol. Surg.* **7**, 180–200.

Katz, J. (1974) Current role of neurolytic agents. In *Advances in Neurology* (Ed. J.J. Bovica). Raven Press, New York, Vol. 4.

Katz, R.L. (1985) Post amputation pain. *Semin. Anaesth.* **4** (No. 4), 332–345.

Larson, A.G. & Marcer, D. (1984) The who and why of pain; Analysis by social class. *Br. Med. J.* **288**, 883–886.

Layman, P.R., Argyras, E. & Glunn, C.J. (1986) Ionophoresis of vincristine versus saline in post herpetic neuralgia. *Pain* **25**, 165–170.

Lipton, S. (1984) Percutaneous cordotomy. In *Textbook of Pain* (Eds P. Wall & R. Melzack). Churchill Livingstone, Edinburgh, pp. 632–639.

Loeser, J.D. (1986) Herpes zoster and post herpatic neuralgia *Pain* **25**, 149–164.

Maher, R.M. (1955) Relief of pain in intractable cancer. *Lancet* **1**, 354–360.

Melzack, R. (1983) The McGill Pain Questionnaire. In *Pain Measurement and Assessment.* Raven Press, New York, pp. 247–254.

Melzack, R. (1984) Acupuncture and related forme of folk medicine. In *Textbook of Pain* (Eds P. Wall & R. Melzack). Churchill Livingstone, Edinburgh, pp. 691–700.

Pagni, C.A. (1984) Central pain due to spinal cord and brain stem damage. In *Textbook of Pain* (Eds P. Wall & R. Melzack). Churchill Livingstone, Edinburgh, pp. 481–496.

Pawl, R.P. (1979) *Chronic Pain Primer.* Year Book Publishers, Chicago, pp. 141–168.

Rees, W.E.S. (1975) Multiple bilateral percutaneous rhizolysis. *Med. J. Aust.* **1**, 536.

Richardson, P.H. & Vincent, C.A. (1986) Acupuncture for the treatment of pain. *Pain* **24**, 15–40.

Scott, W.E. (1982) The continuing problem of pain. *J. Roy. Soc. Med.* **75**, 117–120.

Schreuder, M. (1982) Pain relief in herpes zoster. *S. Afr. Med. J.* **63**, 820–821.

306 | *Chapter 16*

Stjernsward, J. (1985) Cancer pain relief: an important global issue. In *Advances in Pain Research and Therapy*, Vol. 9 (Eds H. Fields, R. Dubner & F. Cervero). Raven Press, New York, pp. 555–558.

Todd, E.M. (1985) Pain — historical perspectives. In *Evaluation and Treatment of Chronic Pain* (Ed G.M. Arnoff). Urban & Schwarzenberg, Baltimore, pp. 1–17.

Twycross, R.G. & Lack, S.A. (1984) Diamorphine. In *Symptom Control in Far Advanced Cancer*. Churchill Livingstone, Edinburgh, pp. 190–198.

Wood PHN. (1976) Osteoarthritis in the community. *Clin. Rheum. Dis.* **2**, 497–502.

Woodrow, K.M., Friedman, G.D., Siegelaus, A.B., Collen, M.F. (1972) Pain tolerance: differences according to age, sex and race. *Psychosom. Med.* **34**(6), 548–556.

Woolf, C.J. (1984) Transcutaneous and implanted nerve stimulation. In *Textbook of Pain* (Eds P.D. Wall & R. Melzack). Churchill Livingstone, Edinburgh, pp. 679–690.

Yates, D.W. (1978) A comparison of the types of epidural injection commonly used in the treatment of low back pain. *Rheumatol. Rehabil.* **17**, 181–186.

17 | Ethics of treatment and research in the aged

M.J. DENHAM

The ethics of treatment

Ethical dilemmas of treatment seldom arises when it is clear that a patient will benefit from proposed medical or surgical treatment and when there are few serious risks. However, there are occasions when the benefits are questionable, the risks are high, the patient is frail and the investigations or treatment involve much 'interference'. Then, it may seem the kindest approach to let nature take its course while keeping the patient as comfortable as possible. Such a decision requires very careful, positive thought and consideration by all those involved in the patient's care.

The caring team needs to be fully informed about many factors before the treatment policy decision is made. These factors include the nature of the patient's illness, the treatment required with its risks and benefit, the presence or absence of other diseases with the risks and benefit of their treatment, the patient's previous quality of life, the patient's and relatives' wishes, the patient's morale, motivation and mental state, the expectation of life, and the patient's age. Even cursory consideration of these factors indicates that an adequate history and patient assessment are mandatory to enable an informed decision to be taken. When necessary, relevant details about the patient may be obtained from the patient's relatives, neighbours, friends, the district nurse or health visitor, home help, care attendant, meals-on-wheels supervisor, social worker, the visiting priest, etc. When an adequate history or assessment is lacking, the patient should always be given the benefit of the doubt and treated.

The following two case histories are given to illustrate some of the ethical dilemmas which may be encountered:

Case 1

> Mr S. was an alert 74 year old man with advanced gangrene of the left leg which needed amputation. However, he was also known to have a proven carcinoma of the bronchus with cerebral metastases, with an average life expectancy of a few months. Consequently, if his leg were amputated there could be too little time to fit him with a pylon and to teach him how to walk.
>
> The dilemma, therefore, was whether to operate and look

to a short-term wheelchair independence, or to allow nature to take its course. The latter course was followed. The patient's strong constitution kept him going, but he became increasingly toxic due to the gangrene, and it was not possible to control the pain with frequent doses of diamorphine. Operation was now considered, but the patient initially refused. Eventually he agreed to amputation. As a result his quality of life dramatically improved due to removal of the dead tissue and reduction in pain, but he was never well enough to return home and he died in hospital a month or so after the operation.

Case 2

Mr W., a 78 year old man living in an old people's home, was admitted with pneumonia, dehydration, septicaemia and extensive osteomyelitis at the site of a total hip replacement performed seven years earlier. He improved somewhat with antibiotics and the correction of the dehydration.

The dilemma was that, on the one hand, anaesthetic and surgical opinion considered him unlikely to survive an operation because of his poor general condition; on the other hand, he would not be cured without the operation.

A major factor in the decision to recommend operation was the expressed desire of the patient to get better. He survived the operation, had a very hectic postoperative course, dying of a pulmonary embolus about two weeks after the operation.

The patient's illness

Detailed knowledge of the patient's illness is mandatory in the treatment policy decision. The natural history of the untreated disease must be understood, the effects of intervention known and problems in establishing the diagnosis considered. Thus, on the one hand, a patient with very slowly progressive disease with minimal symptoms may perhaps be better watched and intervention reserved for later complications, e.g. the development of carcinoma of the breast in the very old and infirm has a good prognosis even untreated, since it is so slowly progressive. On the other hand, if intervention in the early stages of disease improves survival rates, then there is much to be said in favour of intervention, e.g. removal of carcinoma of the vulva which does not involve glands has an 80% survival rate at five years, compared with 30% if the glands are involved.

Doctors are educated to make an accurate diagnosis. However, it is not always possible or indeed necessary to be 100% certain of the diagnosis, especially if the tests needed to prove the point are likely to be exhausting for the frail, older person. Sometimes, clues may be obtained from other non-invasive tests, but acceptability, even of these of tests, needs to be remembered. What may seem to be a simple, acceptable, straightforward test to a younger adult may be quite unacceptable to and be refused by an older person, e.g. non-invasive total body potassium measurements involve being placed in a small, claustrophobic room.

Once the diagnosis is established, the patient and/or relatives should usually be told. There is little difficulty except when the disease is cancer. However, even with this disease, there is a strong case for telling the patient, especially if he or she wants the information, although some may indicate they do not — then their wishes which must be respected. Telling the truth needs to be done tactfully in a series of interviews, to allow the diagnosis to sink in and to allow time for questions and discussions. This approach should allow trust to develop between patient and caring staff, so that further complications, treatment, or management can be discussed openly, allowing the patient to make arrangements for his/her life. Relatives sometimes do not want their loved one to be told about the diagnosis, but this leads to deception, inhibiting truthfulness between family and patient, and between caring staff and patient.

Treatment

The benefit of treatment must be balanced against the risks. Some medical and surgical interventions undoubtedly bring great benefit but sometimes much morbidity results. There is, of course, no dilemma in treating pernicious anaemia, since giving vitamin B_{12} is clearly both beneficial and acceptable, while carrying little or no risk. However, treatment of acute leukaemias in the aged may not only be unpleasant, with side-effects, but also unsuccessful; on the other hand, the condition will be fatal if left untreated.

Surgery in the aged is not without its problems. Emergency abdominal surgery in the aged carries high risk of morbidity or mortality, but conditions requiring such treatment seldom respond to conservation measures. Adelstein & Loy (1979) reviewed coroners' death certificates, which are issued after a medical practitioner has referred to the coroner a death where surgical or other treatment was considered a principal or contributing cause of death. They found that deaths due to surgery increased with age — especially in the presence of pre-existing disease, such as peripheral vascular disease or cardiorespiratory disease. Death rates due to emergency surgery were higher than for elective procedures, but the difference is lessening, mostly due to difficulties in classifying what is an emergency, and also due to improvement in perioperative care. Mental confusion of the patient was a frequent occurrence in the postoperative period.

The role of anaesthesia in perioperative morbidity and mortality has also received attention. The Bedford study (1955) assessed elderly people before and after operation/anaesthesia, and found that 7% developed severe dementia after the operation. This report prompted the Simpson *et al.* study (1961) which found no evidence that anaesthesia had any effect on physical activity, mental ability, or the personality of the patient. However, there were several reasons for the discrepancy in results: the Bedford patients included both emergency and elective cases, and considerable advances had been made in perioperative care between the two studies, e.g. anaesthetic technique, early ambulation, correction of electrolyte inbalance, and the greater use of blood transfusion. In addition, awareness had developed of the great dangers of anaesthesia in older people. However, geriatricians still meet patients who have suffered severe irreversible mental deterioration following admission to hospital with an operation/anaesthesia. Anaesthetic deaths have also been studied by the Association of Anaesthetists of Great Britain and Ireland (Lunn & Mushin, 1982). Although the report has been criticized, it does show that 50% of deaths attributable to anaesthesia occur in those over 70 years of age, and that half of the deaths occurred in elective surgical cases where any adverse risk factors should have been identified, corrected or minimized. However, pre-existing disease such as chronic obstructive airways disease may contribute to these deaths in the old.

The presence of other diseases

The presence of other diseases, their natural history, their effect on life expectancy, and quality of life, their treatment with the risks and benefit, can have a considerable impact on the management of the primary/principal condition. Severe chronic obstructive airways disease in a patient with painful osteoarthritis of the hip may make hip surgery inadvisable due to potential anaesthetic problems and the limitation of mobility after surgery. Then, again, as shown in Case 1, the presence of brain secondaries from carcinoma of the bronchus influenced, perhaps wrongly, the management of a gangrenous leg.

Quality of life

The patient's quality of life is another major consideration in the treatment decision. Yet again, the need for a full, adequate informative history is emphasized. Unfortunately, the concept of quality of life is difficult to define and it can mean different things to different people, who may react in different ways to identical circumstances. Furthermore, a patient's quality of life can be influenced by cultural background, experience and education, which may be quite different from that of the observer. However, quality of life can be assessed by objective or subjective methods (Chapter 15). While objective measures, such as housing and pensions are not subject to observer error, they are insensitive to the feelings of the subject. Subjective parameters, such as satisfaction with life, health and morale, involve subjects making a judgment of their own life, which may not be easy. Although good health, unimpaired mobility, and reduced incapacity seem so necessary to most people as a basis of good quality of life, it is also obvious that many severely handicapped, dependent, housebound people can still enjoy life. For them, and for others, being happy at the present time and looking forward with pleasure to the future are key factors, and this is what the doctor must try to assess.

Potential quality of life after treatment also needs to be evaluated. A patient who has been unconscious for several days due to a massive cerebral haemorrhage will, without treatment, become dehydrated. The ethical dilemma is whether to rehydrate the patient knowing that recovery, if it occurs, is likely to be associated with extensive neurological defects with grossly impaired quality of life, or to allow nature to take its course. One such patient who was rehydrated and recovered consciousness after 10 days, was found to have a severe right hemiplegia with total aphasia. After two years she could just walk with the active help of one person but remained totally dysphasic and totally reliant on others for help to use the toilet, etc. She went to her sister's home, fell down, broke her right neck of femur, was readmitted and never walked again for the remaining two years of her life. Treatment gave her four years of life, but of what quality?

The patient's wishes and mental state

The wishes of the patient must also be taken into account. When the person can make a clear, deliberate, reasoned decision about treatment, and accepts it, the matter is simple. However, if treatment is refused, the reasons should be identified, since, on occasion, it may be possible to overcome the problem and allow treatment to proceed. Otherwise, the refusal must be accepted. On occasion the management decision is taken out of the hands of the caring team. Campbell (1983) relates cases in America where a patient's right to die is decided by the courts on legal grounds which seem lacking in humanity and the true care for the person concerned, e.g. a mentally retarded man of 52 years who, because he was mentally equivalent to an infant, must be offered the rights of an infant, and therefore he has no right to die. Kennedy (1976) indicated that, in such cases, it is a matter of lamentable obscurity whether a legal guardian or other relative can, in law, authorize the withdrawal of treatment.

Management dilemmas occur particularly when, due to confusion, the patient is unable to give a considered opinion. This may be due to a confusional state or dementia. These conditions must be differentiated, since a toxic confusional state is usually treatable and reversible and, consequently, a patient may be able to give a cogent opinion in due course. Dementia is usually not reversible and the mental state is not likely to improve. The disorders are usually fairly easily distinguished on history: a toxic confusional state is characterized by a short history of sudden onset, while a dementia is characterized by a slow onset of long duration. Temporarily confused patients may be expected to do well and may return to a good quality of life, while the demented patient may have more limited horizons and be very dependent on others. Unfortunately, the more demented the patient becomes, the more unrealistic he/she may become about his/her capabilities, all of which emphasizes the need for a detailed history. Sometimes, it can help to assess the degree of cognitive impairment by using a mental questionnaire, e.g. Denham & Jefferys (1972). Those who score highly are usually well able to give consent or refuse treatment, and usually respond well to rehabilitation, while those who score less often cannot give informed consent, are slow to rehabilitate, and are most likely to be incontinent. The test has its limitations: it does not give reliable results in patients who are deaf, dysphasic, depressed, or who have a different ethnic background from those who are UK born citizens. Where it is evident that a patient cannot give informed consent to treatment, the doctor should discuss the situation with the relatives, putting forward clearly the pros and cons of treatment/operation, coupled with thoughtful, considered, informed guidance. Relatives may find it helpful to consider what they think the patient would have decided had he or she been in a position to decide. Where no relatives are available, doctors should discuss the situation with the relevant hospital manager/administrator.

Severe dementia can produce major dilemmas of treatment, even at the most basic level. Feeding is basic care, but it can become impossible to feed patients by ordinary means, especially if they are very ill, disinterested, or refuse food. Caring staff who are close to the patient will find the situation difficult, since death will eventually occur if the patient is not kept hydrated. The problem is how far should the patient be fed by i.v. means, nasogastric tubes, or have food spooned into the mouth. Where feeding causes the patient discomfort, or where quality of life is severely impaired, and feeding only serves to maintain life, the patient should be given as much nutriment as he or she will take, but forced feeding against the patient's expressed actions, feelings or wishes should not be pursued. If death follows, it should not be viewed as defeat. However, when previous quality of life has been good and there is anticipated benefit to the patient, then short-term i.v. or naso-gastric feeding should be considered to tide the patient over.

Motivation

Motivation is hard to define, although it is relatively easy to recognize. In the medical setting it is an obvious active desire to want to get better — a factor most important in rehabilitation. Many severely disabled but well motivated patients will get home in spite of many problems, while a less disabled patient, lacking in motivation, will not. Unfortunately, of course, it is not possible to 'prescribe' motivation, although where depression is a factor, this may be treatable.

Orthopaedic surgeons should consider motivation before offering hip surgery to an old person with severe osteoarthritis of the hip which impairs quality of life due to pain and the loss of mobility. If the patient is likely to co-operate with the rehabilitation team then, all things being equal, the operation is worthwhile.

The patient's age and expectation of life

The patient's actual biological age should be given a low 'weighting factor' in consideration of treatment/non-treatment. Unfortunately, many doctors often tend to dismiss patients over the age of 70 years as beyond treatment. Thus, removal of subdural haematomas in patients over the age of 70 years is often considered a waste of time, but there are examples of excellent results of burr-hole treatment of patients over 90 years old in previously good mental health. Fortunately, cardiologists have not seen age, *per se*, as a barrier to the insertion of pacemakers — centogenerians have been so treated. Furthermore, there are many old people in the community who have a better, healthier more active life than others half their age. Indeed, recently the British Foundation for Age Research launched a campaign called 'Four Score Years and Then', pointing out how active old people can be.

Expectation of life should also be considered. This comprises several factors including not only the patient's age, but also the patient's expected survival in years based on actuarial life scale charts, and the expected survival with or without treatment in relation to the disease under consideration. When expectation of life is long, then this is a pointer in favour of treatment. Where life expectation is short, disease widespread or quality of life poor, then allowing nature to take its course may be the right decision for that person.

The right to die

> Lily was a 76 year old woman who suffered frequent exacerbations of chronic bronchitis, eventually necessitating a tracheostomy and frequent periods of artificial ventilation. One day she said to a nurse looking after her, 'you see I'm up there', casting her eyes heavenwards, 'and me down here — know I'm done for, but them lot', pointing to the Intensive Care Unit, 'won't let me go'. The comment was remembered the next time Lily had a flare-up of her bronchitis, and she was allowed her wish (Robertson, 1978).

The right to die needs to be considered in two situations: firstly, when the patient is ill and has made a conscious, considered decision to refuse further treatment and investigation. Such a decision should be discussed with the patient and, if the decision remains irrevocable, respected and adhered to. Secondly, it must be considered when fit people wish to avoid disease, dementia or disability in the future by taking positive measures to end life, i.e. euthanasia, which is defined as a 'quiet and easy death' (Shorter Oxford Dictionary). This is a sad decision, since research on many debilitating diseases and disorders continues apace, and doubtless improved methods of treatment will be developed. Furthermore, those in charge of continuing care units for the old now take a greater interest in improving quality of life (Denham, 1984).

The subject of euthanasia has been much debated since the 1930s, when the Voluntary Euthanasia Society was formed. All attempts to legalize it have failed and the vast body of medical opinion is against it. Those caring for the aged realize how vulnerable some of their patients would be should such a concept be made legal (Shaeffer & Koop, 1980).

Conclusion

The decision to treat or not to treat must be based on an unhurried, thoughtful, responsible and sensitive judgement, made after considering all the relevant information obtained by the members of the multi-disciplinary team caring for the patient. Hasty decisions must be avoided and no decision should be considered irrevocable — changing circumstances or new information may warrant a reconsideration of an earlier decision. When adequate information is lacking, the patient should be given the benefit of the doubt, and treated, although sometimes this may later turn out to have been unwise. Sometimes a compromise is possible — treatment is given once, but not repeated if unsuccessful.

Ethics of research in the aged

Research in the old can involve not only direct patient involvement and evaluation of drugs, but also assessment of methods of delivery of care, as well as efficacy of equipment and procedures. However, some consider that it is unethical or unjustified to undertake research on the old because of their vulnerability. Others would argue the reverse — research is vital if there is to be a reasonably rapid accurate advance in knowledge of the ageing process and the diseases of old age.

If the need for research is accepted, then there must be discussion on those ethical problems which have special relevance to the old; otherwise, patients and carers may consider that doctors do not give sufficient consideration to their worries and apprehensions.

Standards of research

All research in the old must be of the same high ethical and clinical standards as research in any other group of subjects. Just because the patient is old is no excuse for sloppy, slip-shod research. Consequently each research project must have a clearly defined, reasonably obtainable objective and the design and the methods must be appropriate to achieve that objective — pilot studies require the same standard. Badly designed research is totally unethical since it can subject patients to tests and inconvenience which have no value.

Do the aged need special ethical consideration?

The fact that little is written about the ethical problems of research in the aged suggests that they require little special consideration. However, memories of the abuse of aged ill patients in psychiatric and general hospitals in the UK in the 1960s (Robb, 1967) suggests, from the clinical point of view, that the aged do need special care. Memories, too, of the Jewish Chronic Disease Hospital Case (Katz, 1972) emphasize that the consent procedures for older people can be abused. In that particular case a number of chronically ill old people were injected with cancerous material without their clear consent.

The older person certainly may be vulnerable to requests to take part in research. Firstly, for example, those in longstay institutions become 'institutionalised' and may acquiesce all too easily to requests from research workers without really understanding what is required of them. Secondly, those living alone at home become lonely and might take part in research as a way of obtaining company. Thirdly, there may be an element of *quid pro quo* 'you helped me, so I will help you'.

The problem is really that of consent. The majority of the aged live outside hospital and are of testimentary capacity — they will be able to give consent in the same way as any other person. The real difficulty arises in those old or young people who are confused or who have difficulty in understanding complex studies which may be involved in some research. They certainly require special consideration.

Consent

Consent to participation in research is a complex matter. Some aspects are particularly relevant to the old.

Legal aspects   A few, if any, research workers would deliberately try to trick or deceive a patient into giving consent, but Sir Roger Ormeroyd (1968) has made it clear that consent to research which is obtained by a trick is 'no consent'. Furthermore, research workers will be at fault if they ask *relatives* to consent on behalf of a patient who cannot give informed consent. It is only (legally) possible for a legal *guardian* to give consent for experimental purposes which lead to potential benefit (Pryce, 1978), and legal guardians are unlikely to be available for the old. This clearly has implications for research into severe dementia.

Full or adequate consent There can be little doubt that giving full details of a research project to a subject can induce confusion and anxiety. Epstein & Lasagna (1969) showed that, as the amount of detailed information about a research project is increased, so there is a decrease in the understanding of what is required in that research project. Likwise, a consent form for a breast cancer trial which lists all the possible complications of treatment may well induce worry and compound anxiety already felt.

There is therefore a need to steer a careful, acceptable course between giving excessive detail and giving none at all. Research workers must help to ensure that a person is adequately informed, by being kind, caring, considerate and thoughtful, and using language and terminology which are easily understood. Consent must never be imposed, forced, or obtained under duress. The investigator should always be ready to discuss the proposed research in more detail if the patient wishes it.

Mental capacity Obtaining consent depends not only on the complexity of the information given to the patient, but also on the ability of the patient to understand. This can correlate with his/her mental capacity and ability to grasp concepts and reasoning which may be new and even alien. It may involve using thought processes which have become blunted with age (Chapter 6). Consequently, to help ensure that true consent is obtained, it can be useful to use the two stage consent procedure or assess mental state. Two stage consent involves giving written details of the study (first part) to the patient or volunteer so that he/she can discuss the matter with friends and relatives. The second part consists of a questionnaire to test how well the patient has understood what he/she has been told. This technique had been shown to be effective (Muss *et al.*, 1979), but perhaps not surprisingly it has also been followed by refusal to participate (Ratzan, 1981). Although the method has much to recommend it, logistical problems for the investigator may result. Alternatively, testing the patient's cognitive function, as mentioned earlier in the chapter, can give guidance about ability to understand.

The form of consent The way in which consent is obtained is the source of much debate and, although this is not a specific problem of the old, it does have some relevance for them. Many consider that the explanation and the details of the research should be written and, after time has been allowed for discussions and questions, the patient should be asked to sign a consent form agreeing to participation in the research. However, a person may feel that having signed such a form means that there is no opportunity to withdraw, even though that is not the case. Additionally, the signature may be viewed as a form of protection for the doctor (Cassileth *et al.*, (1980). At Northwick Park Hospital the practice is for the investigator to give a verbal explanation to the patient in the presence of a senior nurse, who ensures that there is an adequate opportunity for questions and that the patient is not forced to agree to take part in the project. When consent has been obtained, a form recording the fact is signed by both the investigator and the nurse and kept with the records.

The content of the written consent form has been much debated — ideally it should list the purpose of the research, the procedures involved, the risks and benefits, the freedom to ask questions and the freedom to withdraw. Such a quantity of information may result, as mentioned earlier, in the patient failing to understand what is required, although a two stage consent procedure might overcome this. Ideally the proposed explanation should be agreed by the local ethical committee.

Randomized clinical trials

There is no doubt that carefully designed drug trials in the aged are especially necessary to evaluate the treatment, to establish the correct dose range and reduce the problems of adverse drug reactions. Ethical committees must be informed of the classification of the drugs to be used, e.g. does the medicine have a product license or a clinical trial certificate or clinical trial exemption? However, the use of placebos in such trials can pose ethical problems. Some consider placebos to be justified in trials where there is no known effective treatment for a particular illness or in the chronic phases of diseases which do have known accepted treatments, but others take the view that placebos will deny patients treatment.

Avoiding harm

Those researching on the aged have a special responsibility to ensure that the volunteer or patient does not suffer harm. The Medical Research Council in Britain (1962/3) has put the matter clearly:

> 'The head of a department where investigations on human subjects takes place has an inescapable responsibility to ensure that practice by those under his control is irreproachable . . . . The progress of medical knowledge has depended and will continue to depend, in no small measure, upon the confidence the public has in those who carry out investigations on human subjects, be they healthy or sick . . . . Mistaken or misunderstood investigations can do incalculable harm to medical progress. It is our collective duty to see that this does not happen, and so continue to deserve the confidence we now enjoy'.

Sometimes the patient does suffer harm. When a doctor has been negligent, it will be possible for the patient to sue that doctor. However, where mishap occurs without negligence, difficulties arise. At present there is no redress for the subject unless the research worker or drug company have some form of insurance. It may be possible to seek 'one off' payment from the Department of Health and Social Security but the matter of 'no fault' compensation is still being debated.

Monitoring research

This subject continues to worry ethical committees. While it seems generally agreed that research should be monitored, there is no agreement about the ideal method. Monitoring research in the aged, as with children, is particularly necessary where there are potential problems of consent, where relatives have been involved, or where the patient is considered vulnerable.

Research may be monitored, at hospital level, by members of the ethical committee visiting wards and questioning staff and patients. Alternatively, research workers may be asked to complete a short annual review form detailing the number of people studied, the details of any consent problems, development in research, and whether the work has been published. Northwick Park Hospital now uses the latter method. Furthermore, it issues to a number of departments — including the pharmacy department, radioisotope department and the ward sisters — lists of approved projects. This ensures that unapproved projects which appear on the wards or elsewhere are immediately recognized and the situation brought to the attention of the ethical committee. Research is monitored at a national level by medical journals which can refuse to publish work considered to be unethical.

Conclusion

Research on the old is necessary, but must be carefully carried out using well designed studies with great care being taken to ensure adequate consent.

References

Adelstein, A. & Loy P (1979) Fatal adverse effects of medicines and surgery. *Popul. Trends* **17**, 17.

Bedford, P.D. (1955) Adverse cerebral effects of anaesthesia on old people. *Lancet* **2**, 259.

Campbell, A.G.M. (1983) The right to be allowed to die. *J. Med. Ethics* **9**, 136.

Cassileth, B.R., Zupkins, R.V., Sutton Smith, K. & March V. (1980) Informed consent — why are its goals imperfectly realised? *New Eng. J. Med.* **302**, 896.

Denham, M. J. & Jefferys, P. (1972) Routine mental testing in the elderly. *Mod. Geriatr.* **2**, 275.

Denham, M. J.(Ed.) (1984) *The Care of the Long Stay Elderly Patient.* Croom Helm, London.

Epstein, L. C. & Lasagna, L. (1969) Obtaining informed consent. *Arch. Intern. Med.* **123**, 682.

Katz, J. (1972) Jewish Chronic Disease Hospital Case. In *Experimentation with Human Beings*. Russel Saga Foundation, New York, pp. 9–65.

Kennedy, I. M. (1976) The Karen Quinlan Case: problems and proposals. *J. Med. Ethics.* **2**, 3.

Lunn J. N. & Mushin, W. W. (1982) *Mortality Associated with Anaesthesia*. Association of Anaesthetists of Great Britain and Ireland, Nuffield Provincial Hospitals Trust.

Medical Research Council (1962/3) Responsibility in investigation on human subjects. HMSO, London, CMND 2382 p. 21.

Muss, M. B., White, D. R., Michielutte, R., Richards, F., Cooper, M. R., Williams, S., Stuart, J. J. & Spurr C. L. (1979) Written informed consent in patients with breast cancer. *Cancer* **43**, 1549.

Ormeroyd, Sir R. (1968) Medical ethics. *Br. Med. J.* **2**, 7.

Pryce, I. G. (1978) Clinical research upon mentally ill subjects who cannot give informed consent. *Br. J. Psychiatry* **132**, 366.

Ratzan, R. M. (1981) The experiment that wasn't: a case report in clinical geriatric research. *Gerontologist* **21**, 297.

Robb, B. (1967) *Sans Everything*. Nelson, London.

Robertson, S. (1978) 'Them lot won't let me go'. In *The Elderly: A Challenge to Nursing*. A *Nursing Times* publication, p. 33, London.

Shaeffer, F. & Koop, C. E. (1980) *Whatever Happened to the Human Race?* Marshall, Morgan & Scott, London.

Simpson B. R., Williams, M., Scott, J. F. & Smith, A. C. (1961) The effect of anaesthesia and elective surgery on elderly people. *Lancet* **2**, 887.

Further reading

Bayliss, R. I. S. (1982) Thou shall not strive officiously. *Br. Med.* **285**, 1373. (Discussion of resuscitation and contrasts the situation in the UK and the USA.)

Bigot, A. (1974) The relevance of life satisfaction indices for research on British subjects before and after retirement. *Age Ageing* **3**, 113. (Adapts American life satisfaction indices to the UK.)

Robertson, G. S. (1983) Ethical dilemma of brain failure in the elderly. *Br. Med. J.* **287**, 1775. (Discussion of patient's wishes in relation to death and euthanasia.)

Index

Page numbers in *italics* refer to figures; those in **bold** refer to tables.

Abbreviated Mental Test (AMT) 73, 97
abdominal surgery, complications 268
absorption, drug 127–8
acid-base disturbances 162–3
  with hypokalaemia 158
acidosis
  with hypokalaemia 158
acupuncture 289, 298
acute assessment wards, defined 110
acute confusional states *see* delirium
adrenoceptors, changes with ageing 139
age-specific gene expression 5–6
aged, defined 169
ageing
  bioenergetic changes with 4–5
  defined 183
  demography 9–25
  physiological changes with 3–4
  theories 5–8
  variability 1–3
airway occlusion pressure technique 64
airways dysfunction 118
  lower 55, 244, 273–4
  upper 57–60
albumin, serum, levels 129, 196–7
  hypoalbuminaemia 124, 173
alcoholism 186–7, 276, 277
alcuronium 209
alkaline phosphatase, levels 125
alpha₁-acid glycoprotein, binding 129
alveolar walls, structure and function
    65–6
Alzheimer's disease 4, 71, 76
anaemia
  diagnosis and treatment 123–4, 198
  pre-operative 170–1
analgesia, profound
  during regional anaesthesia 232
analgesics 232, 291–2, 301–4
  distribution 130
  pharmacodynamics 138–9
  post-operative use 218–19, 244
  pre-operative use 200–1
  see also anti-inflammatory drugs,
    non-steroidal; opiate analgesics
angina pectoris, incidence *189*
antibiotic prophylaxis 179–80, 190
anticholinergic drugs 201, 209–10
  see also atropine
anticholinergic effects, drug-induced
    185–6, 223, 249
anticholinesterases 209

anticoagulants *see* warfarin
anticonvulsants *see* carbamazepine;
    phenytoin
anti-inflammatory drugs, non-steroidal
    251, 291, 298
anxiety states 114
  in cancer patients 300
aorta
  changes with ageing 28, 29–30
  surgical mortality 270
APACHE II (Acute Physiology and
    Chronic Health Evaluation)
    260
apnoea 58, 59
ARDS *see* pulmonary oedema
arrhythmias, incidence
  with halothane 211
  with neuromuscular blockade reversal
    210
arteries, major
  changes with ageing 28
  surgical mortality 270
  see also aorta
artificial ventilation, use 273
  post-operative 218, 268, 270, 271
  weaning from 63–5
ASA score 184–5
assessment, defined 110–11
atelectasis, basal 53, 56, 243
atracurium 208
atropine 139–40, 209
auditory evoked response, use 75
autonomic nervous system, in aged 86–7,
    118
  drugs sensitivity 205

backache, post-operative 220
balance, change with ageing 84
balloon flotation catheterization 272
bed rest, disadvantages 185
benzodiazepines
  metabolism 134, 265
  pharmacodynamics 138
  use 200
  see also diazepam; midazolam
biliary tract surgery, timing 179
biochemical testing 124–5
bioenergetics, changes with ageing 4–5
biological ageing
  versus chronological 1, 314
bladder problems 80, 85

blood flow 233
  and drug distribution 130-2
  cerebral 2, 76-7, 221
  liver 133-4
  renal 146, 222
blood pressure
  measuring venous 40
  systolic changes with ageing 31-2, **33**
  see also hypertension; hypotension
blood transfusions, timing 170-1, 226
blood volume, decreased 147, 214
body mass, lean
  changes with ageing *147*, 274-5
bone disorders 121-2
bowel problems 80, 85
  see also constipation
brain scan (scintiscan) 75
brain structure, changes
  in diseases 71-2
  normal ageing 71
breathing control 60-1
  anaesthesia effect 61-3
bronchitis, incidence 187, 243
burns, patients with
  mortality 178
  surgical preparation 192-3

calcium, levels 124
cancer
  incidence 279
  nutrition and surgery 277-8
  treatment for pain 299-305
  see also carcinoma
cannulation routes
  monitering uses 271
CAPE 98
carbamazepine 82
carcinomas
  and hyponatraemia 153-4
  and pre-operative feeding 173
  colorectal surgery 268-9
cardiac catheterization **43**, 44
  see also balloon flotation
    catheterization
cardiac failure 156, 189, 191
  post-operative 247-8, 249
cardiac output, change with ageing 31, 32
cardiac risk index 171
cardiac structural lesions
  investigations 42
cardiopulmonary resuscitation 279-80
cardiovascular system, in aged
  assessment 36-45, 171, 189
  control changes 30-1
  electrical, biochemical, mechanical
    changes 28-30
  functioning 31-6
  post-operative problems *243*, 247-9
  see also heart
CAT (choline acetyl transferase), levels
  71, 72
cerebral blood flow 2, 76, 221
  after stroke 76-7
chemoreceptor activity 61
chest wall, elasticity 48-9

chest X-ray abnormalities 40-1, 171
cimetidine 136-7, 201
circulatory hyponatraemia 151-2
clinical examination
  cardiac status 40
clinical trials, ethics of 318
Cockcroft/Gault formula 194
cognition 89-91, 101
  assessment 96-8
colorectal carcinoma, surgery for 268-9
coma
  mortality 267
  non-ketotic hyperosmolar 227
communication difficulties, patient 111
complications
  post-operative
    body fluids 250-2
    cardiovascular 247-9, 252-4
    central nervous system 249-50
    mental status 249
    respiratory 242-7
  with regional anaesthesia 238-9
confusion
  acute *see* delirium
  minimizing post-operative 219
consciousness, preservation of
  importance to anaesthesia 231-2
consent, patient
  for research role 316-17
'consequentialism' 282
constipation 80, 123, 303
contraction, myocardial
  changes with ageing 29
Cost Utility Analysis 111
creatinine levels 124, 136, *197*
  clearance rates 2, 194
CT scan (computerized tomography) 75,
  178

day case surgery 201
  anaesthesia in 224
decision making, in aged 113
decubitis ulcers 122
deep venous thrombosis 193-4, 253
dehydration 146-8
delirium
  causes 115, 265, 266, 275
  post-operative 101-2, *243*, 249
  treatment 110, 115-16
dementia 116-17, 290-1
  and depression 114
  assessment 84, 97
  incidence 85
  treatment decisions 313
depression
  and strokes 79, 96
  assessment 80, 98-9
  causes 113-14
  diagnosis and treatment 114, 290, 298
  view of 95-6
diabetes mellitus
  control 120
  diagnosis 119-20
  incidence 197
  surgery on patients with 197-8, 227

diagnosis difficulties, in aged 309–10
diamorphine 302
diaphragm, flattening
    energy expenditure with 49
    surgical importance 49
diazepam 206–7
diethyl ether 212
digoxin, uses 189, 192, 251
dilutional hyponatraemia 150, 151
'disposable soma theory' 6–8
distribution, drug
    extent 128–30
    rate 130–33
diuretic therapy 251
    and hyperkalaemia 159
    and hypokalaemia 157–8
    and hyponatraemia 150, 151, 152
divorce, incidence 14
domestic circumstances, in aged 19–20,
    112
droperidol 200
drug effects, in aged 126–7
    absorption 127–8
    distribution 128–33, **213**
    excretion 136–7, **213**
    metabolism 133–6, **213**
    pharmacodynamics 137–9, 205, **206**
    study difficulties 127
drug interactions 82–3, 185, 276
drug therapy
    and chronic pain 285, 291–2
    and hyperkalaemia 159
    and hyponatraemia 153
    and intensive care 266
    interactions 185–6
    withdrawal 185, 186, 249
DVT 193–4, 253
dysphasia
    and stroke 78

ECG 40, **43**
    pre-operative value 171
echocardiography 42, 43
edrophonium 209
ejection fraction, changes with ageing 31,
    32
elasticity
    larger airways walls 56–7
    lung and chest walls 48–52, 55
elderly, defined 169
elective surgery
    versus emergency 177, 178–9, 269
electrocardiography see ECG
electroencephalography (EEG) 74–5
electromyography (EMG) 75
emergency surgery
    delaying 177–8
    versus elective 177, 178–9, 269
emotional distress 95–6
    assessment 98–100
emotions, in aged 94
    see also emotional distress
emphysema
    and lung volume 50

end-diastolic volume, changes with
    ageing 32
endocarditis, infective
    treatment 190
endocardium
    changes with ageing 27
    treatment for inflammation of 190
endocrine system, in aged 119–22, 197–8
endotracheal intubation 215
enflurane 212
entomidate 208
enzyme activity, intrinsic
    and drug metabolism 134–5
    extrahepatic 135
epidural blocks 233, 235
    for chronic pain relief 289, 299, **304**
epilepsy
    assessment 81–2
    incidence 81
    treatment 82–3
ethics, medical
    for intensive care 280–2
    for research 315–19
    for treatment 308–15
euthanasia 315
evolution of ageing 5
excretion, drug 128, 129, 136–7
exercise
    and cardiac output 31, 32
    and maximum oxygen
        consumption 33–6
exercise electrocardiography 39, **43**
expiratory flow, changes with ageing
    56–7

falls 84–5, 267
fluids, intra-operative administration
    225–6
function, assessment of 74
fundi examination 73

gallstones, surgery 179
gas exchange, impaired
    during anaesthesia 52–3
    post-operative 53
gastrointestinal tract, in aged
    colorectal carcinoma 268–9
    ischaemia of 269–70
    nutrition via 276
    surgical mortality 268
gene expression, age-specific 5–6
general anaesthesia
    and aged diabetics 227
    and patients with pacemakers 226–7
    blood transfusions during 226
    body temperature maintenance 224–5
    breathing control 62–3
    day case surgery and 224
    early post-operative period 217–19
    fluid administration during 225–6
    induction
        agents 204–13, 217, 223
        procedures 214–16
    invasive monitoring 227–8

general anaesthesia—*cont'd*
  maintenance of 216–17
  mortality compared to regional
    234–5, 245, 254
  positioning and handling for 219–20
  tissue oxygen supply maintenance
    220–3
  urine output during 226
  with local 237–8
glycopyrrolate 210
group therapy, advantages 291

haemotological testing 123–4, 198–9
halothane 211–12
Hazard and Griffin formula 163
head
  injuries 267
  positioning for general anaesthesia 219
hearing disabilities 109
  aids for 111
  and nitrous oxide 211
  see also auditory evoked response
heart
  age-related changes 27–31
  arrhythmias 210, 211
  block treatment 192
  clinical examination 40
  failure 156, 189, 247–8, 249
  output changes 31, 32
  rate 31, 33
    during local anaesthesia 239
  status assessment 36–40, 171
  techniques 40–45
heart disease, ischaemic 36
  and anaesthesia 211, 212
hemiplegia 77–8, 147
heparin, dosage 193, 253
hernia, surgery 178–9, *268*
hip surgery
  and DVT 193–4, 253
  regional anaesthesia for 235, 238
  timing and mortality 183
histamine antagonists *see* cimetidine;
    ranitidine
hormone replacement therapy (HRT)
  and osteoporosis 121
Hospital In-Patient Enquiry 106
hospitals
  admissions 106–7, 168
  diet inadequacy 119, 186
hyoscine 210
hyperkalaemia 158–60
hypermagnesaemia 162
hypernatraemia 154–5
hyperparathyroidism 120
hypersensitivity, superficial
  treatment 292, 294
hypertension, causes 192
hyperthyroidism 120
hypoalbuminaemia 124, 173
hypokalaemia 157–8
hypomagnesaemia 161–2, 276
hyponatraemia 149–54
hypoparathyroidism 120
hypophosphataemia 276

hypophysoadrenal axis
  dysfunction 120–1
hypopituitarism 121
hypotension, postural
  and anaesthesia 192, 233, 239
    induced 222–3
  causes 104, 214
hypothermia 86–7, 199
  during surgery 224–5
hypothyroidism 120
hypovolaemia 147, 214

iatrogenic hyponatraemia 151
immune function, in aged 278–9
IMV 273
inappropriate AVP 152–4
incontinence, urinary 85, 123, 305
induction
  inhalation agents 210–12
  i.v. drugs 205–8, 214, 223
  opiate analgesics 212–13
  procedures 214–16
infusion pumps, continuous
  and analgesic administration 302–3
inhalation agents 210–12
intensive care
  admission numbers 258–9
  disease states 266–7
  ethics of 280–2
  interventions 271–80
  patient selection 181, 259–64
  surgical illnesses 267–71
intestinal ischaemia 269–70
intracellular fluid, changes with ageing
    (ICF) 147
investigations, pre-operative 170–3
ischaemic heart disease 36
  and anaesthesia 211, 212
isoflurane 211, 212

jaundice, obstructive
  treatment 175–6, 252
joint diseases 122, 297–9

kwashiorkor malnutrition 172

learning speed, in aged 91
legs, positioning for anaesthesia 220
leukaemias, diagnosis 124
life expectancy 14, 169
  range of mammals 6
life style, in aged *see* quality of life
lignocaine, metabolism 235
lipid soluble drugs
  distribution volume 129, 130
  excretion 136
local anaesthesia 239–40
  complications 238–9, 245, 254
  features 140, 218, 231–5
  mortality compared to general
    234–5, 245, 254
  patient management 236–8, 289–90
  with general 237–8

magnesium, levels 160-1
  abnormal 161-2
malnutrition 171-3, 274, 277
mandatory ventilation, intermittent
    (IMV) 273
marasmus malnutrition 172
marital status, of aged 13-14, 19, 20
mechanical loading, in aged 60-1
mechanoreceptor activity 60
Medical Research Council, quoted
    on research 318
memory
  disturbances 71, 91, 116
  testing 92-4
  types of 91-2
men, pensionable-aged
  chronic pain incidence 285
  creatinine clearance 194
  heart disease incidence 189
  intestinal ischaemia incidence 269
  life expectancy 14, 169
  malnutrition incidence 274
  marital status and life style 19, 20
  metabolic rate 275
  oxygen consumption 32
  potassium levels 156, 157
menopause 7, 148
mental status
  assessment 73, 113-17, 195-6
  post-operative 249
metabolic rate, changes with ageing 2,
    275
metabolism, drug 133-6, 265-6
methadone 302
methohexitone 206
midazolam 207-8, 214, 235
migration flow
  and aged distribution 17-18, 20
Mini-Mental State Questionnaire (MMS)
    97-8
minitracheotomy 273-4
monitoring, patient
  in intensive care 271-2
  of research 319
morale, importance 108-9, 110
morbidity
  and mortality 22-4
morphine 213
  and apnoea 58, 59, 62
  for chronic pain relief 299, 301-2
mortality
  and intensive care 259, 280
  and morbidity 22-4
  and reproduction 6-8
  burn victims 178
  comparison of anaesthesia 234-5,
    245, 254
  decline in late age 14-15
  nutrition and 277
  surgical 183-4, 254, 267-70
motivation, importance 313-14
motor deficits
  and strokes 77-8
mucus, airways 57
  retention 244, 246
multifactorial risk index (MRI) 38-9

multi-infarct dementia (MID) 116, 117
multiple pathology
  and patient management 181, 311
multiple surgical procedures, timing 178
murmurs, heart, examination 40
muscle fatigue, respiratory 63-5
muscle relaxation
  and regional anaesthesia 233
  see also neuromuscular blockade,
    drugs
muscle tone, testing 74
myocardial infarction
  post-operative 247, 248
  pre-operative 189
myocardial ischaemia, diagnosis 191

naloxone 213, 218
National Adult Reading Test 98
nausea, morphine-induced 303
neck
  movements as signs 74
  positioning for anaesthesia 219,
    250
neostigmine 209, 210, 217
nervous system, in aged
  drugs sensitivity 204-5
  neurochemistry and neuropathology 71
  neurological abnormalities
    incidence 72
    investigation 72-5
  post-operative complications 249-50
  surgical decisions 87-8
  see also autonomic nervous
    system; neuralgia;
    neurolysis; sympathetic nerve
    block
neuralgia
  incidence 286
  perineal 297
  postherpetic 292-4
  stump pain 295-6
  thalamic syndrome 295
  trigeminal 296-7
neurolysis
  for chronic pain relief 304-5
neuromuscular blockade, drugs 208-9
  for reversal 209-10, 217
nitrous oxide 211
nomogram, phenytoin 82
non-ketotic hyperosmolar coma 227
nuclear angiography 43
nuclear magnetic resonance (NMR) 75
nutrition
  assessment of state 119
  drug interaction 276
  supplementation
    enteral 173, 276
    parenteral 277-8
  surgery preparation 118
  whilst hospitalized 119
  see also malnutrition

obstructive apnoea 58, 59
obstructive jaundice, treatment 175-6,
    252

oesophageal obstruction, treatment 176
OPCS, projections 16
operative risk, assessment 37-9
opiate analgesics 212-13
    and nitrous oxide 211
    for chronic pain relief **292**
    for post-operative pain relief 218
    pharmacokinetics 138-9, **213**
    see also morphine
osteoarthritis 122
osteomalacia 121
osteoporosis 121
oxygen consumption, maximum
    decline with age 32, 34
    exercise and 34
    medical events and 34-5
oxygen supply, tissue 220-1
    cerebral 2, 76-7, 221
    myocardial 221-2
    renal 222
oxygenation 235
    post-operative 217

pacemakers
    for heart blocks 192
    surgical problems 226-7
Paget's disease 122, 125
pain, chronic 285-7
    causes
        cancer 299-305
        joint diseases 297-8
        neuralgias 292-7
    defined 285
    general management, methods
        drug 291-2
        physical 288-90
        psychological 290-1
    measurement 287-8
pain, post-operative
    relief 219-20
pancreatitis 277
pancuronium 209
paraproteinaemia
    and pseudohyponatraemia 149
parathyroid dysfunctions 120
Parkinson's disease 71-2, 79
    signs and symptoms 79-80
    treatment 81
pathology, senile
    characteristics 105-6
    extent 106-8
    multiple 181, 311
patient preparation, for anaesthesia
    heparin administration 193-4
    nutritive state 186-7, 199
    premedication 185-6, 200-1
    pre-operative evaluation 184, 196-7,
        198-9
    receiving information 101
patient selection
    and psychological status 100
    extent of care 181-2
    for intensive care 259-64
patient wishes 169, 282, 312
    right to die 314-15

perceptual deficits
    and strokes 78
perineal neuralgia 297
perioperative management, patient
    cardiovascular system 39-40
    pulmonary system 52-3, 55
personality, assessment 95
phantom limb pain 295, 296
pharmacodynamics, drug 137-40
    defined 126
    study difficulties 127
pharmacokinetics, drug 265-6
    absorption 127-8
    defined 126
    distribution 128-33
    excretion 128, 129, 136-7
    metabolism 13-16, 265-6
    of opiate analgesics 212
    study difficulties 127
phenothiazines 110
phenytoin 82
phosphate levels, imbalances 276
physical status
    assessment 117-22, 184-5
    disability and depression 114
physiological deterioration
    and ageing theory 3-4
    see also under names of individual
        systems
plasma binding, drug 129, 132-3, 135-6
pneumonia, post-operative
    incidence 243
population, pensionable-aged
    distribution 16-18, 20-22
        global 11-13
    size 10-11, 16
    social aspects 19-20
positioning of patients
    for anaesthesia 219-20, 236, 239
positive pressure ventilation,
    intermittent 214, 273
positron emission tomography (PET) 75
post-amputation pain 295, 296
post-herpetic neuralgia 292-4
post-operative delirium 101-2, *243*, 249
post-operative fatigue 102
post-operative period, early
    management 217-19
potassium, levels 155-7
    abnormal 157-60, 276
preloading, ineffectiveness of 239
premedication
    before anaesthesia 200-1
pre-operative management
    improving cardiac status 39
presbyacusis, overcoming 111
pressure sores (decubitis ulcers) 122
profound analgesia
    during local anaesthesia 282
prognosis, decisions about 174-5
    intensive care 264, 282
propofol 208
prostate surgery, mortality *268*
pseudohyponatraemia 149
psychological status
    abnormal ageing 95-6

and pain treatment 290–1
assessment 96–100
in cancer patients 300
implications for anaesthesia 100–102
normal ageing 89
see also cognition; emotion;
    memory; personality
pulmonary artery catheterization 43, 44,
    227–8
pulmonary embolism
incidence 181
risk 253
signs and symptoms 118
pulmonary fibrosis
and lung volume 50
pulmonary oedema
causes 65–6
diagnosis and management 66–8
pulmonary system, in aged
alveolar functioning 65–6
breathing control 60–3
functioning 48–60
    tests 187, 188, 245
lung elasticity 48–52, 55
muscle fatigue and weaning 63–5
preparation for anaesthesia 187–8
see also artificial ventilation;
    pulmonary embolism;
    pulmonary fibrosis; pulmonary
    oedema; respiratory
    problems, post-operative
pyridostigmine 209, 217

quality of life, in aged
assessment 260, 311–12
social aspects 112

ranitidine 201
rapid sequence induction 216
reading ability test 73–4, 98
recall, memory
versus recognition 92–3
receptor sensitivity
and drug pharmacodynamics 138, 139
recovery, patient
factors affecting 101, 108–9, 313–14
regional anaesthesia *see* local anaesthesia
renal functioning 146, 194–5
and drug excretion 136
blood flow 146, 222
dehydration 147–8
electrolyte control 148, 161, 162
post-operative complications 250–2
reproduction rates
and mortality 6–8
research, ethics 315–19
respiratory problems, post-operative
diagnosis 152, 243
identifying high risk patient 245
incidence 242–3
pathophysiology 152, 244–5
prevention 246–7
respiratory secretions, increase 57, 244,
    246
rewarming
from hypothermia 87, 225

rheumatoid arthritis 122
RNV 42, **43**

scintiscan 75
scurvy, signs of 275
SDAT 116, 117
sedative drugs
during regional anaesthesia 235, 237
for nights 292
sensory deficits
and strokes 78
in aged 109–10
sepsis, prophylaxis 179–80
serum cholesterol, levels 124
sex differences *see* men, pensionable-
    aged; women, pensionable-aged
shivering, stopping 225
Simmonds Sheehan syndrome 121
skeletal system, disorders 121–2
skin fragility 219
sleep apnoea 58, 59
SMI
and airways collapse 244
smoking
and respiratory complications 245
pre-operative banning 187–8, 246–7
social aspects, elderly 19–20, 112
socialization 94
sodium, levels 148
high 154–5
low 149–54, **251**
speech deficits
and stroke 78
steroid administration
abnormal thyroid activity 198
with regional anaesthesia 290,
    298–9
stress
and life expectancy 3
stroke volume, changes with ageing 32
strokes 77–9
and cerebral blood flow 76–7
incidence 77
phenytoin side effects and 82
post-operative 180
stump pain, post-amputation 295–6
subnutrition *see* malnutrition
succinylcholine 210
surfactant
and alveolar funtioning 66
surgical decisions 168–70
elective versus emergency 178–9
extent of care 181–2
investigations for 170–3
prognosis 174–5
prophylaxis 179–80
surgical aims 175–6, 310–11
timing 176–8
sustained maximal inspirations (SMI)
and airways collapse 224
sympathetic nerve block
during regional anaesthesia 233–4
synocopal attacks 87
systolic blood pressure, changes with
    ageing 31–2, **33**

TENS 289
thalamic syndrome 295
thallium scintigraphy 42, **43**
thermoregulation 86–7, 199
   during surgery 224–5
thiopentone
   dosage 206, 215
   drug distribution 130, 131, 138
thirst sensation, changes with ageing 147
thoracic surgery, complications 270–1
thromboembolic problems, post-
         operative 180–1, 193–4, 252–4
thyroid diseases 120
   steroid administration 198
   surgical mortality *268*
timing of operations 176–8
tissue differences, with ageing
   catabolic metabolism 4–5
tolerance, drug 303–4
tone, muscle
   testing 74
toxic confusional state 312–13
transfusions, blood
   timing 170–1, 226
trauma 153, 267
trichloroethylene 212
trigeminal neuralgia 296–7
triple assessment, defined 110
tubocurarine 209
two-phase gas liquid flow, airways 57

urea, blood levels 124
urge incontinence 123
uric acid, levels 124
urine
   incontinence 85, 123, 305
   output during surgery 226
USA
   hip fractures number 24
   mental assessment test 97
   pensionable population number 11
   strokes incidence 77
   surgical numbers 168

valves, heart
   replacement mortality *268*
   structural changes with age 27–8

vascular surgery, mortality 270
vecuronium 208–9
ventilation, artificial 273
   after surgery 218, 268, 270, 271
   weaning from 63–4
   see also mandatory ventilation,
         intermittent
ventricles, changes with ageing 29
visual deficits
   and stroke 78
   hallucinations with 109–10
visual evoked response, use (VER) 75
vitamin deficiencies
   B 275
   B$_{12}$ 211, 275
   C 135, 275
   D 121
   K 276
vocabulary, change with ageing 113
vomiting
   and opiate analgesics 303

WAIS (Wechsler Adult Intelligence
      Scale) 90, 98
warfarin 140
water balance 147–8
   depletion 146–7, 251
withdrawal, drug
   before surgery 185, 186
   delirium due to 249
women, pensionable-aged
   body component changes *147*
   chronic pain incidence 285
   creatinine clearance 194
   heart disease incidence 189
   intestinal ischaemia incidence *269*
   life expectancy 14, 169
   malnutrition incidence 274
   marital status and life style 19, **20**
   metabolic rate 275
   osteoporosis 121
   oxygen consumption 32
   plasma drug binding 129
   potassium levels 156, 157

zoster infections 292–4